A Critical History of Health Films in Central and Eastern Europe and Beyond

The burgeoning scholarship on Western health films stands in stark contrast to the vacuum in the historical conceptualization of Eastern European films. This book develops a nonlinear historical model that revises their unique role in the inception of national cinematography and establishing supranational health security.

Readers witness the revelation of an unknown history concerning how the health films produced in Eastern European countries not only adopted Western patterns of propaganda but actively participated in its formation, especially with regard to those considered "others": Women and the populations of the periphery. The authors elaborate on the long "echo" of the discursive practices introduced by health films within public health propaganda, as well as the attempts to negate and deconstruct such practices by rebellious filmmakers. A wide range of methods, including the analysis of the sociological biographies of filmmakers, the historical reconstruction of public campaigns against diseases and an investigation into the production of health films, contextualizes these films along a multifaceted continuum stretching between the adaptation of global patterns and the cultivation of national authenticities.

The book is aimed at those who study the history of film, the history of public health, Central and Eastern European countries and global history.

Victoria Shmidt is a Senior Researcher at the University of Graz in Austria. Her main interest is to deepen the approaches toward racial thinking in Central Eastern European countries. Recent publications include book "Historicizing Roma in Central Europe Between Critical Whiteness and Epistemic Injustice" (2021).

Karl Kaser is a Professor of Southeast European history and anthropology at the University of Graz, Austria. His research focuses on historical-anthropological issues and encompasses topics such as gender relations and historical visual cultures. His most recent book is *Femininities and Masculinities in the Digital Age*.

Routledge Open History

Routledge Open History provides a platform for the open-access publication of monographs and edited collections across the full breadth of the discipline from Medieval History until the present day. Books in the series are available for free download and re-use according to the terms of Creative Commons licence via the Routledge and Taylor & Francis website, as well as third-party discovery sites such as the Directory of OAPEN Library, Open Access Books, PMC Bookshelf, and Google Books.

Publication will be arranged via a Gold Open Access model. If you have a book proposal for the series, please contact Rob Langham at robert.langham@tandf.co.uk Note that the series is not the only platform for publishing open access at Routledge but the aim is for it to be front and central in our open-access publishing in History.

Islam and the Trajectory of Globalization
Rational Idealism and the Structure of World History
Louay M. Safi

Public and Private Welfare in Modern Europe
Productive Entanglements
Edited by Fabio Giomi, Célia Keren, and Morgane Labbé

East Central Europe and Communism
Politics, Culture, and Society, 1943–1991
Sabrina Ramet

A Critical History of Health Films in Central and Eastern Europe and Beyond
Victoria Shmidt and Karl Kaser

A Critical History of Health Films in Central and Eastern Europe and Beyond

Victoria Shmidt and Karl Kaser

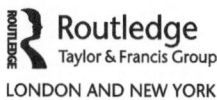

Routledge
Taylor & Francis Group

LONDON AND NEW YORK

First published 2024
by Routledge
4 Park Square, Milton Park, Abingdon, Oxon OX14 4RN

and by Routledge
605 Third Avenue, New York, NY 10158

Routledge is an imprint of the Taylor & Francis Group, an informa business

© 2024 Victoria Shmidt and Karl Kaser

FWF Austrian Science Fund

British Library Cataloguing-in-Publication Data
A catalogue record for this book is available from the British Library

ISBN: 978-1-032-21514-3 (hbk)
ISBN: 978-1-032-22354-4 (pbk)
ISBN: 978-1-003-27226-7 (ebk)

DOI: 10.4324/9781003272267

Typeset in Times New Roman
by MPS Limited, Dehradun

Contents

List of Archives and Their Abbreviations

Academy of Motion Picture Arts and Sciences (AMPAS)
Arhiv Jugoslavije, Archives of Yugoslavia (AJ)
Archiv Masarykovy university, Archive of Masaryk University (AMU)
Bayerisches Hauptstaatsarchiv The archive of the Bavarian State, (BayHStA)
Hrvatski državni arhiv, The *Croatian State Archives* (HDA)
Literární archiv Památníku národního písemnictví, the Museum of Czech
    Literature, Literary Archives (LA PNP)
Národní filmový archiv, Praha, National Film Archive, Prague (NFA)
Slovenský národný archív, Slovak national archives (SNA)
Štátny archív v Košiciach, State Archive in Kosice (SaK)
Centralen durzhaven arhiv, Central State Archives of Bulgaria (CDA)

Figures

Acknowledgments

In writing this book, we have incurred many debts. For providing access to the films, thanks to Kinoteka of the *Croatian State Archives, Zagreb*, the National Film Archive, Prague and Bulgarian Cinematheque, Sofia. Many librarians and archivists have come to our aid: Particular thanks to Jitka Meřínská (AMU), Mirjana Jurić, Nina Kolar and Lucija Zore (HDA), Matěj Strnad and Kristýna Doležalová (NFA), Ondřej Souček (Archive of Czech Television), Alexandar Radojičić (University Library "Svetozar Marković"), Alice Scandiuzz (*Biblioteca della Biennale-ASAC*), Rosen Spasov (Bulgarian Cinematheque), Ivan Stamenković (Jugoslovenska Kinoteka), Genevieve Maxwell (AMPAS) and Igor Stardelov (Cinematique of North Macedonia). We are grateful to Katherine McGilly and Slavoljub Gnjatović on behalf of *Avala Film Way* for permission to reproduce stills from the films, *A two-year-old goes to the hospital* and *Lilika*.

A special debt is owed to John Starkes Bushnell, who has provided access to the unpublished manuscript of a brilliant monograph, *Great nations of the West: Conflicting mind-sets*, by David Joravsky, which was a constant source of inspiration for us. We have had helpful and stimulating discussions with Tamara Bjažić-Klarin, Lucie Česálková, Natascha Drubek, Anelia Kasabova and Chiara Tognolotti.

The research conducted for this text was sponsored by the FWF Austrian Science Fund (M 2674-G28) as part of the project "Die Rassenkunde: Unentdeckte Macht des Aufbaus der Nationen" [Race Science: The Undiscovered Power of Building the Nation]. Financial help for completing this research was provided by the Faculty of Arts and Humanities at the University of Graz.

The publication of the book has been supported by the FWF Austrian Science Fund FWF Austrian Science Fund (PUB 1028-P).

Introduction

Nonlinear historicizing as a method for studying health films

Health films through the lenses of critical heritage studies and critical public health

In this book, we focus on films that can be conceptualized in various ways: Medicine's moving pictures, social-hygienic films, educational, cultural, enlightening, classroom or scientific-instructive films and even propaganda films. We use the overarching term "health films" in order to highlight the central mission behind producing and performing these films: To instruct different population groups on how to embrace new and healthy patterns of behavior in different realms of their lives, from being properly insured to practicing abstinence to avoid venereal diseases or altering daily habits to prevent infections. The films falling under this umbrella were introduced in the 1910s and continued to be a dominant visual method of health education throughout the first half of the twentieth century.

Health films should be seen as a part of the global movement concerning educational films, fueled by frustrations over the destructive influence of a new form of entertainment, the cinematograph. To a large extent, along with accepting the power of this new medium, experts (mainly educators) worried about the corrupting influence of films.[1] The massive interest in producing "proper" films, able to promote desirable patterns of behavior and demandable competencies as a strong alternative to films that threatened morality, can be seen as one of the main driving forces underlying the history of health films.

The production of these films reflected a multilevel structure, from very local filmmaking, creating almost amateur films,[2] to films for the widest possible audience produced within international networks of high-level professionals and experts.[3] Since the early 1920s, enormous efforts had been made to establish, within the League of Nations, a subdivision officially aimed at developing sustainable international collaboration and agreement in questions of teaching, in both the sciences and the arts. The International Institute for Intellectual Cooperation (IIIC), "the cultural arm of the League of Nations, advocated that the League become involved with educational film,"[4] and in 1928, the International Educational Cinematographic Institute, as an IIIC subdivision, was established. In addition, the Red Cross has been

DOI: 10.4324/9781003272267-1

one of the longest-running promoters of health films. Since the early 1920s, the Red Cross has selected "proper" films from around the world and disseminated them through national subdivisions and the international network of the Junior Red Cross. Until nowadays, the Red Cross has supported various regular international events, such as the International Festival of Red Cross and Health Films in Varna, which operated between 1965 and 1991 and was reestablished in 2014.[5] The Rockefeller Foundation not only sponsored the production of health films but also established the film library established at the Rockefeller-backed Museum of Modern Art for promoting educational films.[6] Despite this long and colorful history, health films have undergone systematic scholarly investigation only since the early 1980s.

Explaining the relatively recent increase in interest about these films is the first and most important step toward mapping a continuum of the approaches and methodological lenses applied to the study of health films. Beginning in the 1970s, the convergence of film studies and cinema history sought to reconstruct a rigorous image of cinematography and its powerful but ambivalent role in human life, which "challenged and changed the way people received, disseminated, and thought about information and transmission of knowledge."[7] A concern for the context of the production and reception of films, situated in their historical moment,[8] reverberated with the obsession among film scholars to focus on the role of cinematic authorship in the evolution of genres.[9] This trend was reinforced by embedding cinema history in the rapidly developing field of critical heritage studies, aimed at operationalizing the films' intangibility of cultural heritage "as being produced through sociopolitical processes reflecting society's power structures."[10]

The risks of relegating non-mainstream films to the margins of cinema history and the inevitable oblivion have obliged scholars to revisit the archives of previously underappreciated films and stop "their truncated shelf-life."[11] As nontheatrical films, health films have suffered from a nearly lost legacy due to limited access and archival scarcity.[12] Two interrelated points within critical heritage studies are especially pertinent to health films: 1) the critical revision of heritage as the "best examples of things" relevant to the mission of building a sense of national identity,[13] and 2) exploring heritage as a process of translating the past into new contexts.[14] The enormous interest in films targeted at sexual education and patterns of reproductive behavior most desirable for national interests is one the most visible examples of how critical heritage studies have contributed to historicizing health films.

Along with the motive of preserving and revising the lost legacy of health films, critical heritage studies delineate the difference between films and other types of heritage in terms of the specific "materiality" of films and the predominant role of visual language as a main framework for interpreting a film's history and legacy.[15] Moreover, research on health films has benefited from increasing attention to the role of visual methods in shaping public opinion through metaphors of health and disease.[16] The view on watching films as a manifestation of the essential social habits of an age[17] in the

Western world, which reached the widest possible audience between the 1920s and 1950s,[18] ascribed to the carriers of metaphors in films the status of one of the most compelling arguments in favor of identifying one or another discursive practice as privileged.

Health films as "elite pedagogic media shaped to elaborate the world"[19] have been explored as "evidence of social and cultural history."[20] This trend has stemmed not only from a growing interest in cinema history as a part of *critical heritage studies* but also from the intensive formation of *critical public health* – an interdisciplinary research field aimed at investigating the social and cultural implications of professional medicine and its institutionalization.[21] The long-term challenges of epidemiology aimed at eliminating infectious diseases,[22] the progress of genetics,[23] and the increasing pressure of preventive medicine[24] only reinforce the role of critical public health, which explores "public health as an historical and political construction of a means of restructuring both body and city."[25] Such critical historicizing has aimed at disputing the predominance of an idealized and overly positive view on the progress of medical knowledge. The increased role of physicians and various medical institutions since the last third of the nineteenth century had determined the establishment, rooting and deepening of research that should contribute to a critical reflection of public health as an instrument of state surveillance and the subsequent pressure on individuals.[26]

The resonance of critical heritage studies with the field of critical public health as a main driver for the interest in health films leads to mapping the variety of studies addressing such films through two clusters of questions:

- *Which historical contexts prevail in the narration concerning health films?* Within which historical milieu (e.g., either national, intercountry or international), welfare issues or propaganda, can we place the research on health films? How does research situate health films among other types of related films, including educational films, films for the professional instruction of public health professionals and scientific films? How do variously applied historical models connect the field of public health and critical heritage studies?

and

- *Which position do health films embody in historical narration* – as a structure of public health, propaganda, international relations or its agency (a driving force or a factor)? How do various models explain the role of health films, their development and their popularity? How is the timeline for historicizing health films organized? How has the legacy of health films been explored?

These questions help navigate an in-depth examination of the repertoire of historical models used to study the phenomenon of health films, investigating their explanatory and descriptive possibilities, including options for studying health films in Eastern Europe.

Health films as structure and agency of public policy

Exploring health films as a part of public health history remains the most common framework for revising the U.S. and German cases, which represent the longest history of producing the largest number of health films.[27] The impressive visibility of health films in these countries reverberates with the focus on the embeddedness of public health within the political agenda and its operation as one of the influential tools for managing people. Leslie Reagan and her colleagues synchronize the history of health films with the formation of public health, presenting health films as "more than illustrations" for the past of American medicine.[28] Alexandra M. Lord focuses on the vicissitudes of local and federal politics related to venereal diseases and especially their prevention in the U.S. Armed Forces as a main explanatory scheme for understanding several generations of campaigns that also included health films.[29] Miriam Posner investigates the interrogation of state surveillance and commerce interests as a key explanation for the specifics of the production and dissemination of sexual hygiene films.[30] Lee Grieveson highlights the exploitative political economy and the use of media by elite actors – states, corporations and lobbying and trade groups – for integrating the rural and imperial periphery into a new urban and industrial order and new forms of "corporate liberalism."[31] Among other practices of pedagogic and commercial media, Grieveson analyses health films as a part of a "biopolitical" project that has utilized media in varied ways to facilitate liberal practices of governance and the political economy. In contrast to Grieveson, who exclusively explores educational films as a structure of neoliberal politics, Martin Pernick investigates "the vital role of mass culture in constructing both the meanings and the memory of these [eugenic] movements."[32] In his monumental and revealing book, Pernick focuses on the impact of health films on legitimizing euthanasia as a part of the progressive eugenic movement. He underscores the multilevel interrogation between biology and culture in producing new norms regarding "defectiveness" and "healthy" beauty and recognizes in this connection one of the interrelations between eugenics in the United States and Nazi racial hygiene.

While the history of U.S. health films emphasizes the role of the neoliberal and imperialist pillars of health film production, the exploration of the German case focuses on authoritative regimes as one of the main bases for interpreting the legacy of health films. By focusing on the vicissitudes of sex education films, Ulf Schmidt[33] and Anita Winkler[34] not only shed light on the longue-durée of using films in sexual education in the Weimar Republic, Nazi Germany, capitalist Western Germany and communist Eastern Germany, but also elucidate the continuities and ruptures in the discursive practices regarding reproductive behavior through following the changes in political regimes and their needs as a way to demonstrate the content, planned outcomes and relevance of the films for the priorities of demographic policy. Along with sex education, films that addressed eugenics and its implications, including euthanasia, premarital counseling and sterilization, have warranted the most systematic attention.[35]

Despite obvious difference in political context, the exploration of U.S. and German health films often reproduces the comparable historical model that stresses a set of massive forces or "organic" processes (e.g., the operation of political regimes, especially those authoritative or at the vanguard of global capitalism) that lead to a particular result, as in the growth of an "organism" and its influence.[36] Such a master narrative corresponds not only to the massive legacy of health films but also to the intention to extract health films from historical nothingness through stressing their political importance. This model prioritizes "the values represented, and the style assumed in establishing the composition and mise-en-scène than to the accuracy or authenticity of the images."[37]

Robert Proctor recognizes in such selective memories concerning Nazi medicine strong predilections resulting from particular "ideological gaps," which block the attention of historians to long-term continuities in the campaigns aimed at preventing cancer as well as other important fields of public health.[38] Notwithstanding the critical potential, applying a linear historical model to health films prioritizes politicized explanations and inevitably replaces the films that cannot be directly interpreted as instruments of structural violence, e.g., the numerous cartoons with a focus on elementary hygiene, which not only played a central role in educating the population but also influenced the development of the most popular cartoon series.[39]

Along with the limits of politicizing the linear model comes the irreducibility of events to bodies and states of affairs of ordinary people,[40] excluding from the analysis the role of those who created the films. One of the promising alternatives is reconstructing the professional biographies of the film authors, such as Jean Comandon[41] or Jean Benoit-Lévy, who simultaneously managed the institutionalization of public health and advanced national cinematography.[42] In the focus of applying the *biographical method*, the historians of health films locate the parallel socializing experiences through which those who nurtured the ground for health film production had been constituted.[43] Exploring their professional pathways within the fields of cinematography and public health moves beyond the dichotomy of agency vs. structure and explores health films as a complex phenomenon. The main outcome of applying this method is grasping the intersection of the different socialization frameworks experienced by the authors of health films, in order to reconstruct the authorship of health films as a reflection of an elitist regime of national and transnational authenticities.

Applying a linear model to cross-national, historical comparative analysis aims to differentiate the driving political forces in producing and disseminating health films[44] but does not contribute to the *contextualization* of health films. One of the possible responses to this challenge is the recent trend of stressing the shared emotions and collective practices of consuming films instead of the possessive individualism or behavioral changes that remain in the focus of politicized views on health films as instruments of propaganda. The motif of collective participation in practices around health films brings forward the task of analyzing visual "language" and its recognizability by spectators and emphasizes the active, agentic position of these films. Revealing the obvious differences among various generations of educational films that have addressed diverse target groups inclines us to move beyond exploring the pressures of modernity, nation-building and state surveillance as the main driving forces behind the generation of a "language" of fear or the shame about illness typical of health films.[45] Instead, the univocal interrelation between the mission of health films and the political aims bringing forward the visual language of educational films has made the connections between thoughts, ideas and pieces of data discursive moments that remain understood as nonimportant or disconnected. Exploring educational films stresses the role of the informal urban and rural culture of religious and political street preaching, the music hall and the pub and the style of educational films and health films as a part of cinema-enlightenment derived from the newsreel, the cautionary tale and the joke.[46]

The question concerning the functions of recognition remains at the center of exploring educational films: If educational films have operated as "as visual Esperanto," how universal was this language,[47] and what were the main sources of universalizing and specifying this language? Historicizing educational films has generated various answers – regarding the cultural and social contexts of the research. The recent trend to focus on the international level of educational films has already affected our comprehension of the variety of "visual languages" within health films. A diversity of political philosophies and a broad array of ideologies articulated by international organizations around film education and film studies stress the internally contradictory messages sent by films.[48] They also highlight the ways to solve the dilemma of universalism vs. variety, which translated internationalism, solidarity and friendship as new forms of collective emotions cultivated by the various tools of mass culture, including health films.[49] Recent and current attempts to historicize health films as embedded in the development of educational films illustrate "how simple sequences of events can produce complex consequences and by offering new insights into the dynamics of human interaction."[50]

Which historical model, whether linear or nonlinear, is the most promising regarding the history of health films in Eastern Europe?

The limits and options for historicizing health films in Eastern Europe

Certainly, the historical presence of health films in Eastern Europe is not in question. The materials regarding the activities of the International Educational Cinematographic Institute (housed by the UNESCO Archive) provide a general and specific overview of the involvement of most Eastern European states in producing and disseminating health films during the late

1920s and 1930s. Even a superficial overview of the storerooms and libraries of the National Film Archives in Prague, Sofia, Skopje, Belgrade and Zagreb reveals dozens of health films, along with scenarios of unfulfilled projects aimed at producing health films. Between 1922 and 1939, the School of Public Health in Zagreb produced more than one hundred films of different genres aimed at supplementing and reinforcing various health education campaigns. Between 1921 and 1940, more than 20 films were produced in Czechoslovakia, some in direct cooperation with Yugoslav colleagues.

However, the already-established historical timeline of health films misses the multiplicity of the driving forces that shaped the trajectories of their production and dissemination. Despite the preserved legacy of health films, until now, only a few publications have shed light on their history.[51] Rigorous cataloging, still the main method of historicizing health films produced in Eastern Europe, only reinforces the admiration for these films due to their unique role in the inception of national animated films in Balkan countries[52] and a generally decisive role in the development of national cinematography in Eastern Europe in terms of the professionalization of film production.[53] The rare attempts to revise the legacy of health films have addressed a few issues[54] but they have not contributed to historicizing health films as a social and cultural trend typical of interwar Eastern Europe.

In terms of the Deleuzian differentiation of time within historical narration,[55] the contemporary state of health films in Eastern Europe could be defined as a historical paradox between their central role in the inception of national cinematography in many Eastern European countries and a vacuum in producing recognition of the role of these films in public health and other sociocultural realms. In this disparity, it is possible to locate a more general and multifaceted challenge for historicizing Eastern Europe, especially the complexity of its interwar period – the massive avoidance of processes of analysis that are asymmetrical, irreversible and often unpredictable from the view of linear models.[56]

Our main sources for interpreting health films, namely, critical heritage studies and critical public health, dovetails with such a nonlinear historical model. This approach stands in contrast to the predominant role of medical science and its implications in the Western world that have belittled Eastern European interwar public health and the related ideological movements as eugenics. It further serves as a corrective to the exclusion of such driving forces as the reinvention of an interwar global agenda of demographic policy and the reproduction of international networking among racially minded experts after 1945.

The neglect of such historical continuities simplifies the explanation for the institutional violence typical of public health in socialist countries between the 1960s and 1980s, which concerns the ubiquitous surveillance of socialist authoritarianism. As with public health, the interwar cinematography of Eastern Europe is seen to be "of no importance," except for some recent attempts to introduce the complexities of the driving forces that shaped the development of films and film studies in the region, between the global pressure of progress and local entertainment needs.[57] These shortcomings in interpreting the interwar period can be overcome through new, nonlinear historical models which "no longer assume that small or accidental changes will have minor consequences for human communities or that massive social movements will be of major consequences, because nonlinear processes are not proportional."[58]

The main hypothesis explored within this book posits that health films were not just a manifestation of the ideological transmission of global patterns but rather the repercussion of regional events.[59] The resistance of local populations to public health initiatives, egregious cases of infanticide, the pressure of international bodies on national authorities to present the progress in production and dissemination of educational films, the extreme popularity of films that absorbed the attention of the audience targeted for health films such as *The Kid* by Charlie Chaplin, the appearance of Western health films made using new, attractive artistic techniques such as animation or the emergence of films that translated an ideological message opposed to national interests, like *Frauennot-Frauenglück* (The misery or fortune of women, 1929), are just some of the events that we bring into the focus of our analysis. The inner complexity of events, especially those operating in the "impossible" positions of "minorities" such as interwar Eastern Europe, is often imperceptible from the view of linear models.[60] Even the health films made in Eastern Europe and their dissemination should be seen as still "impossible" for historicizing events.

The epistemic improvement of historical narratives regarding interwar Eastern Europe should be built upon "moving from grouping singular events under basic narrative terms and geo-temporal labels" to *interpretation proper*, "grouping singular events under complex interpretative concepts" and focusing on a rhizome narrative.[61] Our exploration of health films introduces a nonlinear model for redefining the interwar period, launching a process aimed at revising the history of Eastern Europe through aggregating various nonlinear narratives for new explanatory possibilities. We develop a nonlinear model for historicizing Eastern Europe and deconstructing the cultural and historical homogeneity surrounding the predominant role of the experience of authoritative regimes, one of the foundational political myths regarding Eastern Europe[62] that blocks the recognition of the historical role played by many competing or mutually contradictory events such as health films.

In order to achieve multiplicity in narration, we interlink different levels of health film operations to the multiplied narrative: 1) the cases of Czechoslovakia and Yugoslavia, countries with different but the most consistent dynamics of institutionalizing health films among other Eastern European countries; 2) international cooperation initiated by global organizations and intercountry networking targeted with producing shared regimes of authenticity for Eastern Europe, e.g., progressive agrarianism; and 3) the mutual influence of films produced in Eastern Europe, the United States, France and Germany which started to address peripheral and special target groups in interwar period. We aim to overcome the mode typical of master narratives to see Eastern European countries as minor actors, not subjects, but impersonal singularities of global politics.[63] Our nonlinear view aims to historicize health films as a part of "the collective imprint of history on a human community [which] contains complex networks of interactive or feedback loops, which make it possible for a single human act to transform society in unpredictable way."[64]

In line with the frames of nonlinear or rhizome narrative, we first aim to redescribe *the historical time of health films* by placing them into the contexts of specific pathways for institutionalizing public health and cinematography. The main part of the book brings to analytical attention *the event time of health films* through interpreting these films as agents for solving the dilemma of internationalizing Eastern Europe vs. reinforcing the regime of national authenticity, a key concern for historicizing the interwar period in the region.

The historical time of health films in Eastern Europe

An auxiliary task necessary for achieving the objective of redefining the historical time of health films consists of mapping the scope of health films and their production in Eastern Europe. In the early 1920s, the Red Cross had started to recommend to public health experts around the world the use of films for educating the population and the fellows of the Rockefeller Foundation, among other novelties, had learned to use films; meanwhile, in Eastern Europe, there were local attempts to make films a part of the campaigns to address particular health problems. In Trogir (Croatia), the local Institute of Hygiene made a film about malaria strategies to eradicate its carriers, mosquitos.[65] The famous Czech institution for people with physical disabilities, *Jedličkův ústav*, produced a film aimed at promoting the placement of children with physical disabilities to institutions in favor of their rehabilitation (see Part 1, Chapter 2). Jenő Janovics, a famous Hungarian film director, in cooperation with medical experts, made *Világrém* (*Menace*, 1920) as a part of the pre-election campaign in Transylvania[66] (see Part 3, Chapter 8). Another Hungarian film, *Árvák imája* (The prayer of orphans, 1922), promoted cooperation between Hungarian nobility and the Red Cross in favor of rescuing children without parents. Not one of these films promoted a systematic policy or public health initiatives but rather a particular institution attached to a particular location.

In the mid-1920s, both in Czechoslovakia and Yugoslavia, the representatives of the Ministry of Health and Physical Culture and the Ministry of Public Health and Social Policy, respectively, initiated the production of films targeted at addressing the priorities of state policy. In Yugoslavia, at this stage, producing and disseminating health films was connected to the Laboratory of Film, a subdivision of the School of National Health (Zagreb), and mostly documentary films were produced.

Karel Driml, who was responsible for health propaganda at the Ministry, in cooperation with film director Josef Kokeisl, produced his first film, *Procitnui ženy* (Recognizing the Woman, 1925), aimed at promoting new institutional approaches to women's health. In the same year, Kokeisl produced a film chronicle entitled *Počátek nového období veřejného zdravotnictví* (The inception of a new era in public health) in Czechoslovakia, on the opening of the Institute of Hygiene. In another documentary, *Státní epidemická kolona* (The state epidemiological mobile service, 1925) Kokeisl presented the most fashionable decision to bring systematic public health to the periphery – through mobile service.

The Laboratory of Film started its activity when Andrija Štampar was in the prime of his career as a national politician and expert.[67] Two of the first cohort of films, *Lječilište Topolšica* (Sanatorium Topolšica, 1927) and *Dačko ljetovalište Martinščica* (Resort for children Martinščica, 1927), presented new approaches to preventive care for adults and children, and another, *Izmjena liječnika Lige naroda* (The transformation of the physician in the League of Nations, 1928), presented the positive contribution of the international organization in disseminating new, progressive, approaches to protecting people's health.[68]

At this stage, cooperation between healthcare professionals and filmmakers had become systemic and long-term. It is reasonable to recognize in this cooperation one of the most decisive driving forces that made possible the transformation from individual projects to systematic production of health films and their dissemination at national and international levels, one of the hallmarks of health films in Czechoslovakia and Yugoslavia. Another two interrelated practices, namely, rooting the production of educational films in the general development of national cinematography and the involvement of domestic health films in the international movement of educational films, ensured the intensification of the production and distribution of films in the late 1920s and early 1930s.

Czech experts started to become involved at the international level of educational and scientific films in the middle of the 1920s.[69] The participation of Czechs in the international movement reflected the decentralized approach typical of the interwar film industry in the country and the predominance of the model of private business, in line with faith in the free market and the rationality of the public, characteristic of the U.S. approach to educational films in the 1920s.[70] Notably, the transformation from a liberal to a more pro-state approach to producing educational films in interwar Czechoslovakia[71] occurred at approximately the same time that U.S. experts, following their British colleagues (who had already established the British Film Institute), started to make efforts toward institutionalizing educational films.[72] Since the middle of the 1920s, Czechoslovak authorities included health films in events targeted at representing progress in developing public health. In 1924, during their visit to Prague institutions aimed at fighting tuberculosis, representatives of the League of Nations not only conducted research on the medical practices and counseling centers organized by the Masaryková Liga but also watched a documentary about tuberculosis and the puppet show *Začarovaná země* (Enchanted country), produced by Driml.[73] The culmination of the representative function of educational films, including health films, was achieved by the end of the 1920s, when the country started to prepare for its ten-year anniversary. The anniversary represented an opportunity to demonstrate to Czechoslovaks and to outsiders the great progress of humanity as the outcome of creating a new state. In 1927, Kokeisl and Driml produced six films for child audiences,[74] aimed at shaping the "proper" skills regarding nutrition and personal hygiene. These health fairy tales challenged the German puppet shows and the ideology in the background of traditional marionette theater. and the skepticism concerning medicine typical of European marionette culture in the nineteenth century (see Part 2). In 1928, the team produced four fiction films aimed at involving different target groups of adults in the struggle for good health. All these films were included in the program of *Výstava soudobé kultury v ČSR* (Exhibition of modern culture in Czechoslovakia, Brno 1928).

The exhibition, presented in the mass media as "neither Pantheon nor a cathedral but workshop aimed at presenting hands and heads of those who create this state,"[75] was one of the central events in celebrating ten years of Czechoslovakia. Vladimir Úlehla, the Czechoslovak leader in developing scientific films, was the chair of the board responsible for organizing the exhibition, which consisted of four parts: (1) "Man and animate nature"; (2) "Man and inanimate nature"; (3) "State and law"; and (4) "The spiritual life of man."[76] The health films were presented within the first section, shaped by the leaders of the Czech eugenic movement. The anthropologists Vojtěch Suk, Jiří Malý and Jindřich Matiegka[77] developed a section entitled "Man and his race" and Jan Bělehrádek,[78] one of the young leaders of Czech eugenics, made the final decision about selecting materials and events for this section. Driml, who overtly sympathized with eugenics and promoted some of its strategies, including premarital examinations and limiting people with disabilities in their right to have a family, was responsible for the section "Man and his health: The protection of human health, psychology and psychotechnique." On each day of the exhibition, educational films were shown, including the health films by Driml and Kokeisl. The exhibition lasted from May to October 1928 and was attended by more than two and a half million people, including the citizens of Yugoslavia, who were provided with full travel expenses.

The Yugoslav films were shown at international events only in the 1930s, and the leading role belonged to the filmmakers, directly affiliated with the School of Public Health. The non-representation of Yugoslav experts and films at the international level in the 1920s paradoxically played a role in the thrust to intensify the development of educational films, including health films. The pressure of international organizations, reinforced by the desire of national authorities to participate in the persistent movement aimed at using films for educational purposes, became one of the main driving factors for the intensification of film production in Yugoslavia in the late 1920s and early 1930s.

In early December 1929, the Ministry of Foreign Affairs was informed by the League of Nations about a plan to collect information about educational films produced in Yugoslavia. The League of Nations, on behalf of the International Educational Cinematographic Institute, disseminated a questionnaire aimed at measuring the presence of educational films in each of the countries; this research was fully supported by the League, which had made the decision to conduct such a survey in 1929.[79] The Ministry of Foreign Affairs began bombarding the Ministry of Education with letters asking for information about the educational films being produced,[80] which foreign educational films were being shown in the country,[81] and how the Ministry of Education experts viewed the idea of international organizations becoming exempt from taxes on educational films when purchased by other countries.[82]

Replying to the requests by the Ministry of Foreign Affairs took several months and in late August 1930, the Ministry of Education sent a rather pessimistic report about the state of the art in educational films to the Ministry of Internal Affairs: "At least for now, this initiative can be ideologically significant, especially because there is no such thing as a film industry in our country. Private initiatives haven't moved past short advertising films – probably two or three serious attempts."[83] After one more request from the side of the Ministry of Foreign Affairs, the Ministry of Education directly acknowledged the total lack of quality educational films that could be presented at the international level:

> Answering the request to provide information about educational films, the Ministry of Education replied: 'In our country, not one film was produced that would deserve to be presented in an international catalogue beyond the borders of our state. Universities and some laboratories have tried, but the quality does not align with international expectations. For educational purposes, we continue to use films of foreign production.'[84]

Along with admitting the deplorable state of affairs concerning educational film production in Yugoslavia, the Ministry of Education recognized a potential threat to national interests if the distribution of foreign films continued, and the tax on their acquisition was abolished:

> Undoubtedly, the import of foreign educational films would not be commensurate with the export of our films – to our detriment. On the other hand, we would not purchase foreign scientific and health films as long as the Ministry of Finance would not lower the taxes for films of scientific content. In general, the illusion remains to bring the quantity and quality of cinematographic production closer to balance the import and export of educational films.

The main concern of the Ministry of Education was the impact of educational films on shaping a desirable set of collective identities: "Regardless of the dismal state of our film production, it is obvious that educational films carry, to a certain extent, the propaganda of the country in which they are filmed." Later, this answer was extended for more formal use, with the very familiar motif of the opposition between "proper" and "improper" films: "The issue of educational films is one of the most actual and significant when we speak about moral, physical, and mental development of our youth, especially if we consider how devastating and fatal films act for older viewers too."[85]

In these points, the position of both ministries coincided. A few months after the response by the Ministry of Education, the Ministry of Foreign Affairs asked about the possibility to share educational films with international audiences and brought forward the same argument:

France, Germany, England, the United States, Italy, and Japan have already sent films made in their countries; we have been asked by the International Institute to send a list of cultural, educational, and scientific films too. We ask the Ministry to provide this list by the 13th of October, so the catalogue can be published in January of the next year.[86]

In early 1932, the Ministry of Internal Affairs was able to send to the Institute in Rome two lists consisting of 23 films about folk culture, traditions, the royal family, physical exercise, sport and public economy and 27 films about the beauty of Yugoslavia, respectively.[87] How did this become possible?

Milan Marjanović, the author of the plots of the earliest films produced at the School of Public Health, was behind the rapid improvement in the domestic production of educational films: He prepared the lists of films that were sent to Rome. Marjanović was one of those who shaped public discourses concerning the desirable scenarios of developing national cinematography. Not expensive decorations, but entertaining plots and an excellent acting game, according to the politician, should become the basis for the development of Yugoslav cinema.[88] Marjanović consistently criticized the ambitious but unrealistic plans of neighboring countries, Hungary and Czechoslovakia, to achieve success in the export of films and considered it a top priority to focus on films for the population of his country.[89]

Marjanović established *Jugoslovenski prosvetni film* (Yugoslav Enlightening Film), a foundation for which the "mission is to participate, cooperate, and provide sources for developing the domestic production of good films, to propagate Yugoslav films abroad as one."[90] Along with supporting the production of films, *Jugoslovenski prosvetni film* built a 500-seat cinema for promoting domestic production. It was an act contributing to the survival of the reputation of the country but it also helped some Croatian public politicians, like Marjanović and Štampar. who from the beginning of the 1930s had fallen into political disfavor with the country's royalty. It is noteworthy that not only the School of Public Health and *Jugoslovenski prosvetni film*, but also the regional institutes of hygiene, created by the initiative of Štampar, contributed to creating the country's reputation as a film-producing state.

The Institute of Hygiene in Skopje produced five films in 1931: Stevan Mišković, a Macedonian film director educated in Germany, was recruited for this mission. Two films, *Zarazata pobeduva* (When infection wins) and *Malarija* (Malaria) presented the threat of infectious diseases through reminding audiences of the consequences of these epidemics for Serbian troops in 1915 and the heroic role of the physicians who sacrificed their lives in the name of people's health. *Megu idniti domakinki* (Among the future housewives) motivated young women and girls to enter local health schools aimed at equipping them to care for children. *Zemiotres na jugot* (Earthquake in the south) was a documentary that highlighted the role of public health in coping with the consequences of earthquakes. And *Na sonce i vzduch* (In the sun and the air) was a film about health settlements for children.

In 1933, Yugoslavia produced the largest number of educational films, 77 films "about culture and science" as defined in the report. Moreover, among all films produced in the country that year, educational films were dominant; only social advertisements and commercials were produced in higher numbers – 90 in total.[91] The vast majority of films, 61, were produced by the School of Public Health. In 1934, within the Congress of Educational Films held in Rome, Štampar presented the two-part film *Borba protiv bolesti putem filma* (Fighting disease with the help of film), comprised of shorts from more than 30 films produced by the School of Public Health and accompanied by French subtitles for presenting the outcomes and achievements of using health films. In the second half of the 1930s, the health films produced by the Film Laboratory of the School of Health were disseminated around the world. Štampar actively arranged showings of the films as a part of his numerous presentations of a successful model of public health for rural populations, not only in Europe but also in China, Turkey, the United States and Canada.

The event time of health films: The structure of the book

In terms of a Deleuzian approach, the revision of the historical time of health films aims to make connections between thoughts, ideas, pieces of data and discursive moments perceived as quite different, as well as to build "assemblages" of contexts for reconstructing the time of events or the historical role of health films in Eastern Europe. We concentrate these assemblages around the films as main events in cinematic history. We interpret each of the films included in one or another assemblage in terms of historical peculiarities, including a clear and precise definition of the places, events, visual analogies and so on used in the films. This approach aims to nuance our understanding of the message of each film and its acceptance by the audience, which not only prevents historical presentism but also introduces the devices of a visual analysis sensitive to cultural, social and political contexts.

The overall comparative focus of our book serves to redefine the commonalities and differences among health films in Eastern Europe and beyond and to reveal previously overlooked factors such as intercountry cooperation, the interconnection between health films and entertainment activities and the diversity of ideological platforms for producing health films, among others. The assemblages or lines for exploring the formation of health films provide the contexts for applying rhizo-textual analysis of films, which depends on structuring and unifying the plurality of key patterns for storytelling in health films. We explore various ways of juxtaposing the adaptation of already disseminated Western patterns with the establishment of regimes of national authenticity through embedding healthy practices in the relevant cultural and social habitus of the population. Applying rhizo-textual analysis makes visible the hybridization of these discursive practices within and across various clusters.

In line with exploring adaptation as cultural revision,[92] we focus on the changes in the production and dissemination of health films in Eastern Europe in comparison to Western health films, which we see as the hegemonic patterns that were reproduced, refashioned, parodied or, even more, rejected and replaced by novel production elements. The variety of responses to a prior story positions adaptation as (re-)interpretation and (re-)creation[93] and helps to connect production- and reception-oriented practices. We reorganize the space of events in health films produced in different regions into a multifaceted continuum and stress (laterally, not vertically) the coexistence or even the interrelation of multiple versions of cinematic stories.[94] This approach allows us to focus on the films in terms of the audiences targeted by the films: Whole nations, children, men and women and populations in the periphery.

Each of the assemblages consists of films produced in Eastern Europe, interpreted in the context of the Western films offered as possible patterns or, moreover, recommended for dissemination among the populations of Eastern Europe by international organizations. Paraphrasing Henry Giroux,[95] we might say that learning in the interwar period was located in popular spheres, which inclines us to interpret Eastern European films through the historically well-situated possibilities for adapting feature films (both national and foreign) that were the most popular among the people.

In our general understanding of regimes of authenticity, we follow Claud Bremond's idea regarding the rootedness of narrative structures in human social experiences.[96] According to Bremond,[97] the phenomenology of social life shapes the logics of the narrative cycle, as situated between two alternatives: The improvement to be achieved (accomplishment of the task, allied intervention, getting rid of the contender, negotiation, aggression, retribution or reward or vengeance) and the foreseen deterioration (obligation, sacrifice, endured attack and endured punishment). In line with this approach, all health films are targeted with presenting unhealthy habits as predicaments of practical life and opening to the possibility of solving or avoiding these problems. We specify the performance of regimes of authenticity in different clusters of films as the main framework for adapting and modifying global patterns in the production of health films, recruiting a wide range of approaches to investigating these regimes of authenticity and their presentation in culture.

Part 1 elaborates films about "rescuing" children as the future of the nation. We explore these films as part of the inception of the genre of family film – addressing nations and, even more, all of humanity. Noel Brown sees the genre of family films as "a coherent body of films, typically sharing specific ideological overtones, emotive aspects and commercial intent."[98] Health films addressed nations as families in order to include them in the multilevel process of institutionalizing care for children. A number of the films produced in interwar Prague and Zagreb are "rescue" films, designed to convince people of the goodwill of a state that cares for future generations. The neglected child, the protagonist in each of the films, eventually reaches the best possible position by being placed in an institution: A boarding school or professional foster care. The conflict between irresponsible parents and the paternalistic state is shaped by consistent masculinization: Powerful men make decisions, and devoted women implement them. This pattern is reinforced by the consistent combination of the role of the state with the symbols of its historical glory.

We examine the grounding of these discursive practices after 1945 in documentaries and fiction films produced by socialist authorities in the 1960s (e.g., *Dluh – Jedličkův ústav* [Our debt to Jedličkův ústav, 1968]). Finally, Part 1 discusses the films *Lilika* (by Branko Pleša, 1970) and *Neúplné zatmení* (Incomplete eclipse, by Jaromil Jires, 1983) as the systematic negation of the rescue-mission discourse and the revision of the practices of institutionalizing children established by health films and the relevant tools for visualizing these official discourses. Oscar-winning *Kolja* (Kolya by Jan Svěrak, 1996) is explored as a renovation of the rescue film because it highlights the arbitrariness of residential care as a part of the recent totalitarian past and grants families magic powers.

Part 2 focuses on films aimed at teaching children basic hygienic skills such as dental care, proper nutrition and hygienic rules for preventing infectious diseases. We focus our analysis on explaining the interplay of the national traditions of entertainment for children, such as puppet shows and children's literature, and the new, global influence of animation, which emerged in Eastern European countries during the middle of the 1920s. Two Czech films, *Kašparek a Bodulínek* (The clown and Bodulínek, 1927) and *Kašpárek kouzelníkem* (Magic medicine, 1927), and one Yugoslav animated film *Campek nevaljalac* (Naughty Champek, 1929) are examined as reinforcing the priority of health for future men from the middle class – the main protagonists in each of the films.

Part 3 speaks to the question of why health films made in Eastern European countries often appealed to men, considered sons of the nation, who became husbands and fathers and embraced a responsible attitude toward their own health as an integral part of growing up. Imposing an active position regarding one's own health exclusively to men is one of the most visible specifics of the health films produced in Yugoslavia and Czechoslovakia. Part 3 aims to explore the driving forces that coined this specific gender-based disparity and how the films for men promoted the idea of "proper" male behavior, including the prevention of alcoholism and venereal disease, good models of fatherhood and so on. We reconstruct this part of the history of health films through the theory of narratives by Rick Altman and his classification of narratives into dual-focus, single-focus and multi-focus types, which provides a better understanding of how different approaches to negating one's own subaltern past shaped the discursive practices of public health propaganda targeted at men.

We continue with the historical reconstruction of women and their specific status in nationalist movements, as "stepdaughters of the nation." We trace the transformation of disciplining practices such as the female *Bildungsroman* disseminated in the late nineteenth century in the plots and artistic devices of health films aimed at persuading women to accept not only new practices of care but also being institutionalized throughout their lives by public health surveillance. Historically, the films produced in Prague and Zagreb address women in cities and rural areas, respectively. We explore the specifics of visualizing the mission of surveillance as determined by this difference.

In Part 4, the several waves of campaigns against infectious and sexually transmitted diseases are reconstructed as multilevel projects that reflected the very first model for providing global health security, which divided the world into developing countries, where the early warning of potential outbreaks of infectious diseases was to be provided, and the rest of the world, developed countries that should be protected. Such a model was easily adopted by Eastern European states for legitimizing themselves and the politics of internal colonialism regarding their peripheral regions. We bring the different obstacles into analytical focus, especially the resistance of local populations, reevaluating health films as tools aimed at involving people into practices of prevention and timely medical treatment. Part 4 reconstructs the history of health films for the periphery as one of the most extreme and consistent performances of "otherness" – even in contrast to women, seen as alien to the fledgling nations. The films for the periphery produced between the end of the 1920s and 1930s established a specific genre of health film, as a cultural institution aimed at connecting different collective singulars: The population of peripheries, national governments and the global agents of health security interested in practicing public health as a tool of political surveillance.

To conclude the book, we revise the methodological tools that we have applied for the historical reconstruction of health films as a possible answer to the grip of the binary opposition historians face, between the global and the national. We discuss the options for the epistemic improvement of historical narratives regarding interwar Eastern Europe, which should be built upon "moving from grouping singular events under basic narrative terms and geo-temporal labels" to *interpretation proper*, "grouping singular events under a complex interpretative concept" and focusing on a rhizome narrative.[99]

Notes

1 Between the 1910s and 1920s, educators from various countries carried out surveys aimed at highlighting the increasing importance of the cinematograph for youth formation. Mostly, these surveys warned the public about the corrupting effects of the cinematograph and called for introducing strict regulations regarding access to the films and control over production.

2 Elizabeth Lebas (2011) *Forgotten Futures: British Municipal Cinema 1920–1980.* London: Black Dog Press.

3 Zoë Druick (2007) The international educational cinematograph institute, reactionary modernism, and the formation of film studies, *Canadian Journal of Film Studies*, 16, 1, pp. 80–97; Marina Dahlquist and Joel Frykholm (2019) *The Institutionalization of Educational Cinema: North America and Europe in the 1910s and 1920s* Bloomington, Indiana: Indiana University Press.

4 Kenneth Garner (2012) *Seeing is Knowing: The Educational Cinema Movement in France*, 1910–1945 Doctoral Thesis, University of Michigan, pp. 153–154.

5 Pictures in the service of the Red Cross (1982) *International Review of the Red Cross* 4 pp. 120–126.

6 Victoria Cain (2011) "An indirect influence upon industry": Rockefeller Philanthropies and the development of educational film in the United States, 1935–1953 in Devin Orgeron, Marsha Orgeron, Dan Streible (eds) *Learning with the Lights Off: Educational Film in the United States* Oxford: Oxford University Press, p.239.

7 Devin Orgeron, Marsha Orgeron, Dan Streible (2011) Introduction in Devin Orgeron, Marsha Orgeron, Dan Streible (eds), *Learning with the Lights Off: Educational Film in the United States* Oxford: Oxford University Press, 3–15 p. 11.

8 John O'Connor (1990) *Image as artifact The historical analysis of film and television* Florida, Malabar Robert E.Krieger Publishing Company; Jeffrey Richards (2000) 'Rethinking British Cinema', paper given at 'Cinema, Identity, History: An International Conference on British Cinema', held at the University of East Anglia in July 1998. Published in Justine Ashby and Andrew Higson (eds), *British Cinema, Past and Present* (London 2000), pp. 21–34.

9 Rick Altman (1999) *Film/Genre*. London: BFI.

10 William Logan and Gamini Wijesuriya (2015). The new heritage studies and education, training, and capacity-building. In William Logan, Máiréad Nic Craith, Ullrich Kockel e (eds.), *A Companion To Heritage Studies*, Malden, MA: John Wiley and Sons. 557–573. p. 569.

11 Anna McCarthy (2011) Screen culture and Group discussion in postwar race relations in Devin Orgeron, Marsha Orgeron, Dan Streible (eds) *Learning with the Lights Off: Educational Film in the United States* Oxford: Oxford University Press 397–423 p. 398.

12 Dan Streible, Martina Roepke and Anke Mebold (2007) Nontheatrical Film *Film History*, 19, pp. 339–343; Orgeron et al. Learning with the lights off, p. 7.

13 Rodney Harrison, (2013). *Heritage: Critical approaches*. New York: Routledge. p. 98.

14 Andrea Witcomb and Kristal Buckley (2013). Engaging with the future of 'critical heritage studies': looking back in order to look forward. *International Journal of Heritage Studies*, 19 (6), pp. 562–578.

15 O'Connor *Image as artifact*, p. 4.

16 Sabine Schlegelmilch (2017) Film als medizinhistorische Quelle / Film sources in medical history Author(s): Medizinhistorisches Journal, 2017, Bd. 52, H. 2/3 (2017), pp. 100–115; George Lakoff (1987) *Women, Fire, and Dangerous Things What Categories Reveal About the Mind Chicago:* University of Chicago Press; Dedre Gentner, Keith J. Holyoak and Boicho N. Kokinov. Kokinov (2001) The analogical mind: perspectives from cognitive science Cambridge MA MIT Press.

17 Alan J.P. Taylor (2001) *English History 1914–1945* Oxford: Oxford University Press, p. 313.

18 Richard Howells and Robert W. Matson (2009) *Using Visual Evidence.* Berkshire Open University Press.

19 Lee Grieveson (2017) *Cinema and the Wealth of Nations: Media, Capital, and the Liberal World System.* California: University of California Press, p. 3.

20 O'Connor Image as artifact p. 7.

21 David Armstrong (1995): The Rise of Surveillance Medicine, *Sociology of Health and Illness* 7, 3, pp. 393–404; Borowy, I. (2009) *Coming to Terms with the World's Health: The League of Nations Health Organization 1921–1946,* Frankfurt a. M. 2009, pp. 13–15).

22 Nancy Ley Stepan (2012) *Eradication: Ridding the World of Diseases Forever?* London: Reaktion Books.

23 Robin Bunton and Alan Petersen (2002) Genetics, ethics and governance, *Critical Public Health,* 12:2, 95–102.

24 Dietmar Jazbinsek (2000) *Gesundheitskommunikation:* Medien in der Medizin - Medizin in den Medien! [Communication within public health: Mass media in medicine and medicine in mass-media] VS Verlag für Sozialwissenschaften.

25 Dittmar Machule, Olaf Mischer, Arnold Sywottek (1996) *Macht Stadt krank?: vom Umgang mit Gesundheit und Krankheit* [Does the city make sick? Treating Health and disease] Hamburg: Dölling und Galitz Verlag p. 146.

26 Martin French and Cavin Smith (2013) 'Health' surveillance: new modes of monitoring bodies, populations, and polities, *Critical Public Health,* 23:4, 383–392.

27 More than 500 health films were produced in Germany in the first half of the twentieth century, and approximately 1,000 were produced in the United States.

28 Leslie J. Reagan Nancy Tomes, Paula A. Treichler (eds.) (2007) *Medicine's Moving Pictures: Medicine, Health, and Bodies in American Film and Television.* University Rochester Press.

29 Alexandra M. Lord (2010) *Condom Nation: The U.S. Government's Sex Education Campaign from World War I* Baltimore: The Johns Hopkins University Press.

30 Miriam Posner (2018) Prostitutes, Charity Girls, and The End of the Road: Hostile Worlds of Sex and Commerce in an Early Sexual Hygiene Film in Bonah C, Cantor D, Laukötter A (eds) *Health education films in the twentieth century* Rochester, NY: University of Rochester Press, pp. 173–187.

31 Grieveson *ibid.*

32 Martin Pernick (1999) *The Black Stork: Eugenics and the Death of "Defective" Babies in American Medicine and Motion Pictures since 1915* Oxford: Oxford University Press, p. 14.

33 Ulf Schmidt (1995): Der medizinische Film in der historischen Forschung. *Mitteilungen aus dem Bundesarchiv* 3, 82–84; Schmidt, U. (2000): *Medical Research Films, Perpetrators, and Victims in National Socialist Germany 1933–1945.* Husum.

34 Anita Winkler (2015) Debating Sex: Education Films and Sexual Morality for the Young in post-War Germany, 1945–55, *Gesnerus.* 72(1): 77–93.

35 Karl-Heinz Roth (1988): Filmpropaganda für die Vernichtung der Geisteskranken und Behinderten im "Dritten Reich" [Film propaganda for extermination of mentally disabled people in the Third Reich] In: Gütz Aly, Karl Friedrich Masuhr, Maria. Lehmann (eds.) *Reform und Gewissen. Euthanasie im Dienst des Fortschritts*

20 *Introduction*

[Reform and conscience: Euthanasie in the service of progress] Berlin: Rotbuch Verlag *pp.* 125–193; Karl Ludwig Rost (1987) *Sterilisation und Euthanasie im Film des "Dritten Reiches"*[]. Husum; Karl Ludwig Rost (1988): Propaganda zur Vernichtung "unwerten Lebens" durch das Rassenpolitische Amt der NSDAP [Propaganda for extermination of unvaluable lives through the Race polotic Department of NSDAP]. *1999* 3: 46–55; Jutta Philips-Krug and Cecilia Hausheer (1997): *Frankensteins Kinder. Film und Medizin.* Zurich: Hatje Cantz Verlag; Ulf Schmidt (2000): *Medical Research Films, Perpetrators, and Victims in National Socialist Germany 1933–1945.* Husum).
36 Randolph Roth (1992) Is History a Process? Nonlinearity, Revitalization Theory, and the Central Metaphor of Social Science History, *Social Science History* 16, 2, 197–243, p. 200.
37 O'Connor 1992, p. 115.
38 Robert Proctor (1999) *The Nazi War on Cancer.* Princeton: Princeton University Press p. 248.
39 Valérie Vignaux (2011) Entertainment and Instruction as Models in the Early Years of Animated Film: New Perspectives on Filmmaking in France in Animation, SAGE Publications, 6, 177 – 192.
40 Paul Patton (2006) The event of colonialisation in Ian Buchanan and Andrian Parr (eds.) *Deleuze and the Contemporary World* Edinburg: Edinburg University Press 108–124 p. 112.
41 Lorenzo Lorusso, Thierry Lefebvre and Béatrice de Pastre (2016) Jean Comandon Neuroscientist, *Journal of the History of the Neurosciences,* 25:1, 72–83; Sonia Shechet Epstein (2019) The way they move, available online https://lareviewofbooks.org/article/the-way-they-move/
42 Valérie Vignaux (2007) *Jean Benoit-Lévy ou le corps comme utopie* [Jean Benoit-Lévy or the body as utopia] Paris: AFRHC.
43 Bernard Lahire, B. (2019) Sociological biography and socialisation process: a dispositionalist- contextualist conception, *Contemporary Social Science,* 14:3–4, 379–393.
44 Christian Bonah and Anja Laukötter (2015), *Screening Diseases. Films on Sex Hygiene in Germany and France in the First Half of the 20th Century* (Themenheft), Gesnerus 72, 1.
45 Bill Marsh (2010) Visual education in the United States and the 'Fly Pest' Campaign of 1910, *Historical Journal of Film, Radio and Television* 30 1 21–36; Anja Laukötter (2021) *Sex – richtig!: Körperpolitik und Gefühlerziehung im Kino des 20. Jahrhunderts* [Sex – right! Bodypolitics and education of feelings in the films of the twentieth century] Göttingen: Wallstein Verlag.
46 Elizabeth Lebas (1995) 'When Every Street Became a Cinema'. The film work of Bermondsey Borough Council's Public Health Department, 1923–1953, *History Workshop Journal,* 39, 1, 42–66.
47 Miriam Hansen (1991) *Babel and Babylon: Spectatorship and American Silent Film* Cambridge, MA: Harvard University Press p.77.
48 Druick ibid pp. 83–84.
49 Ilaria Scaglia (2020) *The Emotions of Internationalism: Feeling International Cooperation in the Alps in the Interwar Period (Emotions in History)* Oxford, Oxford University Press.
50 Roth Is History a Process? p. 217.
51 Vjekoslav Majcen (1995) *Filmska djelatnost škole narodnog zdravlja "Andrija Štampar": (1926.–1960.)* [Films "activities of the School of Public Health Andrija Štampar" 1926–1969] Zagreb: Hrvatski državni arhiv; Nadezhda Marinchevska, N. (2001) *Bylgarsko animacionno kino 1915–1995* [Bulgarian animation between 1915 and 1995] Sofia: Kolibri; Željko Dugac (2010) *Kako biti čist i zdrav.*

Zdravstveno prosvjećivanje u međuratnoj Hrvatskoj [How to be clean and healthy. Health education in interwar Croatia] Zagreb: Srednja Europa pp.109–114.

52 Zlatko Sudović (1978) Pedeset godina crtanog filma u Hrvatskoj 1922.–1972 [Fifty Years of Cartoon Film in Croatia, 1922–1972] Zagreb; Ivo Škrabalo (1998) 101 godina filma u Hrvatskoj, 1896.–1997. [101 years of film in Croatia] Zagreb, Nakladni zavod Globus.

53 Aleksandra Milovanović and Mila Turajlić (2017) Balkanski film na raskršću: Evropeizacija vs. regionalizacija [Balkan film on the crossroad: Europeanization vs. regionalization] *Casopis Instituta za pozorishte, film, radio i televiziju 32*, pp. 119–137.

54 For example, the Czech film *Procitnutí ženy* (Recognizing the woman, 1925) has undergone gender analysis within the recent project "Civilized woman: Ideals and paradoxes of the visual culture of the First Republic," implemented at Charles University in Prague.

55 Patton The event of colonialism, p. 117.

56 Roth Is history a process? p. 212.

57 Karl Kaser (2018) *Hollywood auf dem Balkan Die visuelle Moderne an der europaischen Peripherie (1900–1970)* Wien: Böhlau Verlag; Lucie Česálková (2012) Cinema outside cinema: Czech educational cinema of the 1930s under the control of pedagogues, scientists and humanitarian groups, *Studies in Eastern European Cinema*, 3:2, 175–191.

58 Roth Is History a process? p. 214.

59 Félix Guattari (2009) *Soft subversions: Texts and interviews 1977–1985* Los Angeles: Semiotexte pp. 37–38.

60 Nickolas Thoburn (2006) Vacuoles of Noncommunication: Minor Politics? Communist Style and the Multitude *in* Ian Buchanan and Andrian Parr (eds.) *Deleuze and the Contemporary World* Edinburg: Edinburg University Press. 42 –56 p. 44.

61 Juan Fernandez (2020) Story makes history, theory makes story: developing Rüsen's *Historik* in logical and semiotic directions, *History and Theory*, 57 1 75–103, pp. 91–92.

62 Michael Walzer (1987) *Interpretation and Social Criticism*. Cambridge, Mass.: Harvard University Press; Rosi Braidotti (2006) The becoming-Minoritarian of Europe *in* Ian Buchanan and Andrian Parr (eds.) *Deleuze and the Contemporary World* Edinburg: Edinburg University Press, 79–94, pp. 79–81.

63 Gilles Deleuze (1998) *Essays critical and clinical* Verso p. 42.

64 Roth Is history a process? p. 200.

65 Andrija Štampar (1925) *Socijalna medicina. Uz saradnju jugoslovenskih socijalnih lekara* [Social medicine: From the experinece of Yugoslav physicians] First volume Zagreb: Institut za socijalnu medicinu p. 282.

66 Zsuzsa Bokor (2017) Kihez szól a? Egy egészségügyi kampányfilm a 20. század elejéről [Who is it for? A health campaign film from the early twentieth century]. Available online https://www.filmtett.ro/cikk/4746/a-vilagrem-egy-egeszsegugyi-kampanyfilm-a-20-szazad-elejerol

67 Željko Dugac (2005) *Protiv bolesti i neznanja: Rockefellerova fondacija i meduratnoj Jugoslaviji* [Against Disease and Ignorance: The Rockefeller Foundation and Interwar Yugoslavia] Zagreb: Srednja Europe.

68 Majcen *ibid* pp. 103–104.

69 The presence of Czech experts at the international educational film conference in Paris, in 1926, was modest, but five years later, three of six boards established during the Third International Educational Film Conference in Vienna included Czech experts. Bohumil Milič, a teacher affiliated with the Masaryk Academy of Labour, joined the Commission of Pedagogy and Psychology, aimed at developing

expertise in the field of the influence of films and especially educational films on child development. Vladimir Úlehla, a professor of botany at the Masaryk University, in Brno, the Czech leader in developing scientific and ethnographic films, obtained the position of an expert within the Commission of Film in Science (for research and teaching). And Anton Matula became a member of the Commission on Photographs, with a particular focus on photographs for disseminating competencies as a medium of education and their relevant influence on humans. More in Adolf Hübl (1931) *Dritte internationale Lehrfilm-Konferenz in Wien* [The Third conference of educational film in Vienna] Wien: Österreichische Bildspielbund.

70 Cain An indirect influence upon industry: p. 231.

71 Antonie Doležalová and Hana Moravcová (2020) Czechoslovak film industry on the way from private business to public good (1918–1945), *Business History,* DOI: 10.1080/00076791.2020.1751822

72 Victoria Cain "An indirect influence upon industry."

73 Co nového v cizině [News from abroad] (1924) *Zdraví lidu Zdravotnický měsíčník Čsl. Červeného kříže* 2 3 p. 23.

74 In the National Film Archive, four of these films were preserved, but according to the information published in mass media, the partnership of Driml and Kokeisl produced more fairy tales such as *Prach náš vrah* (Dust is our enemy), *Divotvorný lék* (The miracle remedy), *Nová perníková chaloupka* (The gingerbread house): Nové české filmy se zdravotní tendenci (1927) [New Czech films with the tendence to promote health] *Zdraví lidu Zdravotnický měsíčník Čsl. Červeného kříže* 8.p. 270.

75 Wilhelm Bisom (1928) Expozice vědy, duchové a technické kultury a školství vysokého na Výstavě soudobé kultury v Brně in Expozice odboru vědy, duchové a technické kultury a školství vysokého Publikace č.1 [Exposition of Science, Spiritual and Technical Culture and Higher Education at the Exhibition of Contemporary Culture in Brno in Exposition of the Department of Science, Spiritual and Technical Culture and Higher Education Publication No.1] Brno p. 19–24.

76 ibid.

77 These scholars contributed to the longue durée of race science in Czechoslovakia, more in Victoria Shmidt (2020) Race science in Czechoslovakia: Serving segregation in the name of the nation Studies *History and Philosophy of Science Part C: Studies in History and Philosophy of Biological and Biomedical Sciences,* 83.

78 Výstava soudobé kultura v Československu: Odbor pro vědu, duchovou a technickou kulturu a školství vysoké [the Exhibition of Contemporary Culture in Czechoslovakia: The Board of science, spiritual and technical culture and higher education] Vladimir Úlehla Personal collection B 57 box 18 folder 888 AMU.

79 Ministarstvo inostranih dela Kralevine Srba, Chrvata i Slovenaca [Ministry of foreign affairs of the Kingdom of Serbs, Croats, and Slovenes] Miniserstvu Prosvete [The letter to the Ministry of education] 29.01.1930 Arhiv Jugoslavije fond 66 fascikle 92.

80 Ministarstvo inostranih dela Kralevine Srba, Chrvata i Slovenaca [Ministry of foreign affairs of the Kingdom of Serbs, Croats, and Slovenes] Miniserstvu Prosvete [The letter to the Ministry of education] 30.01.1930 Arhiv Jugoslavije fond 66 fascikle 92.

81 Ministarstvo inostranih dela Kralevine Srba, Chrvata i Slovenaca [Ministry of foreign affairs of the Kingdom of Serbs, Croats, and Slovenes] Miniserstvu Prosvete [The letter to the Ministry of education] 30.04.1930 Arhiv Jugoslavije fond 66 fascikle 92.

82 Ministarstvo inostranih dela Kralevine Srba, Chrvata i Slovenaca [Ministry of foreign affairs of the Kingdom of Serbs, Croats, and Slovenes] Miniserstvu

Prosvete [The letter to the Ministry of education] 30.05.1930 Arhiv Jugoslavije fond 66 fascikle 92.

83 Ministerstvo prosvete Kraljevine Yugoslavie [Ministry of Education of the Kingdom of Yugoslavia] Ministarstvu inostranih poslova [The letter to the Ministry of foreign affairs] 24.08.1930 Arhiv Jugoslavije fond 66 fascikle 92.

84 Ministerstvo prosvete Kraljevine Yugoslavie [Ministry of Education of the Kingdom of Yugoslavia] Ministarstvu inostranih poslova [The letter to the Ministry of foreign affairs] 12.12.1930 1930 Arhiv Jugoslavije fond 66 fascikle 92.

85 ibid.

86 Ministerstvo inostranih poslova Ministerstvu prosvete Mezhdunarodni institut za vospitni bioskop: izdanje mezhdunarodnog kataloga pouchnich filmova [Letter to the Ministry of Education: International Educational Cinematographic Institute: Publication of the international catalogue of educational films] 08.09.1931 1930 Arhiv Jugoslavije fond 66 fascikle 92.

87 Jugoslovenski prosvetni film [Yugoslav enlightening film] Ministerstvu prosvete opshte odelenie [Letter to the Ministry of Education. The department of general issues] 29.09.1931 1930 Arhiv Jugoslavije fond 66 fascikle 92.

88 Milan Marjanović (1927) Filmska tehnika [Film techniques] *Vijenac* 6 pp. 155–157.

89 Milan Marjanović (1927) Filmska Industrie [Film industry] *Vijenac* 3–4 pp. 85–88, p. 88.

90 Vojin Đorđević (1933) *Filmski almanah* [Film Year Book] Belgrade: Arfa p. 91.

91 Drzhavna filmska centrála [The State film Board] (1934) *Izveschtaj drzhavne filmske centrale o prometu i snimanju filmova i broju bioskopa u Kraljevni Yugoslavii u 1933 god.* [The report of the state film Central Committee about the dissemination and production of films and the number of cinemas in the Kingdom of Yugoslavia] Kinoteka of the State Archives of Croatia, Fond of Škola za narodnog zdravja, box 3.

92 Linda Hutcheon (2006) *A theory of adaptation* London: Routledge p. 170.

93 ibid p. 172.

94 ibid p. 169.

95 Henry Giroux (2002). Neoliberalism, corporate culture, and the promise of higher education: The university as a democratic public sphere. *Harvard Education* 72, 2.

96 Claude Bremond (1966) La logique des possibles narratifs, *Communications*, 8, pp. 60–76.

97 Claude Bremond (1973) *La Logique du récit*, Collection Poétique, Éditions du Seuil.

98 Noel Brown (2012) The Hollywood family film A History from Shirley Temple to Harry Poter London New York I.B.Tauris p.12.

99 Fernandez Story makes history, theory makes story.

Part 1

Child and nation in the focus of rescue-mission health films

1 The interwar obsession with family

Eugenic pathos vs. humanistic skepticism

The (im)possibility of the mission to rescue the child in interwar discursive practices

In *Kariéra matky Lízalky* (The career of mother Lízalka, 1935), first published as a serial novel in *Hvězda československých paní a dívek* (The star of Czechoslovak women and girls)[1] *and* then as a separate edition, Karel Andres describes the main female protagonist, Marie Lízalová, as "a typical figure of the outskirts of the city, thin, quarrelsome, but with a kind heart, which in the morning you will find on the porch (*pavlač*[2]) violently quarreling with a neighbor, and in the evening, crying, sobbing in the cinema because of the story of an abandoned child."[3] It is unlikely that the choice of such a popular genre as a film about an orphan to represent an example of obsession with cinema was coincidental. Along with the many other shadowy sides of moviegoing as a primary form of entertainment, *Kariéra matky Lízalky* emphasizes the danger of over-obsession with films concerning family well-being.[4] Ironically, the film adaptation of *Kariéra matky Lízalky* in 1937 reinforced the elements of humorous family chronicles, one of the most popular genres of the interwar period, in favor of achieving better reception and a larger female audience addicted to cinematography.

Kariéra matky Lízalky remains one of many testimonies of the interwar obsession with the healthy family. The film can be seen as one of multiple attempts by various actors to shape the idea of "proper" family life as a pillar of national, or even global, welfare, as well as an example of the systematic attempts by other actors to resist the pressure of this eugenics-based movement. Since the 1910s, eugenics at the national and global levels has started to devote more attention to families as entities for selecting those suitable for "healthy breeding." Multiple competitions among families with children and spousal pairs aimed at involving young generations in pre-marital counseling and preparation for healthy parenthood, along with the general practices of positive eugenics, including the very first initiatives in sexual education, special training for future mothers and so on. While expert knowledge aimed at rationalizing approaches to family life, new discursive practices within public life posited "good" families, especially mothers, as sacred.

DOI: 10.4324/9781003272267-3

In the 1920s, a few Central and Eastern European countries, including Czechoslovakia and some parts of Yugoslavia, adopted the celebration of Mother's Day, first proclaimed by U.S. President Woodrow Wilson, one of the most consistent proponents of positive eugenic measures. From the very beginning in the United States, this holiday connected motherhood and nationhood: Public expressions of love and reverence toward mothers included displaying the U.S. flag on all government buildings and private houses as well.[5] Kathleen W. Jones convincingly shows how Mother's Day fulfilled social functions beyond the purely personal mother–child relationship and advanced the mission of uniting the American nation.[6] Specifically, Mother's Day offered a unique option for bringing together traditional religious values and new, eugenics-based rhetoric concerning the role of mothers in preventing the "race suicide" of the nation.[7] In Yugoslavia, Mother's Day started to be celebrated on different days in the first decade of the twentieth century, with active participation of both the Orthodox and Catholic Churches. In Serbia, during the week before Christmas, spontaneous placement of children without parental care was practiced, when orphans tried to catch the eye of childless couples.[8] In Croatia, the celebration of Mother's Day on the second Sunday in May from the second half of the 1920s was patronized by the *Hrvatska katolička ženska sveza* (Croatian Catholic Women's Union). In Slovenia, Mother's Day was celebrated on March 25, the same day as the Annunciation of Mary and it was accompanied by charity actions for children in orphanages.

Among other aims, celebrating Mother's Day was used for fighting against infanticide in Central and Eastern Europe. In Moravia, one of the long-term mottos in the annual ceremony directed at rewarding mothers with many children was "*Svátek matek – děti musí žít*" ("Mother's day – children must live").[9] Timely placement of "illegitimate" children in institutions was seen as the main strategy for overcoming one of the intractable social "diseases," namely, murder by one's own mother. In her short essay aimed at persuading the public of the necessity to encourage institutional care for children born outside of marriage, Josefina Sobotková, a social worker at the local board in Kroměříž, juxtaposed sentimentalized stances such as, "Instead of breast-feeding, poor little creatures receive a blow to the head or the constriction of a tender throat," with arguments about the special vitality among "children of love," who "often have outstanding talent because they were conceived in a moment of passion or extraordinary tenderness."[10]

After this romantic introduction, Sobotková turned to a utilitarian argument, verging on the eugenic:

For the insignificant money that the state allocates to professional caregivers (*řemeslné pestounky*), from whom children will receive neither education and upbringing, nor even basic needs, we will not purchase a healthy future generation of people capable of working. As long as we do not strive to take better care of illegitimate children, they will join the ranks of criminals and the backward instead of joining the ranks of full-fledged members of the young state.[11]

Instituionalizing care for those children who could not be brought up in families reached the top position among state priorities for child protection: Not only those women who brought up ten or more children were rewarded on Mother's Day but also the caregivers of residential care institutions.

The dual status of residential care as equal to family care in terms of its meaning in educating new generations for the nation and opposing inadequate parental care aligned with a eugenics-based approach rooted in interwar North America and Western Europe. Such an approach was targeted at isolating not only people (including children) "improper" for family life but also children of "improper" parents: Migrants, people with disabilities or those who were seen as suffering from social diseases such as tuberculosis, alcoholism and venereal disease. The segregation of people with disabilities and the socially disadvantaged became a welcome institutional solution in North America and Europe before the First World War and escalated to one of the central tasks during the interwar period, along with the practice of forced sterilization. Between the late 1910s and 1930s, campaigns for promoting residential care were directly related to the eugenics movement and its representatives at the level of national governments and ministries in different parts of the world.[12]

Traditional family values in the eugenic and anti-eugenic rhetoric of Hollywood family films

In the first third of the twentieth century, family was the focus of not only scholars, experts and social welfare practitioners but also filmmakers who were interested in shaping a new type of entertainment, namely, family visits to the cinema. Hollywood "was a 'family' institution, an amusement in conjunction with its growth as a near-universal cultural institution with reorientation to the successfully cultivated the middle classes' social respectability."[13] Family films easily adopted a diversity of views on "proper" parenthood and family life – also because of the historical role of literature and theater in promoting both eugenic and anti-eugenic stances concerning spousal life and parenthood, even before the institutionalization of the eugenics movement.[14]

The outstanding theatrical potential of hereditary theory[15] was easily embraced by filmmakers. The leaders of the eugenics movement invested much effort into making eugenic ideas visible, especially with regard to "invisible" (but decisive for eugenics) objects such as genes, carriers of disease or heredity itself. And they accepted the new visual medium of film with great enthusiasm. The engagement of Western literature, theater and then cinematography with evolutionary ideas and a rational approach to marriage reverberated with the eugenic goal of bringing reproductive issues and, especially, the role of women as selectors and vessels, to the fore.[16] Many of the pro-eugenic, semi-documentary and semi-feature films like *Eugenics baby*

(1914), *Where are my children?* (1916)[17] or *Birth* (1917) directly addressed women and were expressly advertised to female audiences.[18] Unsurprisingly, the most common cinematic and anti-eugenic response abused this focus and reestablished the priority of men's common sense; the comedies *Nell's eugenic wedding* (1914), *Eugenics vs. love* (1914) or *Jerry's eugenic marriage* (1917), among others,[19] ridiculed women as mindless followers of eugenics.

Instructive messages and righteousness often operated as the main positive characteristics of eugenic films[20] while anti-eugenic comedies presented the struggle between two flows of influence on young women: The elderly single female relative devoted to eugenic ideals and the loving man who opposes genuine feelings in trying to control an inexperienced young soul. *Bunny backslide* (1914) by George D. Baker, with the popular American comedians John Bunny and Flora Finch, presents the story of a love triangle among a widow who professes eugenics and tries to control others with the help of medical authorities, her obese groom and a cheerful young plump woman. The triangle is resolved through the careless marriage of the latter two and the widow's subsequent disappointment in science. In these types of comedies, it is possible to recognize the earliest attempts to construct family films that would address a wider audience than the pro-eugenic films targeted at female audiences.

These anti-eugenic comedies aimed to "respond to cultural requirements for optimistic, comforting narratives that provide reassurance and reaffirm often conservative social values; and on the other, to innate desire for spectacle, escapism, and release from everyday pressure and anxieties."[21] The sensitivity of such criticism toward the eugenic film can be judged by the numerous attempts among supporters of positive eugenics to justify themselves in front of the public and even demonstrate a willingness to compromise between "rational" and "emotional" approaches to marriage and parenting: "What eugenicists want is to make health the only consideration that restricts romance."[22] Both cohorts of films struggled for acceptance by the middle-class audience, whose expectations and desirable patterns directly shaped a new genre – the family film.[23]

Along with the gender-based interrelation between eugenics and cinematography as mass entertainment for the middle classes and those who dreamed of belonging to it, some films deepened the argument against eugenics and introduced social injustice as the breeding ground for eugenic ideas. The film *Their mutual child* (1920),[24] based upon the novel *The coming of Bill* (1919), by Pelham Wodehouse, a consistent critic of eugenics and the rational scientific-like approach to family planning, was lost, but the reviews and the novel reveal the intention to attack both patterns, namely, the pro-eugenic instructive approach and the masculine-based critique of eugenics. Through the vicissitudes of the love relation between wealthy Ruth and unaffected Kirk, both Wodehouse and the film question the core of middle-class morality, such as affiliation with higher classes, the predominance of financial success and, even more, hygienic skills as the grounds for children's health. To achieve their own happiness, Ruth and Kirk struggle against Ruth's aunt, Mrs. Lora Delane Porter, who embodies the ideals of eugenics, and Bailey, Ruth's brother, whose personality resembles the male characters of anti-eugenic comedies. For Wodehouse, both the aunt and the brother present the different sides of the same middle-class hypocrisy, incompatible with true intimacy and attachment. In *The kid* (1921), Charlie Chaplin has moved further in the critical deconstruction of the eugenic view on family audiences of popular films as symbolizing respectability, profitability and mass cultural acceptance.[25]

The deconstruction of residential care in *The kid* by Charlie Chaplin

By the 1920s, Chaplin had attained the reputation of a consistent critic of eugenics and political practices aimed at performing eugenic ideals. Ewa Barbara Luczak underscores the role of the eugenics movement as a kind of negative driving force that led Chaplin to deconstruct nativism and the eugenic dislike of migrants in *The immigrant* (1917) or to ridicule eugenic surveillance over the reproduction of the population in *Dog's life* (1918). Chaplin was clearly unsatisfied with conservative critiques against eugenics. His film, *The cure* (1917), can be easily interpreted as challenging not only the practices of Dr. Kellogg, one of the influential proponents of eugenic ideals for healthy individuals and healthy families,[26] but also the comedy *Bunny backslide* (1914).

According to Luczak, "[B]y attacking the discourse of eugenics Chaplin in fact waged a war over American identity."[27] *The kid* indicates that Chaplin deconstructed not only the fundamental values of American identity but also the general idea of Westernness or Europeanness and its core, the belief in the progressive nature of development toward human perfection and the necessity to move from the "primitive" stage of childhood to human maturity – adulthood. Moreover, Chaplin directly links his doubts about sacralizing childhood as the preparation for a fruitful adult life with his skeptical view on any institutionalized forms of assistance to people. While eugenics stemmed from recapitulation theory, with its strong division of coming-of-age into the stages of "savageness," "barbarism" and the desirable "civilized" individual, *The kid* aligned with the phenomenology of a split-self divided into a True, like-child, Self and a False, like-adult, Self, inviting us to find our wise child, calls to the internal child and the replacement of the false, adult, self with the return of the child-body into adult flesh.[28] Challenging the utilitarian meaning of childhood questions the role of institutions such as those directed at public health, social protection or education.

Like Chapin's earlier films, *The kid* does not skimp on sarcasm toward the disciplinary society and its leaders, doctors, social workers and police officers. Instead of helping the sick John, the doctor calls the local authorities responsible for collecting orphans and placing them into orphanages. Two men come to the Tramp to remove young John. Their belief in their own superiority is only reinforced by the apparent hierarchy between the senior manager, who communicates with the Tramp through the junior manager. One of the remarkable details is the open condemnation of the practice of seizing children by ordinary people – three women are watching with poorly concealed anger during the removal procedure and do not interfere with Chaplin's character to save the child.

Nell Hurley (1960) underscores the mission of the Little Tramp as a witness of injustice who should "detonate the very structure of conventional society amid an explosion of laughter."[29] *The kid* responds to the multiple campaigns in favor of residential care for children from asocial families, as well as to Chaplin's personal experience with such care, one of the most consistent experiences of injustice. Furthermore, Chaplin's comic principle of contrast, setting the Little Tramp against the world,[30] highlights the art of survival as inevitably negating the concept of morality as slippery and relying on the vulnerability of human beings as a paradoxical strategy for being rescued from the pressures of the external world and its institutions.[31]

The films by Chaplin reached a very special position in interwar Central and Eastern Europe, and not only because of their "very ability to reach mass audiences internationally to unify audiences not merely on a national but a global level."[32] Representatives of avant-garde art borrowed Chaplin's esthetics of minimalism and mechanism, followed his deconstruction of bourgeois values, tried to reproduce sophisticated stylizations of primitivism[33] and actively discussed these innovations in periodicals. This acceptance by intellectuals only reinforced the acceptance of Chaplin's esthetics by mass audiences – who attended *The kid* more and more, making it one of the most popular family films produced in Hollywood. The attractiveness of Chaplin's films for the mass audience reflected the increasing popularity of moviegoing as family entertainment, as well as the acceptance of Chaplin's films as a historically proven antithesis to the defeated Habsburg monarchy, where his comedies were banned.[34] The Little Tramp started to be seen as a Balkan because of his adventurism, balancing between legality and illegality, and fatalism.[35]

The popularity of Chaplin, an honored member of several artistic groups in Central and Eastern Europe,[36] developed hand-in-hand with worries from the side of those who promoted the interests of newly established states and desirable national identities. The Czech philosopher Zdeněk Smetáček, who shared Bergson's view on observing comic situations as an efficient tool for "preventing us from undesirable behaviour which is not accepted by social order," directly underscores the controversial effect of Chaplin's comedies and especially *The kid*:

[T]he reaction to Chaplin's films is a testament to how empathy, as in other cases, suppresses laughter. More sensitive viewers stop laughing earlier, those who resist empathy later. The truth is that where the comicality of Chaplin's film ends, his works get their moral meaning. Chaplin is not only and not so much the giver of laughter, but the awakener of our dormant conscience.[37]

While psychological plausibility and the power of emotional attachment in *The kid* were not the subjects of doubt, Chaplin's "imagined paradise in the slums"[38] was seen as a utopian view on care for children that should be debunked. The very first feature health films produced in Prague and Zagreb turned the incredible popularity of *The kid* toward the aim of promoting institutions providing for the welfare of children and especially residential care as the only suitable option in contrast to unreliable care from the side of asocial caregivers, whether biological or substitute parents. The deconstruction of the main messages of *The kid* was embedded in the consistent promotion of "proper," institutionalized, childhood for the next generations of citizens.

Notes

1 *Hvězda československých paní a dívek* was one of the most popular periodicals in interwar Czechoslovakia until the middle of the 1940s.
2 *Pavlač* is a projecting structure protruding in front of the load-bearing wall, which serves as an access path to individual apartments on one floor. At the end of the nineteenth century and the beginning of the twentieth century, such construction was used mainly for lower-category housing in many countries of Central Europe, including Czechoslovakia.
3 *Hvězda československých paní a dívek*, 22.6.1935, No. 25, p. 2.
4 Marie Vintrová (2004) Rodinná krnonika z periferie (žánrová inovace v nejrozšířenějším ženském týdeníku První republiky [Family chronicle from the periphery (genre innovation in the most widespread women's weekly of the First Republic] in Michal Jareš, Pavel Janáček, Petr Šámal *Povídka, roman a periodický tisk v 19. a 20.století* [Short story, novel and periodical in the 19th and 20th centuries] Sborník příspěvků ze sympozia pořádaného oddělením pro výzkum literární kultury ÚČL AV ČR v Praze 13–14.11 2004 [Collection of the contributions to the symposium of the research of literal culture of the Institute of Czech literature, Academy of Science, Prague], 194–200.
5 President Woodrow Wilson's Mother's Day Proclamation, source: U.S. National Archive and Records Administration https://www.archives.gov/global-pages/larger-image.html?i=/historical-docs/doc-content/images/mothers-day-proc-l.jpg&c=/historical-docs/doc-content/images/mothers-day-proc.caption.html
6 Kathleen W. Jones (1980) Mother's Day: The Creation, Promotion and Meaning of a New Holiday in the Progressive Era, *Texas Studies in Literature and Language*, pp. 175–196.
7 Jones, ibid., p. 185.
8 Biskup Nikolaj i Arhiđakon Ljubomir Ranković *(2012) Srpske slave i verski običaji [Serbian religious celebrations and traditions]* available online: https://svetosavlje.org/srpske-slave-i-verski-obicaji/?pismo=lat
9 The postage stamp with this motto was issued by the local authorities of Kroměříž in 1947 to celebrate Mother's Day: Sociálně právní ochrana: Den matek [Social protection: Mother's day] 1949 box 6 folder 423/49 State Regional Archives in Kroměříž.
10 Josefina Sobotková (1928) Nemanželské děti [Children born outside of marriage] in *Výroční zpráva o činnosti okresní péče o mládež a ostatních humanních spolků v*

Holešově [Annual report about the activities of local authorities concerning youth care and other charity unions in Holešov], Halašov: Tiskarna Balatka a Šrámak.
11 Ibid., p. 11.
12 David Braddock and Susan Parish (2001) An institutional history of disability. In Gary L. Albrecht, Katherine D. Seelman, and Michael Bury (eds), *Handbook of Disability Studies*, London: Sage, 11–68.
13 Noel Brown (2012) *The Hollywood family film A History from Shirley Temple to Harry Poter*, London, New York: I.B. Tauris, p. 17.
14 Donald J. Childs, in his *Modernism and Eugenics: Woolf, Eliot, Yeats, and the Culture of Degeneration* (Cambridge University Press 2001), underscores the role of intellectuals in promoting eugenic ideas before eugenics became one of the most influential social movements globally in the twentieth century.
15 Tamsen Wolff (2009) *Mendel's Theory: heredity, eugenics, and early twentieth-century American drama,* London: Palgrave, p. 5.
16 Kirsten Shepherd-Barr (2015) *Edwardians and Eugenicists. In theatre and evolution from Ibsen to Beckett.* Colombia: Columbia University Press, p. 168.
17 Kim, Grace, "Where Are My Children? (1916)". Embryo Project Encyclopedia (26.05.2017), available online: https://embryo.asu.edu/pages/where-are-my-children-1916. 19.12.1919, p. 19.
18 Martin S. Pernick (1996) *The Black Stork: Eugenics and the Death of "Defective" Babies in American Medicine and Motion Pictures since 1915*, Oxford: Oxford University Press.
19 Ewa Barbara Luczak (2021) *Mocking eugenics: American Culture against Scientific Hatred*, London: Routledge, p. 23.
20 The *Baltimore Sun* describes one of the eugenic photoplays, filming a theatrical performance entitled "Temptation, the Eternal Combat," about the coming of age of a young man who has inherited the best possible physical, moral, and intellectual qualities. It presents his preparation for the mission of reproduction as follows: "While it is a frank handling of a vital theme, it is done in a way that will not be offending to anyone. It is an allegorical screen production, based on eugenics, teaching the value to youths and maidens alike of moral and physical purity. It is a warning and plea to all persons of marriageable age," Tells of Life's pitfalls *The Baltimore Sun (Baltimore, Maryland)*, · 29.06.1919, p. 54.
21 Brown, *ibid.*, p. 10.
22 Evening Public Ledger (Philadelphia, Pennsylvania), 27.10.1921, p. 11.
23 Wolff *Mendel's Theatre.*
24 Comedy and eugenics feature films: *Their mutual child* The Omaha Daily News (Omaha, Nebraska) 21.04.1921, p. 4; The Morning Post (Camden, New Jersey)· 10.03.1921, p. 3.
25 Brown, ibid, p. 17.
26 Luczak, ibid, p. 26.
27 Ibid p. 41.
28 Karmenlara Seidman (2004) The call of the wise baby in Chaplin's The Kid Women and Performance, *A Journal of Feminist Theory*, 14 1, 117–136, pp. 131–132.
29 Neil Hurley (1960) The social philosophy of Charlie Chaplin, *Studies: An Irish Quarterly Review*, 49 165, 313–320, p. 316.
30 Surya P. Verma and Binod Mishra (2021) The art of survival: Understanding Charlie Chaplin's The Little Tramp through the Lens of little narrative, *Quarterly Review of film and Video*, 38 5, 400–413, p. 402.
31 Ibid., p. 403.
32 Brown, ibid., p. 3.

33 Bojan Jović (2018) *Avangardni mit Čaplin* [Avantgarde-Mythos Chaplin] Beograd: Službeni glasnik, pp. 236–237.
34 Ivan Motýl (2018) Tulák Charlie a jeho české stopy [The Tramp Charlie and his Czech traces] *Týden* 25, 2, 02.01.2018, p. 38–41.
35 Jović, ibid., p. 241.
36 In Czechoslovakia, Chaplin accepted the invitation of the *Devětsil*, the group of Czechoslovak avangardists.
37 Zdeněk Smetáček (1925) Bergson a Chaplin [Bergson and Chaplin], *Přítomnost*, 12.03. 136–138, p. 138.
38 Seidman, ibid., p. 121.

2 Collective care vs. the "backward" family in *Jak Vašíček přišel k nohám*

The brotherhood of the disabled captures Czech screens and hearts

> On Friday, an original propagandist film, *"Jak Vašíček přišel k nohám,"* was shown for the first time in cinematograph Sanssouci with unusual success. After a short speech by principal Bartoš, the film was shown, and, from the very beginning, it was accompanied by spontaneous applause, which culminated after the end of the film and turned into a standing ovation for the little hero. We lacked neither tears nor enthusiasm.[1]

In autumn 1921, the review, among many others, documented the great success of a small film studio in Prague, *Atroposfilm*, with the film *Jak Vašíček přišel k nohám* (How Vašíček got his legs, 1921) about dramatic destiny of young Vašíček.[2] The film begins with a scene of boys who compete in running across the tracks in front of a train. The most courageous and decisive, Vašíček, wants to be the last to run across and win, but he loses both legs. Now he should transform his passion for thrills into an intense adaptation aimed at approaching the level of "productive individual." Only placement in an institution, *Jedličkův ústav*, therapy and new friendships with children like him, other students of the institution, make the option for coming of age and coping with his impairment possible.

Critics directly opposed the catharsis of the film to the "artificial" and "dirty" influence of many other, mostly foreign, feature films that "only play on selfish and false sentimentality":

> The audience loves films that transport them into a different world than the one in which they live their daily life. The filmmakers soon recognized this weakness in the audience, and the flow of films from the social life of the ancestral and monetary aristocracy, or, again, from the atmosphere of the pubs and the demi-monde, is still dense and abundant. Of course, such flow does not work fertile soil, but only multiplies mud, especially when its drops are usually not pure water, but some artificial fluid. The film presented this week in cinematograph Sanssouci introduces the public to

DOI: 10.4324/9781003272267-4

the mostly unknown part of life, but more importantly, the part of real life not constructed but totally authentic, the life of pupils in *Jedličkův ústav*.[3]

The call for reality and the necessity to accept this call contributed to the success of *Jak Vašíček přišel k nohám* as an embodiment of national aspirations. In his later numerous publications, August Bartoš, the author of the plot and the main educator at *Jedličkův ústav* between the 1920s and 1940s, often reiterated the film's motto: "I would like a house where unfortunate and weak children could come and exit into life, confident and capable people."[4] This stance could be addressed not only to people with disabilities but also to the entire nation, which was expected to be emancipated from the pressures of an unhealthy past. The tasks that would empower disabled people as a particular group and the nation as an entity were intertwined through an understanding of freedom as a health instinct. "[O]ur ancestors at one time breathed so much air of freedom, and we yearn for their freedom,"[5] Bartoš said in one of his manuals for the educators of people with disabilities, systematically providing the analogy between becoming mature citizens and functionally healthy individuals.

Establishing communities of students able to support each other during their stay at the institution and especially after finishing the vocational training comprised the main pillar of rehabilitation in *Jedličkův ústav*. The community or, even more, the "brotherhood" was seen by Bartoš as a resource equally important to professional assistance and scientific progress in the rehabilitation of people with disabilities. Not parents but children themselves and educators were those who made decisions about release from the institution (see Figures 2.1 and 2.2). In the film, there were many scenes targeted at demonstrating children's ability for self-government and cohesion in learning, work and leisure activities. The scenes of the outside activities of children are complemented by nicknames that reflect a self-ironical attitude

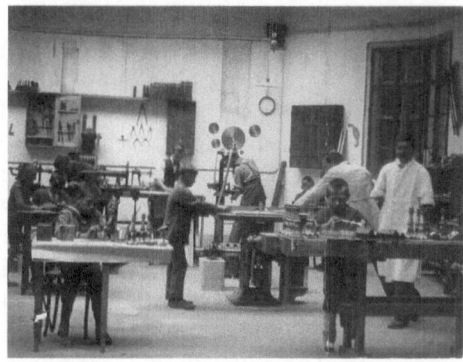

Figure 2.1 Brotherhood of disabled boys in *Jak Vašíček přišel k nohám* (How Vašíček got his legs, 1921).

Source: NFA, ©OOA-S, Prague 2021.

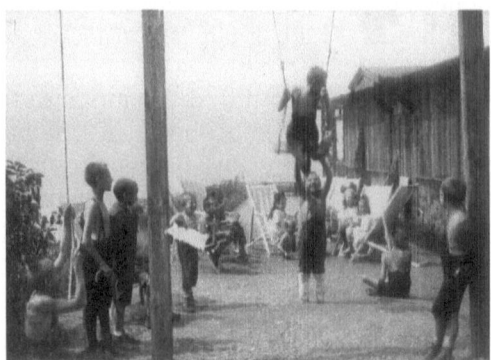

Figure 2.2 Brotherhood of disabled boys in *Jak Vašíček přišel k nohám* (How Vašíček got his legs, 1921).

Source: NFA, ©OOA-S, Prague 2021.

toward impairment and the readiness to accept it, aligned with Chaplin's self-ironic mode: The young girl with legs deformed by rachitis is called "Mařenka without a horse," and the boy without hands who loves painting is the "handy painter."

Although Bartoš often denotes "children," his focus is primarily on boys. The majority of his stories, as well as the characters in films, are boys and young men. The central message of empowerment through successful vocational guidance can be comprehended only through storytelling that addresses boys more than girls. The major part of the film is about the choice of profession; while Vašíček likes painting, he makes decision to become an orthopedic prosthetist and to continue his cooperation with an older alumnus of *Jedličkův ústav.* Embedding the self-government so important for educating disabled children in the preparation for political participation (in the film, young boys read newspapers that present different political views) should be seen as practicing the idea of citizenship as a kind of manhood, a central point in the ideology of *Jedličkův ústav.*

Without a doubt, not the young boy but rather the *Jedličkův ústav,* one of the first institutions in the Czech lands established for Czech people with disabilities, should be seen as a main "character" in this film, a clearly masculine symbol of the newly established state and its readiness to accept the task of care for the weak. The film included not only a coming-of-age story but also a very detailed description of the different sub-departments within *Jedličkův ústav,* including the workshop for making prostheses and fitting them for children, the system of medical rehabilitation and, above all, the various options for vocational training. The film directly promoted the preferability of institutional care for socializing children with disabilities against family care, due to insurmountable parental limitations. Although the film was lost, the surviving stills of the film and its description, as well as numerous statements by Bartoš, reveal the consistent opposition of insufficient parental care and the ideal options provided by institutions.

One of the stories from Bartoš's collection, titled *Zachraněný* (Rescued), presents the comparable case of Lojzík, whose mother has died and his father works in the mines. Due to cerebral palsy, Lojzík is limited in his ability to move and spends his days in bed, instead of going to school or playing with his peers. The emotive description of the physical pain and weakness that Lojzík experiences is accompanied by a recounting of his loneliness and inability to improve his life, despite his brave and consistent attempts:

> The wheelchair broke when he fell on it. Well, it needs to be repaired. No sooner said than done. So, here's a saw. Here is a hammer and nails. But what is it? His hand shook, twitched and … aah, how colitis, how colitis, how painful. Lojzik looks frightened in front of him. Where does all this pain come from?[6]

His father is the only one who makes up Lojzík's community and who teaches his son everything. One day, the father perishes in a mine collapse, and the boy is sent to a boarding school, at first under terrible conditions, but "his repressed passion for life awakened and began to control his actions. His legs were amputated and he did not die; on the contrary, he felt a new strength in himself and was looking forward to the opportunity to go on the first excursion in his life."[7] While begging was the only option until Lojzík would be trained, he makes the decision to go to *Jedličkův ústav*, where, despite his age and the late start, he graduates from school in a few months and becomes "a new man who is not sentenced to be sick" or "remain a useless burden to his homeland."[8]

Bartoš emphasizes the isolation of people with disabilities from the "healthy" as a pre-condition for providing "the space of equality among their own kind that emancipates people with disabilities from the derogatory sympathy in the eyes of the healthy."[9] Isolation from parents, in favor of becoming a part of the community of a residential institution, is another pillar of Bartoš's approach, which questions the self-giving love natural for pelicans but not for humans. Bartoš mentions *The Pelican* by August Strindberg as a cruel but fair irony that fights against an illusive and romanticized view on parental love. Ignoring the moral roughness of parents from lower social classes, who employ an overly utilitarian approach to their disabled children, is one of the main motifs in Bartoš's texts. He shares Strindberg's transformationalist ideals that shaped a pessimist view on the "backward" and uneducable lower classes[10] and stresses the role of society and state care as guarantees for children from lower-class families.[11] The cascade of short examples of selfish parents who force their disabled children to beg, steal and prostitute themselves serves not only the aim to persuade the audience about the unique role of residential care but also the "naturally limited ability of people to love children with disabilities, and instead social obligations to care."[12] According to the shots in the film, Vašiček's parents also resist but after visiting their son and observing the hopeless life of a disabled vagabond and former militant and the humiliating pity for him, they accept the rightness of the institutionalized approach.

Jak Vašíček přišel k nohám as a model of public politics concerning people with disabilities

The generally positive attitude toward residential care, especially for those who were seen as coming from a "backward" social space, reverberates with the ironically incredulous view on charity and the religious grounds underlying its practice. In his extremely anti-religious pamphlet, *Na soudě božím* [At God's ordeal], published as an annual pre-Christmas text in 1933, Bartoš consistently deconstructs each of four world monotheistic religions as limited in the ability to provide ideological grounds for the empowerment of people with disabilities. The book was accompanied by cartoons, and one of the largest on the cover of the book represented the adoration of the Magi – three boys, one blind, one on crutches and one without hands, who have turned to the infant Jesus. The pamphlet concluded with a plea not to spend money on charity but to donate to the development of institutions such as *Jedličkův ústav*. This attack against traditional religions demonstrates Bartoš's situatedness within the pro-state movement in favor of replacing Christianity, especially Catholicism, with the civil religion of public health and new, healthy cults that promote citizenship.[13] Many of the reviews of the film *Jak Vašíček přišel k nohám* opened with statements such as "Every day, hundreds and hundreds of requests to accept a child come to the institute, which remain without a positive answer due to a lack of available places."[14] Moreover, the showings of the film in Prague in 1921 were orchestrated to collect money for developing this type of institution across the country.

The film enjoyed a long public life as "the best educational Czech film,"[15] "uncritically and positively received by journalists of different political affiliations,"[16] which underscores its supra-political and national meaning. The film was purchased by the Ministry of Education for disseminating in schools and factories – among working parents, and until the end of the 1930s, it was screened, for instance, in the Bata shoe factory. The film accompanied a majority of national and international events aimed at promoting the institutionalization of care for people with disabilities, such as the "Exhibition of the social care for youth," held in 1922 in Prague or the exhibition *Výstava soudobé kultury* ("Exhibition of contemporary culture"),[17] at the ten-year anniversary of new Czechoslovak state in 1928. The long echo of this approach reverberated in the socialist period as well.

In 1968, Czechoslovak television launched an unprecedented charity action, collecting funds for *Jedličkův ústav*.[18] The 45-minute documentary consisted primarily of interviews with the staff and young people with disabilities, entitled *Dluh*, which in the Czech language connotes "debt" and "obligation" simultaneously. The film begins by following a four-year-old girl through the streets of Prague, who has a minor disability in her legs and another girl with cerebral palsy, who learns to walk under the supervision of a rehabilitation nurse at the institution. The visual difference between the ability to walk is noted: "[A]nd she will be once an adult, and she really wants to resemble others who are healthy. Who knows how she will be accepted … ?" A close-up follows, with the purposeful face of a girl who moves under the command of rehabilitation nurse: "Foot forward, forward."

The major part of the film consists of interviews with young men who share their doubts and thoughts regarding their future and the role of institution. Each of the cases is accompanied by the comments of the social worker responsible for their post-institutional placement. An unnamed man, 24 years old, placed in the institution for seven years, is featured. He has finished eight classes of secondary school and *střední odborná škola zdravotnická* (secondary vocational medical school) and has entered a medical university, representing the most successful pathway of placement. Remarkably, neither he nor the social worker attribute his success to the institution but to his will and industriousness. To the question, "What should be done for making this path possible for others?" the young man answers: "We need a team of psychologists who would accompany and correct the mental development of each of our students."

The film introduces the issue of "forced integration" – the cohabitation of those educable with those at a level of "imbecility," due to the limited number of available places in special institutions: "[T]hey must encounter each other, play with each other, and these children aggravate the development of normal children. Additionally, can you imagine that they sleep in a common room?" The catastrophic consequences of late intervention into disability and the necessity to start rehabilitation as soon as possible represent one of the central motifs of the film: "Despite all the dedication of the nurses, it is a house of despair, and we put these children in that house."

The film ends with a scene of playing football, one of the visual similarities with *Jak Vašíček přišel k nohám*, narrated by the journalist Libuše Hájková: "People who are lucky and born healthy have no right to consider others a burden. They have no right." The premiere of *Dluh* took place on December 9, 1968, during the Advent period traditional for motivating the public to take part in charity. The account *Akce Dluh* (Action *Dluh*) had been set up to help children from the institution and the development of the institution overall. The collected funds were spent on building a new workshop for seamstresses and for separating incontinent children and youth in a pavilion next to the school building, segregating them from those children seen as potentially having "functional health." Until nowadays, the history of *Jedličkův ústav* is a matter of public pride, rarely engendering a critical view of its role in shaping the politics of segregation against people with disabilities.

The longue-durée of residential care for those disabled in the Czech lands was not limited by the national borders – in interwar Central and Eastern

Europe, Czech experts in substitute care reached the position of internationally accepted experts. In 1933, Đorđe Žužić, an expert at the Ministry of Health and Social Policy of Yugoslavia, responsible for the reform of care for "abnormal" children, was sent to Prague to study the Czechoslovak experience in institutionalizing care for disabled children. While the development of residential care for children in Yugoslavia was slow[19] and met numerous obstacles, the experience of Czech educators was seen as the most desirable model. Among the many institutions he visited, he characterized *Jedličkův ústav* through the production quality of its carpets, "which were of such quality that they could be produced by the best masters, who should be completely physically healthy."[20] This admiration of the ability to achieve perfection entered into a contest with the critical view on the idea of the utility of people as a main desirable result of the efforts of education: "Those who think only about the benefits of education do not think about evil and forget about insane asylums, hospitals, and prisons, whose inhabitants are most often men, women, and children from the same area in which we live."[21]

This controversy was not resolved, but was overshadowed by the idea of a new, totally different form of residential care that would fully correspond to the humanistic message of the newly created state:

> Moving through Czechoslovakia means moving through people for whom their children are the symbol and object of social care, who, from workers to intellectuals, feel themselves proud when they pass along Masaryk House[22] where innocent members of future civilization spend their days learning and working.[23]

In the three films produced by the School of Public Health, *Zapušteno dijete* (Neglected child, 1930), *Pomoć u pravi čas* (Help at the right time, 1930) and *Spas male Zorice* (The rescue young Zorka, 1929), the contradiction was transformed, presenting multiple institutionalization of the child, including substitute family care as the perfect solution to the intergenerational conflict of those old and unable to be reeducated and those young who are open to new healthier and more useful life than their less "civilized" caregivers.

Notes

1 Bouřlivý úspěch filmu *Čech: Politický týdenník katolický*, 21.11.1921, No 320.
2 Remarkably the protagonist was named Vašek, by the Czech analogy of John, the main character of *The Kid*.
3 Jak Vašíček přišel k nohám *Čas*, 23.11.1921, No 274, p. 3.
4 August Bartoš (1925) *Cestou k životu: Feuilletony vychovatelovy* [On the way to life: Feuilletons from the educator], Brno, p. 53.
5 Ibid., p. 49.
6 Ibid., p. 8.
7 Ibid., p. 10.
8 Ibid.

9 Ibid., p. 19.
10 Shepherd-Barr *Theatre and Evolution.*
11 The positive attitude among experts and popular writers toward residential care for the socially vulnerable was part of the mainstream in the public life of interwar Czechoslovakia. One example is the novel *Dětský domov Jany Rajnerové* [The orphanage of Jana Rajneorvá] by Maryna Radoměrská, about a wise female principal of an orphanage who rescues young souls from being corrupted by life in big cities. It was published in *Hvězda československých paní a dívek in 1938.*
12 Bartoš, ibid., pp. 37–38.
13 More about this path of dependence on public health as civil religion can be found in Victoria Shmidt (2019) *Politics of disability in interwar and socialist Czechoslovakia: Segregation in the name of the nation,* Amsterdam: Amsterdam University Press.
14 Večer lidový denník *Jak Vašíček přišel k nohám: film o nejubožejších a nejzapomínanějších* [Jak Vašíček přišel k nohám: a film about the poorest and most forgotten] 20.07.1921, No 162, p. 12.
15 This definition was often used in advertisements for the film in newspapers and magazines.
16 *Jak Vašíček přišel k nohám* Školní kinematografie časopis pro uvedení filmu jakožto výchovné učební pomůcky [School cinematography magazine for the introduction of film as an educational teaching aid] 26.11.1921, p. 11.
17 Výstava soudobé kultura v Československu: Odbor pro vědu, duchovou a technickou kulturu a školství vysoké [Exhibition of Contemporary Culture in Czechoslovakia: Department of Science, Spiritual and Technical Culture and Higher Education] Vladimir Úlehla, Personal collection B 57 box 18 folder 888 AMU.
18 In the 1950s, *Jedličkův ústav*, like many other residential care centers for people with disabilities, underwent an attack from the side of the Ministry of Health, which was interested in expropriating the buildings of these institutions in favor of services for mothers and children. Although many institutions were forced to move, *Jedličkův ústav* defended its right to stay in Prague and even expand; more in Victoria Shmidt (2015) *Child welfare discourses and practices in the Czech lands: the segregation of Roma and disabled children during the nineteenth and twentieth centuries,* Brno: MUNI PRESS.
19 Only in the late 1930s did the Yugoslav authorities make a decision about establishing special institutions for children with "mental retardation" – *duševno zaostale dece* – under the pressure of experts from the Central Hygienic Institute. The capacity of these institutions (they accepted no more than 40–50 children) could not satisfy the need for care among these target groups: Inspekcioni izveshtaj: Odelenje za smeshtaj duševno zaostale dece Velika Gorica Fond 39 Ministarstvo socijalne Politike a narodnog zdravlja 1919–1945, FAS 7 AJ.
20 Đorđe Žužić (1934) Ministarstvu socijalnoj politiky i narodnogo zdorovjy Alexandrovi Zemun Referentu za abnormalu decu [To the Ministry of Social Policy and National Health Alexander Zemun Referent for abnormal children] folie 475–484 Fond 39 Ministarstvo socijalne politike a narodnog zdravlja 1919–945, BOX 7 AJ.
21 Ibid.
22 Part of the complex of services offered to young women by the Masaryk House included a shelter for temporary placement of children with working mothers.
23 Žužić, ibid.

3   The institutionalized child as a precondition for the healthy nation in the films of Mladen Širola

Zapušteno dijete, Pomoć u pravi čas and *Spas male Zorice*: Three trajectories for institutionalizing children

Zapušteno dijete, Pomoć u pravi čas and *Spas male Zorice* could be analyzed as a film trilogy that connected two tasks, to promote basic hygienic skills aimed at preventing infectious diseases and to ingrain an unconditionally positive attitude toward the pro-state institutions of substitute family care. Generally, both messages reverberated with the call for the nation to attain maturity, including the ability to accept a rational view on efficient parenting and the ability to be aligned with hygienic skills. The three films represented the debut of Mladen Širola as a film director at the School of Public Health. Širola, who led the Marionette Theatre in Zagreb at that time, wrote short performances aimed at disseminating hygienic skills for local amateur puppet theaters organized by the Sokol movement across Yugoslavia.[1] A few of these performances, such as *Ivin zub, Macin nos* (Iva's tooth, Masa's nose, 1928) and *Campek nevaljalac* (Naughty Champek, 1929), had already been filmed for the School.

Širola started filming stories about "rescuing" children in the period when the position of the School of Public Health and his leader, Štampar, had lost much of their official status. Štampar had been forced to retire because of his dispute with the authorities, namely, King Alexander, and Štampar's refusal to support the dissolution of the Constitution.[2] The appeal of the genre of a film about saving a child can also be considered an attempt to maintain the ambition to influence Yugoslav healthcare. This intention can be reinforced by the political crisis of 1931, determined by the election law that factually limited the options for political participation for the *Hrvatska seljačka stranka* (Croatian Peasant Party), with which the School of Public Health and its workers had started to be closely associated in the quest to advance the welfare of the rural population. Širola himself, along with his father and brother, shared the political agenda of the Party.

Furthermore, Širola can be compared with two other film directors, controversial politician and writer Milan Marjanović, who not only produced a dozen of documentary health films including films about physical culture in

DOI: 10.4324/9781003272267-5

Sokol movement but also established the company *Jugoslovenski prosvetni film* in Belgrade, and Kamilo Brössler, who efficiently adapted and modified the method of contrasting the two destinies of two characters, healthy and unhealthy, adapted from American and French health films.

Širola sought to find his own style of attracting the attention of the public and gaining popularity. He chose intertextual pleasure, consistently employing visual similarities in the main characters of *Zapušteno dijete*, *Pomoć u pravi čas* and *Spas male Zorice* to the characters of the most popular and well-known family comedies. In all three films, the child protagonist was performed by Ada Širola, a daughter of Mladen Širola. One can speculate about the reasons for such casting (either due to the absence of a tradition of casting children[3] or because of the reliability of family connections), but the consequence was the construction of an unambiguous image of a child, a cheerful, intelligent, open heart, who may find herself in different life circumstances, requiring the efforts of various institutions and even institutional networks.

The constellation of these films aligned with the position of international bodies, including the Save the Children Foundation, which promoted institutions for children targeted at ensuring substitute care could be divided into such categories as "open," "semi-closed" and "residential."[4] This approach was seen as especially suitable for Balkan countries in which the "population mainly rural was not in the habit of using social and health insurance as a strategy for getting the guarantees of their welfare."[5] The films were replete with reminders on how to care for the hands to avoid infections ("Wash your hands properly"; "Trim your nails regularly"), how to use a handkerchief or spittoon and how to eat correctly. Alongside such prompts, the films translated meta-skills for those obliged to educate children, their parents, for example, how to teach children – in the form of various plays and non-boring comments, rather than punishment. The question of how deliberate the message against physical violence was presented in the films as a part of the "backwardness" of caregivers remains open but it was seen as a relic of the past incompatible with the modern approach to education.

Zapušteno dijete exploited a whole range of visual analogies and associations with *The kid* (1921) by Chaplin but inverted the motif of rescue, from being placed into an institution, to the impossibility of being rescued from diseases and a hopeless future in any other way. One of the possible explanations for such a negative adaptation could be the fact that *Zapušteno dijete* was the only urban-situated film produced by the School of Public Health, and Širola tried to align it with the expectations of the urban public. By adding the adjective "neglected" to the word "child" in the title, *Zapušteno dijete* questions the main message of Chaplin's film about attachment and unconditional love. The film tells the story of blind Tomo and his son Janko, relegated to begging. At the beginning, Janko is dressed like John in *The kid*, in oversized boots, a cap with a large visor and a torn jacket far beyond the size of the boy, which aggravates his ability to move. It is noteworthy that, in the next scene, after being placed in a boarding school, Janko changes into clothes more suitable for sports and games: Shorts and a comfortable shirt with short sleeves.

Spectators remain uninformed about whether the appearance of Janko is the result of his father being blind or the (presumed) lack of a mother, but this uncertainty inclines the audience to think about Janko's parents in eugenic frames, as "improper." Not only blindness but also missing knowledge about its cause highlights the social helplessness of Tomo. The major part of the film follows the wanderings of father and son around Zagreb, their occasional meetings with ordinary, intact and healthy city dwellers, until a police officer arrests Tomo and Janko for begging in a prohibited zone. The judge decides to place both in different institutions. After a heartbreaking scene of separation, Tomo is sent to an *invalidski dom* (institution for adults with disabilities), and Janko is sent to a boarding school, where he is not only taught the rules of hygiene, but also treated for infectious diseases. The film presents the police officer who arrests Janko and Tomo and accompanies them to the institutions in a completely opposite way than the brutal and stupid police officer in *The kid*. The officer is sensitive enough to give father and son the time to say goodbye, and he accompanies Janko and shows him Zagreb and its attractions: A new promenade, the statue of Josip Juraj Strossmayer and, finally, his new home, the massive multi-stored orphanage in the city center. In the finale, the son and his father meet again. A kind nun who teaches Janko leads Tomo to the boarding school, where the father has an opportunity to share the success and happiness of his son.

As in most films produced by the School of Public Health, the action of *Spas male Zorice* takes place in a village, where the old drunkard Jitrićka abuses Zorka, a young orphan for whom she cares because she receives a small sum from the community for doing so. Despite the consistently negative image of the abuser, the performance of Jitrićka can be easily interpreted as aligned with the canon of slapstick comedy, on the verge of clowning, one of the favorite genres of the mass public, including rural Yugoslavia. The film touches upon the issue of abusive behavior from the side of guardians as important but avoids any possible accusations of vilification of the biological mother. Jitrićka exploits the girl by sending her to collect food and alms. Like Tomo and Janko, they beg together – they even visit the Marija Bistrica, one of the main places of pilgrimage in Croatia, on the Feast of the Assumption of Mary for begging. The emphasis on begging as consistent evidence for the irresponsible behavior of caregivers resonated with several anti-begging campaigns initiated in Yugoslavia in the late 1920s.

Being a part of these public campaigns, *Zapušteno dijete* and *Spas male Zorice* presented beggars as those who suffered from trachoma and syphilis, two diseases that inhabited a special position in health propaganda, ascribing the late calls for medical help as verging on a crime against the people. This argument was closely linked with the intention to introduce public health as available to all, even for the poor, one of the central points of the political agenda of the School of Public Health.

The young Zorka contracted a skin rash because she had sifted through the garbage to find cigarette butts for Jitrićka. Instead of following the instructions of the physician and applying medicine, Jitrićka employs the signs of the sickness for better begging. She grows furious at the interference of the neighbors and pours out her anger on the girl: She brutally beats Zorka and leaves her in the yard for the night – in late August. The next morning, the humiliated Zorka escapes to another village, where she has been accepted by a new, substitute family, whose parents and two children wear national costumes and efficiently use national customs for promoting new, healthier patterns of nutrition and entertainment.

This turn of events aimed at presenting the public with a new form of placement for children without parents – foster care had been adapted by experts in Zagreb after learning about this form of care from the French experience. The main reason behind promoting family foster care was the limited options for placing children into residential care, largely the domain of private charities. Among 102 residential care institutions, only 18 were public, mostly organized in cities such as Belgrade and Zagreb. *Spas male Zorice* was thus part of a campaign to popularize foster care throughout the country. At the beginning, in the early 1930s, only several Croatian villages in Sava Banate[6] were involved in this experiment. By the end of the 1930s, the practice of foster care had taken root: 37,216 children had been cared for in this way.[7] In official reports, a decrease in child mortality in the villages that practiced foster care was the key positive outcome, but in the film, the transformation of Zorka from a "savage" child to a well-educated young girl represented the most impressive recommendation for foster care. Step-by-step Zorka gives up her unhealthy habits, and the film ends with the death of Jitrićka, which occurs while trying to capture Zorka. Her death, despite all its drama, is the price for emancipating Zorka from her past.

Pomoć u pravi čas tells the story of collective efforts to stop the dissemination of diphtheria among the children of one Yugoslav village. The choice of this disease was determined by the intractably high mortality rate among children from infectious diseases such as measles, scarlatina and diphtheria all across the country: The share of those who died due to these diseases exceeded 20 percent among all infected (only the share of death from dysentery and smallpox was higher).[8] Children represented a large majority of these cases and their fatalities until the end of the 1920s, when treatment with antitoxin serum became available. It is possible to think that Širola, like many other Europeans involved in health propaganda, was excited by the recent history of the magical rescue of children in Alaska from diphtheria, well known as the Great Race of Mercy. News of this campaign was spread widely across the world in the late 1920s.

The film begins with a scene from the boy's funeral, in which the whole village participates. The audience witnesses close-ups of mournful faces and the backs of parents bent over from grief, followed by a procession. The main character, young Marica, is infected by her own mother, who has given her daughter a kiss after returning from the funeral. The next day in school, the teacher explains the symptoms of diphtheria, and Marica with horror discovers she has all the described symptoms. The teacher sends the children home, and Anica accompanies her friend and asks why her parents do not want to call the doctor. Viewers recognize that Marica's father has no trust in physicians, only interested in "making money off poor villagers." Even the mother's pleas do not move the father.

Anica cries and shares her worries about her friend the next day in school, and the teacher sends her to the doctor, who immediately visits Marica, gives her anti-diphtheria serum and instructs her mother on how to care for the girl and prevent the dissemination of disease. The father's attack on medical intervention was countered by the doctor's prognosis that Marica could die due to infection and the fact that the treatment was free of charge. Through this scene, the film aims to promote Štampar's intention to create a system in which medical care would be accessible to as much of the population as possible, not just the wealthy.[9] The doctor then, in cooperation with the teacher, tests all the children[10] and makes the decision to declare a quarantine due to the number of susceptible and infected children. The doctor's assistant instructs Marica's parents how to apply hygienic rules and moreover involves the father in caring for his child. Marica is on the way to total recovery, and the very last scene in the film depicts her return to school and her participation in collective plays.

All three films were disseminated throughout Yugoslavia. *Spas male Zorice* was the first film by the School to be shown to the rural public in Bosnia at the initiative of the local Sokol movement in Mostar. This first experience was so successful that in the following years, the use of films in health propaganda became the main strategy in many Bosnian regions. Mica Trbojević, a pediatrician from Zagreb, who presented on the experience of foster care at the first Balkan child-welfare congress in Athens in 1935, of course mentioned the film, which was then purchased by other Balkan countries. *Pomoć u pravi čas* became the most-screened health film in Slovenia, Bosnia and Macedonia between 1931 and 1935, and more than 60 copies of the film were used for regular performances in each of the parts of Yugoslavia.[11] To the spectators who lived in different conditions, whether in cities or in rural areas, the films provided new regimes of authenticity, more "civilized" and European, through revising views on "proper" childhood, "improper" care for children and the indispensable role of experts and institutions such as schools, public health or residential care to meet the needs of the child. In this turn, Širola blurs the boundaries between the child as a symbol of the nation and the child as one of the most powerful metaphors for human progress and development. What were the main artistic techniques for translating this message?

Gender, religion and class in film metaphors about irresponsible parenting

Imaginative understanding, one of the main features of Chaplin's films, inclines viewers to practice recognition of various characters of *The kid*. The trilogy by Širola forces the audience to explain and evaluate the film's motifs and the emotions experienced by children and their caregivers to promote a particular message, namely, about the indispensable role of institutions in ensuring the "proper" development, health and welfare of children. especially those in poverty or living in poor conditions such as peripheral rural areas. In the films, an unhealthy mutual dependency between the child and the irresponsible caregiver represents the main obstacle to a happy move toward the future. Širola consistently counterposes the idea of the artificial, unnatural character of such attachment, in contrast to the naturalness of a "real" childhood ensured by various institutions.

The emotional affinity of a child to socially incapable parents manifests not only in the "pure child's soul that does not know the sin of neglect" but also in the inevitability of such attachment and the necessity of strong measures to limit the negative influence of caregivers. When Zorka, who has been given a dinar by her stepfather for her assistance, decides to buy something ostensibly good for her new siblings, according to her previous, unhealthy life – bonbons. At the moment she has given the bonbons to her brother and sister, the stepmother intervenes with the words that bonbons are unhealthy; she offers them oranges instead. The short lecture about the utility of fruit ends with the children playing ball with the oranges before eating them. This scene can be easily interpreted as opposing artificial, bonbon-like, attachment to a natural, and literally fruitful, relationship with substitute parents.

Janko is described as "wild child," followed by a scene in which he wanders around the city market and gazes with surprise at things that are familiar to any city dweller: Toys, bicycles and so on. The boy is trapped in this "savageness" by his affinity for Tomo. Their attachment is inseparable from slovenliness and it causes mixed feelings, if not disgust. Janko shares bread with his father, reminiscent of the several scenes in *The kid*, feeding John or John making pancakes. But along with this tender moment, Janko picks his nose immediately after giving half of the bread to his father, which nullifies any sentimentality. Remarkably, John picks his nose too – during a scene in which he receives a toy dog from his mother. However, Chaplin does not underscore the inappropriateness of this gesture. Picking one's nose symbolizes a social barrier, which, if overcome, ensures acceptance by society. This action thus prevents Janko from being accepted by other children, who overtly laugh at him, as well as the parents of children, who observe Janko's attempts to engage in the collective activities of children in the city garden.

The films attribute an outstanding role to childhood and the specific activities of this period that place the child among peers under the supervision of experienced educators. Along with various forms of abuse and neglect from the side of irresponsible caregivers, there is one highlighted in particular: The neglect of games and healthy entertainment for children. The films directly provoke emotional response from the side of viewers to the lack of such activities: Janko with longing watches his peers play in the park and with no less sadness peers at children's bicycles in the shop window. Zorka watches her peers who participate in the collective procession with envy. Furthermore, Janko and Zorka are not accepted by their peers as long as they do not behave themselves in alignment with the normal regularities of a happy childhood. Being placed in the new conditions of the institutions, both protagonists are happy to be a part of a children's community. *Pomoć u pravi čas* stresses not only the acquisition of hygienic skills by Marica's parents but also the obvious change in the attitude of the father toward the friendship of his daughter with Anica. At the beginning of the film, he does everything possible to interfere with their friendship and games, including a scene in which he tramples a bouquet presented by Anica to her friend. At the end, he not only brings flowers to his recovering daughter but also looks upon the girls' games with affection. Širola stresses the naturalness of children's play, accompanying the scene with a short moment of play between a cat and her kitten. Each of the films is finished by scenes of collective play: The protagonists are leading round dances or playing hide-and-seek.

All three films are constructed as stories of transformation from an unhappy, "backward" world of disability, addiction, poverty and prejudice to a new, meaningful and happier one. Children return from being forcibly placed in the unhappy world of hopeless adults to a "proper" childhood, in the cradle of future generations of the nation. Širola consistently works with the metaphor of movement for presenting institutionalized care for children as a sustainable road toward a better future. If "the 'Little Tramp' always seemed to find a door in the walled-up cubicle of society" and to make "his escape from social restrictions,"[12] the child characters in *Zapušteno dijete*, *Pomoć u pravi čas* and *Spas male Zorice* accept more and more social regularities that help them overcome the obstacles to a healthy childhood that should bridge them with the nation.

At the beginning of *Zapušteno dijete*, it is late evening, and Janko stands before an advertisement featuring goods for children. Then, without waiting for the one he was waiting for, he sits on the ground and picks his nose. This very first scene combines gloom and the impossibility to move to create a feeling of hopelessness. The subtitles inform the viewer that beggars start their day by going to the city. The next scene conveys the main idea of the film, namely, the impossibility of equal and mutual love between Tomo, the blind father, and Janko, his son, because of the father's disability that forces too many duties upon the son. Viewers observe the feet of both protagonists as they climb the hillside, witnessing the boy's unsteady steps as he supports his father and his father's even less confident movements. The motif of seeing from a perspective that moves from downwards to upwards represents the impossibility of the disabled father rise to his feet. In several following scenes, viewers see the feet and legs of the "civilized" representatives of the middle classes who give to beggars, with their confident, rapid and purposeful gait, as well as their modern clothing, but no faces.

In *Pomoć u pravi čas*, the immobility of a corpulent father, a consistent opponent of public health, is contrasted with the easy-going Anica, who always manages to evade Marica's father, in his attempts to catch and punish the overly nimble girl. A very similar unsuccessful attempt to catch Zorka fatally ends Jitrićka's life; she is unable to move properly due to her alcohol addiction. The same actress performs the role of Marica's mother and the substitute mother of Zorka, but the dynamic is different. In *Pomoć u pravi čas*, the actress moves slowly and often pauses to sigh heavily, cry or sink to the floor without strength, but in *Spas male Zorice*, she moves quickly and gracefully.

The metaphor of stagnation and deadlock as a potential risk to children that remain attached to "backward" caregivers is reinforced by opposing the active participation of the healthy and already "civilized" in reproducing national traditions and being "inside" the nation to the alienation of asocial caregivers from being an active part of the community, or "outsiders," the subjects of Catholic charity or assistance. *Pomoć u pravi čas* questions the role of religion as a potential agent of resistance to public health and a brake on the "civilizing" process, with a view of disease and death as "God's will." It is notable that during the disinfection of the room in which Marica lies, the doctor's assistant washes the crucifix over the girl's bed with creosote after taking away all icons as potential collectors of infection. This gesture seems to hint at the need of a medical upgrade in everyday religious practices. It occurs one day after the physician has asked "to take away all unnecessary things." The film translates for viewers the possibility to juxtapose religion and medicine. This scene and some others, for instance, family praying in *Spas male Zorice* clearly evidence the different approach to religion among the Yugoslav filmmakers in contrast to their Czech colleagues who mostly aimed to replace Christianity especially Catholicism by civil religion.

The impossibility of the "backward" caregivers to "catch" the progress of their already institutionalized children reverberates with the gender-based inequalities fixed in the films. The films deepen the difference between men and women in embracing desirable and undesirable patterns of behavior regarding health and disease. The fathers seem to be more educated than the mothers in the films: Janko teaches his father new hygienic skills and Marica's father learns several lessons from the experience of his daughter's illness, including the change in his attitude toward his daughter, from disdain for one who will soon leave home to tender acceptance of her as an only child. The sarcastic image of the patriarchal father in the first half of *Pomoć u pravi čas* transforms into a humorous picture of an overly sentimental man who is ready to blow the dust off his daughter. Moreover, the viewer does not observe any change in the patriarchal order of the family: The father remains the head. Disciplining humor accompanies the character of Jitrićka, who, during the entire narration, is never quite sober – even when her condition shifts from getting drunk to dying, it appears comical. But laughing at Jitrićka distances the viewer from the feeling of superiority of "proper" women – for instance, the new substitute mother of Zorka.

The films exploit a wide range of analogies between the state as father and the nation as mother - this division is reinforced by the consistent gender-based imbalance in these films. In *Zapušteno dijete*, the father and his son are touched by a state institution, and the rescue of the young Zorka and Marica can be seen as a return to the fold of the nation, to a family that follows national traditions and adapts them to a new mission. In *Pomoć u pravi čas*, the male physician and the female teacher symbolize the different flows in the institutionalization of children in favor of a healthy nation – stricter and more focused on surveillance from the side of public health, and flexible, community-based care organized by educators.

In *Pomoć u pravi čas*, viewers can trace multiple oppositions between "backward" and progressive women. Marica's mother is unable to provide for the vital needs of her daughter because she is obedient to her "backward" and patriarchal husband, while the more educated teacher and a more independent young friend are able to do so. Apart from highlighting this difference, the film does not promote the idea of making women more independent. It is not the mother, but rather Marica's father who becomes more educated and changes his parenting stereotypes. This internally contradictory attitude toward the role of women was a part of the ideology of the Sokol movement as well: "The Yugoslav woman, who is still dependent on her husband, has an uncorrupted, selfless soul, which enables her to make the greatest sacrifices."[13] Presenting the most important roles of women as mothers, homemakers and workers is a predominant motif within health propaganda, including health films that attributed to women the function of caregiver in the early stages of child development.[14] The institutions of education, social protection and public health should accept this function in the late stages of the child's growth. This view on childhood and parenting has long been entrenched in public opinion and social policy practices.

Notes

1 Mladen Širola (1927) *Marionetsko kazalište u službi zdravstvenog prosvjećivanja* [Puppet theatre in serving the mission of health enlightenment], Zagreb: Tisak Jugoslovenske štampe.
2 Sara Silverstein (2013) Man of an Impossible Mission? Andrija Štampar's Separation of Politics and Healthcare in Yugoslavia and the World Health Organization. Available online: https://www.issuelab.org/resources/27898/27898.pdf?download=true
3 The group of child artists, *Dječje carstvo* (The Kingdom of children), was established by Tito Strozzi and Mladen Širola in 1935; before that, there was no tradition of recruiting children as actors.
4 International Union Save the children "Vergleichende Übersicht über einiger Ausdrucke der Kinderfürsorge." [Attachment to the letter to Yugoslav Union for Child Protection] of 22.08.1935 Fond 39 Ministarstvo Socijalne Politike a narodnog zdravlja 1919–1945 box 7 folder 2 AJ.
5 Alojzia Štebi (1935) Les devoire et la collaboration des *banovinas*, des districts, et des autres institutions administratives et autonomes pour la protection des enfants de la campagne [The oblugations and collaboration of banovinas, districts, and other administrative and autonomous institutions for the protection of rural children]. Resume to the presentation at the First Balkan Congress on Child

Development Fond 39 Ministarstvo Socijalne Politike a narodnog zdravlja 1919–1945 box 7 folder 2 AJ.

6 Milica Trbojević who was a niece of Nikola Tesla was one of the main promoters of family foster care in rural area: Mica Trbojević (1935) La paysanne – gardienne de l'enfant éntranger [Peasants as guardians for alien children] Congrès *balkanique* de *protection* de l'Enfance [The first Balkan child-welfare congress] Fond 39 Ministarstvo socijalne politike a narodnog zdravlja 1919–1945 [Ministry] box 7 folder 2 AJ.

7 Andrija Štampar (undated document) Maternal and child welfare in Yugoslavia the draft of the presentation, Undated document HR-HDA-831 Andrija Štampar, box 3.

8 Statistički podaci o stanovništvu: skarlatina, variola vera, morbilli, dysentiria, difteria et croup, typhus abdominalis, typhus exanthemanticus [Population statistics: scarlet fewer, measles, dysentery, diphtheria and croup, abdominal typhus, asthmatic typhus], Fond 39 Ministarstvo Socijalne Politike a narodnog zdravlja 1919–1945 box 6, folder 15, AJ.

9 Željko Dugac (2010) "'Like Yeast in Fermentation': Public Health in Interwar Yugoslavia" in *Hygiene, Health and Eugenics in Southeastern Europe to 1945*, Christian Promitzer, Sevasti Trubeta and Marius Turda. Budapest (eds), New York: CEU Press, 193–232, pp. 201–204.

10 The film shows in detail the two types of test: the Schik test, a skin test for indicating people susceptible to diphtheria, and a test that swabbed the back of the throat.

11 Zdravstveno-prosvjetni rad [Health education] *Kniga za sokolsko selo [Book about Sokol village]*, 1935, 1 8–9, p. 29.

12 Hurley, ibid., p. 319.

13 Elza Skalarjeva (1934) Jugoslavenska žena u sokolskoj organizaciji [Yugoslav woman in the Socol organization] *Sokolska prosveta*, 4, 3–4, 125–129, p. 125.

14 Đura Brzaković (1934) Prosvećivanje žene u selu [Enlightenment of women in the village] *Sokolska prosveta*, 4, 3–4, pp. 122–125.

4 Central and Eastern European film in the search for deconstructing the institutionalized child

The critical reception of residential care for children within global and national campaigns for family care

After 1945, criticisms of residential care for children started to emerge. Mistrust of the institutions providing care stemmed from an argument supported by attachment theory, which stressed the extremely negative consequences for child development in the early years. John Bowlby prepared his report, "Maternal care and mental health,"[1] which fostered long-term debates concerning the role of emotional ties between mother and child. Along with the report, a campaign in favor of reorganizing public health and child protection in line with protecting attachment spread first in the United Kingdom and then across the world. James Robertson, a psychiatric social worker, produced several documentaries aimed at collecting data about the psychological processes and personal responses of children concerning separation from their parents and placement into one or another institution. Robertson intended to introduce to the public the feelings of young children whose limited verbal capacities might otherwise limit our recognition of their circumstances.

The 40-minute documentary, *A two-year-old goes to the hospital* (1952), depicts the suffering of a little girl, Laura, who is admitted to the hospital for eight days for a minor operation (repairing an umbilical hernia). This common type of hospital stay has been criticized by proponents of attachment theory as one of the most consequential for young children. Donald Winnicott, a leading member of the British Psychoanalytical Society, commented:

> The film was definitely about a real problem. The effect of separation of small children from their mothers was so often serious, even producing irreversible changes, that every time when a child is to be taken into hospital there ought to be a careful weighing up of the value on the physical side against the danger on the psychiatric side.[2]

The film documents the increasing passivity and unresponsive behavior of Laura, amid attempts by hospital staff to involve her in play and during the visits of her parents, especially her mother. Indirectly, the film portrays

DOI: 10.4324/9781003272267-6

"correct" parenting models, such as role-playing games, the use of special books, etc. Furthermore, it depicts the desired demographic scenario – Laura's mother is pregnant, one of the goals of public campaigns aimed at women in the United Kingdom of the 1950s.

Other films by Robertson presented a typical scenario of the child's behavior over the few first days in institutional care. Such a short-term perspective created space for a positive and hopeful view on the possibility to cope with the consequences but at the same time, it warned viewers that longer placement into institutions was irreversibly negative for the child. Although the purpose of collecting data on the emotional responses of young children to separation can be interpreted as purely scientific, this approach undoubtedly subjectivizes children and tries to underscore the need to consider not only their basic needs, but also their feelings. Robertson sought to challenge the widespread attitude of doctors who preferred to ignore the influences of emotional attachment, and his films launched wider debates among international audiences.[3]

Yugoslav and Czech experts were at the vanguard in advancing attachment theory in the socialist world. Štampar was one of the experts in the World Health Organization in the early 1950s and strongly recommended the report by Bowlby as well as the films by Robertson. Along with an intensive struggle against maternal and infant mortality, since the early 1950s, the Czechoslovak government had started investing in studies targeted at comparing children in families with those placed into residential care institutions. Marie Damborská and Jiří Dunovský, Czech pediatricians, introduced to the public the very first results of studying multiple disorders of development among small children placed into institutions.[4] The *Sociodiagnostický ústav* (Social Assessment Centre) in Prague started to monitor the development of children younger than one year old in special settings – *kojenecké ústavy* (infant institutions), a relatively new type of care for infants. Psychologist Zdeněk Matějček, along with Josef Langmeier, became the members of research team in 1952, and between 1954 and 1960, under the authority of The Children's Mental Health Hospital, they conducted several surveys among children placed into institutions for various target groups: Orphans, children with the difficulties in behavior and those with mental disabilities.

The height of popularity for attachment theory in Czechoslovakia arrived in the early 1960s. Cultivated by the power of Antonín Novotný, the President of Czechoslovakia between 1957 and 1968, the familialization of social policy served multiple political tasks. It would help to cut the expenses on pre-school care by attributing the indispensable role in the early development of children to the mother. Prioritizing care for children also operated in favor of replacing women from many of the labor market niches. Overvaluing maternal care helped to legitimize the political authority of Novotný, who efficiently opposed his own politics to the previously "inhuman" placement of children in kindergartens and nurseries during the presidency of his predecessor, Antonín

Zápotocký, the President of Czechoslovakia between 1953 and 1957. These motifs significantly transformed the message of attachment theory.

In contrast to the activities by British promoters of attachment theory, who highlighted the necessity to redistribute power between professionals and parents for the good of the child, Czechoslovak scholars focused on the consequences of an upbringing in residential care settings. One of the central points of the Czech version of attachment theory was the division of children (but not parents) according to their ability to develop healthy emotional ties; those who were delinquent, possessed mental disabilities or had experienced long-term residential care were seen as unsuitable for family placement. Proclaiming the superiority of socialist psychology, Matějček and Langmeier propelled their studies into international contexts, recognizing four stages of development in attachment theory: (1) empiric – the first third of the twentieth century; (2) alarmist – marked by Bowlby's report for WHO; (3) critical – after the first wave of popularization; and (4) current – theorization with Czech psychologists at the vanguard.[5] The promotion of family placement and the struggle against deprivation did not enter into a contest with the consistently positive image of residential care for children with disabilities, who were seen as limited in their ability to develop emotional affinities with parents.

This background is reflected in the documentary *Děti bez lásky* (Children without love, 1963) filmed by Kurt Goldberger, one of the leading film directors of the *Studio populárně vědeckých a naučných filmů* (Studio of Popular Science and Educational Films). Goldberger had extensive experience in studying Western, mainly British, educational films, as well as international acceptance of his *Před startem do vesmíru* (Before launching into space, 1960) aimed at introducing a wide audience to the global agenda of conquering space. Goldberger had the opportunity to watch Robertson's films and to consult with Matějček, who had become one of the leading figures in the production of films. Like *A two-year-old goes to hospital,* Děti bez lásky addressed the public and aimed at educating it about more responsible parenting (see Figures 4.1 and 4.2). Despite multiple visual similarities, the film by Goldberger emphasized the view on attachment theory developed by Matějček and Langmeier, with a focus on blaming mothers and underscoring the limited options for recovery among children exposed to residential care.

Děti bez lásky opens in a psychiatric counseling center for young people and children, where dozens of teenagers, together with adults, are waiting for an appointment. The cascade of short stories that follows links the vulnerable circumstances of residential care or systematic neglect in the parental family in young children with a wide range of asocial behaviors. Each of the stories is ended by the same diagnosis, *deprivační syndrome* (deprivation syndrome). In the next several scenes, viewers can grasp the meaning. They observe the application of various psychological projective tests,[6] which portray the children's views on their experience of being alienated from emotional affinity with their mothers. Then, in-depth interviews with a mother who placed her newborn son into a children's home until the age of five are featured. She has

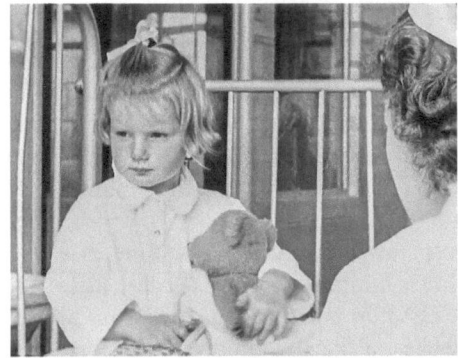

Figure 4.1 Teddy bear as a broker between child and nurse, *A two-year-old goes to hospital (1952)*.

Source: Concord Media, ©Katherine McGilly.

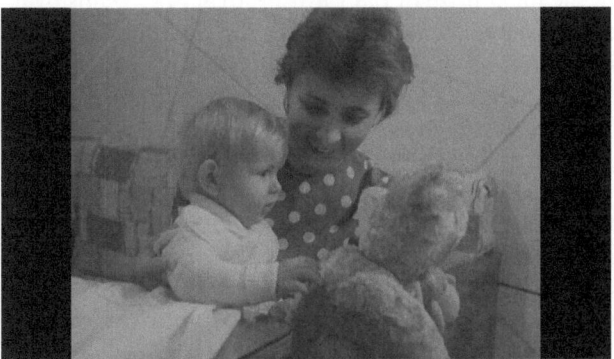

Figure 4.2 Teddy bear as a symbol of closed emotional ties in *Děti bez lásky* (Children without love, 1963).

Source: NFA.

taken him back only after she marries. An interview with the boy connects the absence of an emotional tie between them to multiple forms of deviant behavior, including a knife attack against his sister and systematic theft.

Aligned with the tradition in health films to oppose "proper" to "improper" behavior, the film charts the difference in the development of a child in a "normal" family and a child placed into an institution. First, viewers observe two infants: One who grows up in a family and is happy in a boundless world of love, and another who lives in an institution, where love and care are measured, at the disposal of a nurse taking care of 12 children. The film then stresses the presence of the mother as the grounds for safety and the ability to develop cognitive activities, counterposing the strict limits of such development among toddlers in residential care, who experience mistrust and uncertainty from the very beginning of life.

The narrator underscores the increasing ruptures in mental development and the children's ability to express themselves. The child raised in a family moves on to become a "real hero of our days" but those in residential care are pictured as a "barbarian tribe without any respect for things." It is remarkable that this part of the film is narrated on behalf of the children – Kurt Goldberger presents the children as if they could speak. To those who are placed into institutions, the narrator attributes the ironic tone of a disillusioned people; for instance: "Our life is unpredictable; yesterday, I drove a car and today I could only cry ... ." The film ends with a discussion about the similarity in the negative consequences of placing children in residential care and spending more than a few hours in kindergartens. The conclusion is univocal: The normal development of the child depends on emotional ties with the mother. It is further crucial to realize the point of no return with regard to deprivation, as its consequences are devastating for children's mental development.

In 1963, the film won the main prize of the Fifth Festival of Czechoslovak short films[7] in the category of popular science films "for a persuasive social analysis of the problems connected with pre-school education."[8] And in 1964, the film participated in the 25th Venice Film Festival and won *Targa Leone di San Marco per il miglior film di vita contemporanea e di documentazione sociale* (Lion of San Marco for the best film of contemporary life and social documentation). The idealized attitude toward family care and toward the unique role of mother–child emotional ties became engrained in public discourse, labeling the children placed in institutions as inevitably sentenced to deprivation and "retardation." In his next film, *Lidé* (Humans, 1964) Goldberger tells stories of adoption, stressing the importance of adopting children at an early age to avoid the risks of deprivation. After the invasion of the Warsaw Pact troops, Goldberger moved to Western Germany, where he continued his career as a documentarist. Among other social projects, he participated in the *Die Fernsehe-Elternschule* (TV School for parents), for which he produced a four-part film *Drei entscheidende Jahre* (Three decisive years, 1971) aimed at presenting the role of early development and "proper" and "improper" parental approaches to children of this age. Goldberger had produced several similar films for other TV campaigns, including ARD.

Děti bez lásky was welcomed by a wide audience and launched wider debates concerning care for children without parents. Around the same time, several initiatives for developing substitute family care were undertaken. Czechoslovakia established several SOS-*kinderdorfes* as an alternative to large-scale residential care. Journals and newspapers started posting information about children suitable for adoption, in hopes of involving people in substitute family care. The journal *Vlasta*, which represented *Svaz žen* (The Union of Women), was among these periodicals, opening discussions among experts and local practitioners aimed at presenting different arguments in favor of limiting the placement of children in institutions and extending the options for substitute family care instead. The outcomes were published as an article titled "*A přece budou mít rodiče*" ("And yet they will have parents"),[9] which presented multiple strategies targeted at breaking the predominance of residential care. Matějček remained a regular contributor to *Vlasta*, publishing several interviews dedicated to various issues concerning the emotional ties between mothers and children, adoption and raising adopted children.

Lilika: An Eastern European response to the issue of youth in social policy and culture

The increasingly intolerant attitude toward residential care reverberated with more general disappointment in social policy concerning families and children as inefficient in the context of demographic crisis in a major part of socialist Europe. The political and scientific redefinition of parenthood echoed in the call for critical revision of the images of families and children in mass culture, including films and television that had started to compete for acceptance by the public since the late 1950s. The seismic industrial development of the 1960s called for profound changes in Western film style, and one of the important results was to create space for independent filmmakers who could introduce new topics and artistic solutions.[10] The ongoing emergence of the teenager as a social entity and a consumer group reached its multiple reflections in film production and consumption. Some films supported the waves of moral panic against teenage delinquency, some used youth culture for creating a new, attractive, type of entertainment and some established New-Wave film movements in different countries.

The question of how to depict adolescents and youth influenced not only Western film but also Eastern European cinematography, which, along with fears and hopes concerning new generations, revised the role of residential care and, more generally, the system of child protection. Since the late 1960s, a new cohort of films, mostly presenting the conflicts of young women and institutionalized care for children, started questioning not only the efficiency of child protection but also general approaches to understanding childhood and family life. *Lilika* (1970), the directorial debut by Branko Pleša, can be seen as the first among this cohort.

The 12-year-old Lilika lives with her mother and her mother's partner and spends her life caring for her little brother, whom she loves deeply, and communicating with one of her aunts, who makes money as a prostitute with the guests of a luxury hotel, and another aunt, who is only a hotel maid "because her ankles are not that pretty." Due to constant complaints about Lilika's antisocial behavior (she steals fruit and skips her lessons), the mother's partner forces Lilika's mother to send a request for placing the girl into boarding school. When the social worker (performed by Pleša) has arrived, Lilika tells how she loves her family without even hiding the asocial life of her loved ones. She is clear in her intention to stay with her mother, her "new father" and her little brother. But her caregivers have another opinion. The girl's behavior has not improved, which leads social worker to Lilika's school, where he marshals evidence in favor of placing her into a special school.

While the wheel of institutional care is spinning, Lilika dreams of the social worker – in her fantasies, he, dressed in a national costume, takes her on horseback to a distant, but bright and happy place. In reality, Lilika is friends with Peca, a silent boy who has already experienced boarding school and after graduation, remains with his mother. Peca loves Lilika and is horrified at the prospect of her being placed in a boarding school. During the night before the court that should make the decision about placing Lilika into the school, they escape together and walk in the city center. Peca smashes the window of a fruit seller's shop so that a stream of oranges, her favorite fruit, spills onto Lilika. Lilika distracts the police to let Peca hide, while she herself, with her head held high and eyes of complete contempt for the adult world, marches to the court, one of the multi-story buildings that she admires, among other signs of fashion and modernity. Lilika gracefully and easily moves between the benches of the court and not only looks defiantly at those who have gathered to make a decision and who look like frozen mannequins but plays in front of them with a stolen orange. In the very last scene, when Lilika is already sitting in the police car, which is supposed to transfer her to the special school, she looks up, even if there is no way to see the social worker looking down on Lilika.

In *Lilika*, Pleša questions the unconditionally positive attitude toward institutions of child protection: The film begins with the citations from "The Brothers Karamazov" by Fyodor Dostoevsky, about the unatoned tears of a child and the priceless harmony of the world.[11] Pleša pictures the system of child protection as a bulky and unwieldy machine that would rather crush children than carry them into better conditions. It is reasonable to interpret *Lilika* as an interrogation of the approach to the institutionalizing child and childhood entrenched in the films by Širola and Bartoš.[12]

Instead of devaluation of attachment, a central motif of rescue-mission films, *Lilika* focuses on the vacuum of attachment and mutual affinity – only the friendship between Lilika and Peca exhibits the energy of mutual recognition and acceptance. Neither relatives nor helping professionals have enough sympathy to prevent the removal of Lilika. Pleša admits that he was inspired by Albert Camus and his novel "The Stranger," when he was conceptualizing the film, in the "absurdity and dullness of feelings" as a reaction to institutionalizing the ordinary life of people.[13] He directly compares the destiny of his main protagonist with the dramatic history of Meursault: "Lilika is not a 'child' film; it is a story of kind girl who lives with her mother, a former prostitute, on the outskirts of the city and who is sacrificed by her family for their comfort."[14] Her ability to love and be devoted to those whom she loves looks like an exception, for which the girl pays with her alienation.

Lilika opposes a young girl to the head of the local social protection board, a handsome man and tells the story of Lilika's emancipation from her fantasies about a strong man who is able to rescue her. This scenario is obviously shaped under the influence of mass culture. The film could not be attributed to *Bildungsroman* but the emancipation of Lilika from gender-based stereotypes and prescriptions plays an important role in her coping strategy and coming of age. Pleša doubts the understanding of childhood as an important period in preparing children for adult life; moreover, he does not portray Lilika as a "ruined child."[15] *Lilika* presents the main protagonist as a young female, not a naïve innocent child; she is full of curiosity and prone to provocative behavior. In the finale, it's difficult to think of Lilika as a victim of the system – she's well-armed to resist institutional arbitrariness and deal with imminent trauma.

Pleša deconstructs not only the main messages concerning child protection, "proper" parenting, family life and childhood but also the metaphors and analogies of "proper" childhood, among other mediums introduced by rescue-mission films. In *Lilika*, the "naturalness" of a "proper" playful childhood meets the poverty and informal activities of those children who are not under the pressure of parental expectations. Lilika does not have her own toys but she encounters them when she helps her other, not beautiful, aunt to clean the hotel rooms. Instead of "normal" children's toys and entertainment, Lilika observes different female scenarios – even when she helps her mother or aunts to undress, she looks as if she is playing with them as dolls.

Pleša underscores dirtiness and forbiddances as two main forces that shape Lilika's milieu. Because of poverty and neglect, Lilika looks sloppy, and her school uniform is particularly untidy, small in size, too short and old. The camera often opposes disorderly Lilika to her neat peers who gaze upon Lilika with wide open eyes. The school scenes add more to the dirtiness of Lilika's world – the main part of the action occurs in the toilet, where Lilika shares her stolen fruit and her fresh knowledge about sexual life. It is remarkable that in response to the teacher's question about why she has missed school, Lilika is in the habit of replying, "I had to wash."

The spectators may be tempted to compare Lilika with Cinderella: Lilika even has a speck of soot on her cheek at the beginning of the film and her position could be easily interpreted as Cinderella. But the intention of Pleša is not to victimize her but to stress her ability to resist and the incompatibility of this coping strategy with the expectations dictated by the idea of "proper" childhood. In many reviews, Lilika is defined as "rowdy" or as Gavroche,[16] who "knocks on our conscience,"[17] but Pleša rejects such a romantic view by questioning the options for child protection to rescue a child who has been already objectified by traditional childhood discourses. The film was shown to psychologists, sociologists and educators in order to discuss the options to help children "like Lilika" or, even more, to cut the number of "juvenile delinquents" like her.[18] The oranges, her favorite fruit all along, that Lilika likes so much, are forbidden for her because of their price, but she does not wait for someone to give her an orange, with a lecture about its usefulness, like Zorka from *Spas male Zorice* – she takes it in her own way (see Figures 4.3 and 4.4).

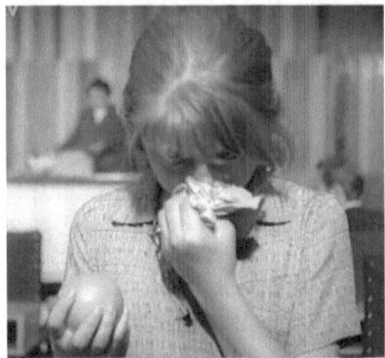

Figure 4.3 Lilika takes her orange (Lilika, 1970).
Source: Avala Film Way.

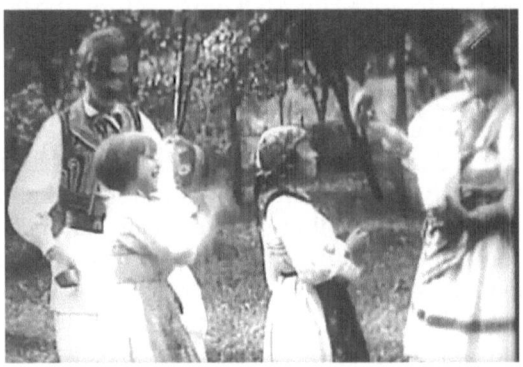

Figure 4.4 Zorica gets her orange, *Spas male Zorice* (Rescue young Zorka, 1929).
Source: Kinoteka, HAD.

The individualistic loneliness of a child vs. collective care in late socialist Czech films

Lilika garnered international attention and won several prizes. While official media in socialist Czechoslovakia were very modest in presenting *Lilika* to the public,[19] a copy of film was purchased by the *Filmová a televizní fakulta Akademie múzických umění v Praze* (Film and TV School of the Academy of Performing Arts in Prague)[20] and attracted the attention of Czech film-makers.[21] Two films, *Neúplné zatmení* (Incomplete eclipse, by Jaromil Jireš, 1983) and *Kukačka v temném lesu* (Cuckoo in a dark forest, by Antonín Moskalyk, 1985), play on the main hermeneutic codes of *Lilika* but within specific cultural and historical Czech contexts, including the longue-durée of an uncritically positive attitude toward residential care institutions. Both films were produced by film directors affiliated with the New Wave, who easily introduced in these stories the motif of individual protest against collective pressure.

The 14-year-old Marta Rezková is rapidly losing her eyesight. After overhearing a conversation between her mother and one of the doctors, Marta is sure that her younger sister is to blame, because of whom Martha fell and hit her head. This accusation absorbs Marta, who decides that sooner or later she will commit suicide, but before that, she will tell her mother about her sister's guilt. The film, full of flashbacks to the time when Marta could see, presents the girl as eidetically sensitive and even endowed with the ability of synesthesia: Experiencing seeing through other senses. Marta is placed in a boarding school for children with visual impairment, and there her gift attracts the attention of Moš, a psychologist who studies synesthesia among children and youth with visual impairment.

While the girl works through the inevitable distancing from her family and mixing feelings of guilt, sympathy and fury toward her mother, her life becomes more and more institutionalized. These two processes remain separated for Marta, who lives her internal life more than she adapts to the space and rules of the boarding school. Even though the viewers witness the internal life of the girl in detail, including regular depictions of her eidetic perception, they do not have a chance to comprehend her feelings and their dynamics. For instance, catharsis, coping with loneliness and rejecting the idea of suicide are observable but not explainable. Moš is juxtaposed against this complex internal life. His motives as well as affects are easily interpreted: He is led by his hypothesis and would like to prove it. His crash is one more option for Marta to indicate the meaning of loneliness and independence or distant attachment.

Falling is one of the central metaphors in *Neúplné zatmení:* Marta plans to end her life by jumping off the balcony, and one of the skills she is afraid to master under the supervision of educators is the ability to fall. Moving from light, clarity and ease to darkness, uncertainty and complexity is another central metaphor of the film. Generally, shifting from falling to moving to darkness is a kind of key message of the film: Coming of age means more and more uncertainty, and this understanding of becoming an adult is diametrically opposed to the traditional view fixed in the rescue-mission films (see Figure 4.5). The choice between the ability to fall, which she is offered to learn in the boarding school, and movement into the darkness is impossible. Marta remains in a zone of incomplete eclipse – with full understanding of this state of growing up.

Jireš includes in the film detailed portrayals of hospitals and boarding schools, not necessarily to attribute to them special meaning or for devaluating them as Miloš Forman did in *One Flew Over the Cuckoo's Nest* (1975) – but for emphasizing their very premise, namely, not to help us to move up and develop but to teach us to fall down and accept it. In *Kukačka v temném lesu*, Moskalyk moves further in deconstructing the role of institutions in the

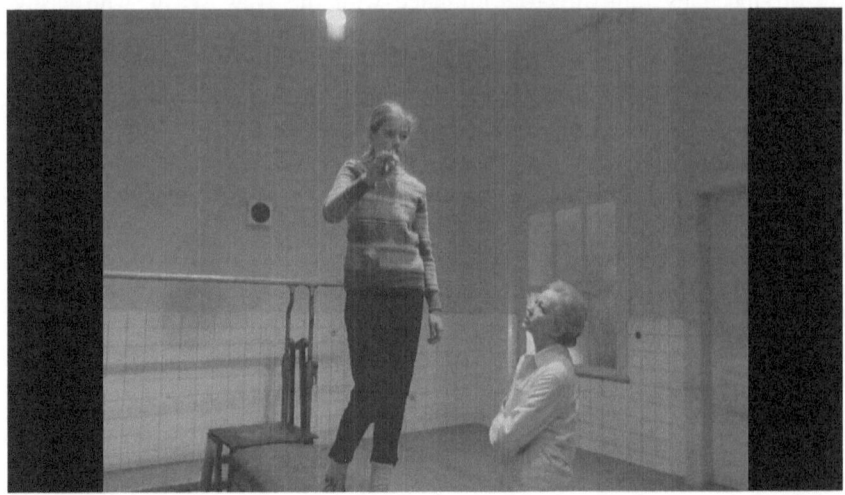

Figure 4.5 Marta measures darkness, *Neúplné zatmení* (Incomplete eclipse, 1983).
Source: NFA.

lives of children. In his film, all the institutions, orphanages, substitute families and medical boards serve the aims of a totalitarian régime – the Third Reich. It offers the possibility to present these institutions as a conveyer of thanatopolitics (see Figure 4.6). Emilka loses her parents – her father was

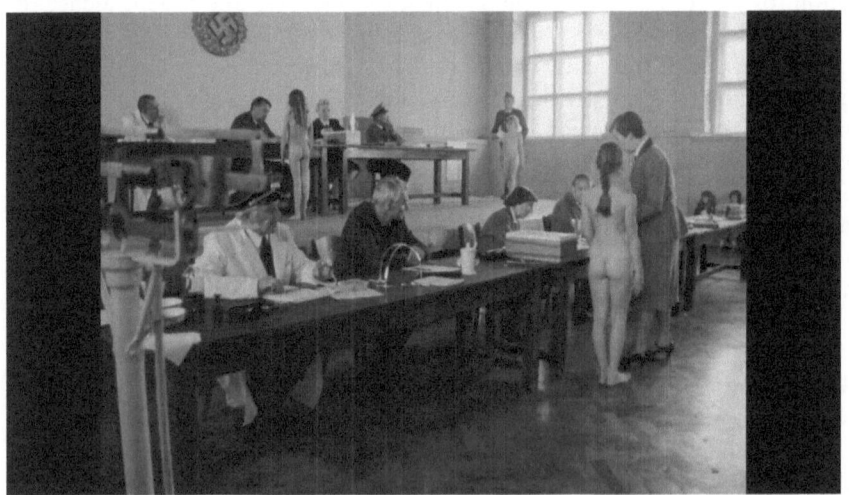

Figure 4.6 A conveyer of thanatopolitics: Selection of children for the Lebensborn Program in *Kukačka v temném lesu* (Cuckoo in a dark forest, 1985).
Source: NFA.

shot, and her mother was sent to a concentration camp for helping partisans. Because of her ideal Nordic type, indicated by the Board of the Lebensborn Program, Emilka, like a few other children, is sent to the orphanage at the monastery where she should be prepared for placement in a new, Aryan but childless family. Emilka not only practices physical exercises and German, but also she is taught to play new games and take part in the amateur theater, the typical entertainment for Aryan children. During one of the perform-ances, she is chosen by the commander of concentration camp, who does not have children due to his wife's disability; she cannot walk. While the new stepfather unconditionally accepts Emilka, her stepmother starts hating her. Moreover, she is bullied at school, where German children tease and insult Emilka for her less-than-ideal pronunciation and unclear origin. The teacher and the father help Emilka to cope with it; she also receives a dog who guards her.

Her stepfather teaches Emilka how to swim and spends time with her – but she is also taken to the camp, and she observes his cruelty to the prisoners. Emilka withdraws more and more into herself and even en-tertains thoughts of suicide. But the war approaches its end and her stepmother dies in an air raid. The stepfather pretends to be a former prisoner and escapes with Emilka, but he is exposed and executed. In the final scene of the film, Emilka returns to her mother, and a bouquet of red carnations is presented to the mother, who is still in a hospital bed. Moskalyk, who filmed the two very dramatic books by Holocaust survivor Arnošt Lustig, *Dita Saxová* and *Modlitba pro Kateřinu Horovitzovou*, shared his fear of any institutionalization as a very strong step toward structural violence. He pictures the coming of age of Emilka in a very similar manner to Jireš – the institutions that we are in the habit of defining as serving thanatopolitics saved Emilka. This easily prompts the question of the balance and imbalance between biopolitics and thanato-politics of child protection institutions.

Lilika, Neúplné zatmení and *Kukačka v temném lesu* expose social institutions (including those charged with child protection) as misogynistic and seriously question their positive role as a part of coming of age. Each of the three films embodies a consistent anti-eugenic message regarding the expectations from children as future generations and the role of prepa-ration for adult life. The opposition of a girl and a man presented in each of the films as a quasi-father includes the psychoanalytical motif of attachment as an indispensable experience in challenging the patriarchal world and its institutions. Practicing disobedience to such institutions empowers the girls in the films, not in terms of achieving social success but through developing a more authentic "me." Along with casting doubts on institutions, these films pose the issue of collective identity as a part of symbolic violence from the side of the nation. This radical humanism is not the only possible answer to the issue of child protection and its role in nation-building.

A renaissance in rescue-mission films after 1989 with the aim of delegitimizing the socialist past

After 1989, dozen of films portrayed the legitimacy crisis of diverse institutions including child protection in post-socialist Central and Eastern Europe. Mental health clinics, children's homes and boarding schools were presented as an integral part of a totalitarian regime and a testimony to its arbitrariness. *Děti bez lásky* received its second life after 1989, presented as a part of the myth about the systematic resistance from the side of psychologists against the communist regime and its intention to replace family care with residential institutions: "In the 1950s, communist Czechoslovakia plunged into various attempts at social engineering. The experiment with children was one of them. The family stopped being taken seriously, and collective education began instead."[22] The history of the film was full of numerous legends about its banning by the Women's Union, its multiple triumphs at the Venice Film Festival in 1964, where the film would have been secretly taken by Miloš Forman, etc.

The debut film of Filip Renč, the full-length *Requiem pro panenku* (Requiem for a maiden, 1991), presented, in a historically inaccurate manner, the case of forced placement of a young Romani girl into a mental health institution when she experiences arbitrariness and violence.[23] *Marian* (Petr Václav, 1995) is another example of exposing the cruelty of the socialist regime through narrating the story of a Romani boy placed into various institutions.[24] Václav directly applies attachment theory to explaining the delinquent pathway of Marian, removed from his family at an early age and then moved from institution to institution until he committed suicide. It is possible to reveal visual similarities with the film *Děti bez lásky* and *Lilika* as well. *Kolya* (Svěrák, 1996), which won an Oscar in 1996, should be seen as the most well-known film in this cohort.

Kolya can be read as an adaptation of *The kid.* Like Chaplin, Svěrák seeks to tell a story about "the art of survival in the darkest time."[25] Like *The kid,* Kolya tells the story of the accidental paternity of an old and, apparently, unlucky bachelor who, despite his initial reluctance to take responsibility, rescues the boy from the hell of institutional care and eventually returns him to his biological mother. Among the other clichés about late Central and Eastern European socialism, the Oscar-winning *Kolya* exemplifies the insensitive cruelty of socialist child protection. *Zubatá* (literally, "Toothy"), a social worker, arrives late by half a year upon the request of a Czech cellist, *Franta Louka* (literally, "Meadow"). The cellist is a single man, and under life's pressure, desperate and unemployed, he meets and accepts an offer of mock marriage to a young Russian beauty, who dreams of a German fiancé. After acquiring Czechoslovak citizenship, she united with her actual fiancé. However, she leaves Kolya, her five-year-old son, in Franta's care. Not speaking Russian and lacking the skills to raise a child, Franta asks social services for help. By the time the social worker finally visits, Franta and

Kolya have overcome their cultural gap and developed strong emotional bonds. Unsurprisingly, Zubatá ignores what Franta says and what Kolya wants. She offers only one possible solution for authoritative child protection: The removal of Kolya from Franta's care and placement in an institution akin to a Soviet shelter. Franta and Kolya are left with no other option than to escape and hide. The Velvet Revolution – the transition of power – finally rescues not only Franta and his Czech friends but also Kolya – who reunites with his mother.

Like *The kid, Kolya* highlights the negative role of the adult protagonist's sexual desire and sublimation as a way of establishing deep mutual affection with the adopted child. Both fathers offer their children a lifestyle bordering on antisocial behavior. The Tramp teaches his kid to break windows and then offers to repair them. Louka plays in a funeral band and Kolya plays at funerals – using the lace panties forgotten by one of the many girlfriends for draping a toy coffin.

Ultimately, both films contrast informal care for children as a source of vitality to formal residential care, seen as a source of inevitable deprivation. But along with the visual affinity and multiple resemblances of the plots, one of the driving forces that led *Kolya* to win the Oscar for best foreign language film, the father and the son in the films espouse totally different messages. While *The kid* constructs dichotomies stemming from class antagonism, *Kolya* replaces the contest between the poor and those who serve the interests of the higher classes with national tensions. For rescuing Kolya, Louka withstands those who are seen as the main historical enemies of the Czechs, namely, Russians and Germans. Replacing classes with nations orchestrates a totally different view on identity and belonging. In the final scene, the Tramp retreats into obscurity, uncertain about his future, but he is open to deep unconditional love. But Louka and Kolya return to the "folds" of their nations, Kolya to his mother, who is happy in Germany, and Louka becomes father to the child of Klara, performed by Libuse Safránková, who had already obtained the position of the female symbol of the Czech nation.

The liberation of Louka from the impossibility of serving his people with words, music and deeds should symbolize a new life for the entire nation – without the Soviet invaders but with the hope of a new generation. The occasional care for a Russian boy represents a kind of unique opportunity to invest in the moral superiority and self-righteousness, strategically proper (according to Svěráks) behavior in favor of surviving the Czech nation in face of totalitarian pressure. Escaping with Kolya, Louka prepares him for a new life full of freedom. In this way, the Czech film promotes desirable collective identity and celebrates the triumph of liberation.

Utopian motifs, one of the main tools for creating the narrative in both films, serve mutually opposing messages. The parenting by the Tramp, full of creativity and patience, embodies an anti-modernist radical leftism and provokes us to wonder if human dignity and goodwill are the exclusive privileges of the poor and tests our own limits of unconditional love. The transfer of Louka from substitute paternity to true, inside-the-nation, fatherhood, feeds the myth about the revival of the Czech nation and blocks any critical historical reflections of the socialist past through the inversion of the story about Czech and Russians to a moralizing parable about redeeming freedom by saving the enemy's child.

Notes

1 The first edition was published in 1961, and the extended, second edition, *Maternal Care and Mental Health/ Deprivation of Maternal Care*, was issued in 1966.
2 A Two-Year-Old Goes to Hospital: A Film Shown By John N Bowlby, and James Robertson (1952), in Proceedings of the Royal Society of Medicine, Section of Paediatrics, Vol. 46, pp. 425–426.
3 Michal Shapira (2013) *The War inside: Psychoanalysis, total war and the making of the democratic Self in postwar Britain.* Cambridge: Cambridge University Press, pp. 212–213.
4 Iveta Jusová and Jiřina Šiklová (eds.) (2016) *Czech Feminisms: Perspectives on Gender in East Central Europe*, Indiana: Indiana University Press
5 Josef Langmeir and Zděnek Matějček (1963) Psychická deprivace [Mental deprivation]. Prague: SZN.
6 The film depicts in detail the application of the Thematic Apperception test and Kinetic family drawing. Clearly, these scenes aimed at preparing audiences for very probable psychological counseling, which had started to be disseminated in Czechoslovakia in the second half of the 1950s.
7 This annual event reflected the structure of the state-organized production of educational films, divided into several categories including popular science films; more in Lucie Česálková et all (2015) Film – náš pomocník: studie o (ne) užitečnosti českého krátkého filmu 50. Let [Film – our assistant: a study of the (un) usefulness of Czech short film in the 1950s] Praha: NFA.
8 Fifth Festival of Czechoslovak short films (1964) *Československý film* No 4 pp. 14–18, p. 17.
9 Vlasta 1964 18 13, pp. 10–12.
10 Brown, ibid., pp. 97–98.
11 The full quote reads: "It's not worth the tears of that one tortured child who beat itself on the breast with its little fist and prayed in its stinking outhouse, with its unexpiated tears to 'dear, kind God'! It's not worth it, because those tears are unatoned for. They must be atoned for, or there can be no harmony … ."
12 According to personal communication with an archivist from the National Archives in Zagreb Lucija Zora on 27.07.2021: "In 1969, the entire collection [of films and equipment of the School of Public Health] was taken over by Jugoslovenska kinoteka in Belgrade. They made 35 mm copies and films were used from that period on, to a certain extent." It is reasonable to assume that Pleša had an opportunity to watch these films, especially those made by Širola, who had the reputation of a popular children's author. Moreover, it is reasonable to imagine that he may have seen these films as a child – growing up in Bosnia.
13 Lilika Branka Pleshe dobar posao [*Lilika* by Branka Pleše does her job well] Јутарње новости Београд 18.VII. 1970.
14 Ibid.
15 M. Kyjundžić Gledamo u bioskopima. Tuga iygublenog detinstva [We look at lost childhood in cinemas] *Dnevnik Novi Sad* 16.10.1970.
16 *Gavroche Thénardier* is a fictional *character* from the novel *Les Misérables* by Victor Hugo, a cocky, independent, sharp-tongued street boy, one of the most

disseminated literary analogies for heroizing children who struggled against capitalist injustice in socialist countries between the 1960s and 1980s.

17 Čudovita "Lilika" [Beautiful Lilika] Tedenska tribuna Ljubljana 17.12.1970.
18 Za Liliku specijalne predstave [Special performance of Lilika] *Veherne новости
    Београд* 5.06.1971.
19 In the early 1970s, only the journal *Kino* had published a very short anonymized
    review of the film, with the main idea of the "sinking of a young girl in modern
    life": Kino, 1970 25 19, p. 14.
20 The copy of the film is in the Film Archive in Prague.
21 In 1986, a student of FAMU, Slobodan Ščepanović, filmed a remake of *Lilika* as a
    tribute to the film by Pleša.
22 Jitka Polanská (2017) *Děti bez lásky*: film, který změnil pohled na jesle [Children
    without love: a film that changed the way we look at the nursery]. Available
    online: https://www.eduzin.cz/skola-a-ucitele/predskolni-vzdelavani/laska-na-
    pridel/.
23 Victoria Shmidt (2019) When National Female Bildungsroman Meets Global
    Fantasies about Nazis: Historical Roots and Current Troubles in *Lída Baarová*. 4
    pp. 61–78, p. 63.
24 Victoria Shmidt and Bernadette Nadya Jaworsky (2020) *Historicizing Roma in
    Central Europe: Between critical whiteness and epistemic injustice* London:
    Routledge, pp. 36–37.
25 Verma and Mishra, ibid.

Part 2

Health films for teaching children

5 The complex legacy of early animated health films in Eastern Europe

Picturing germs in animated health films

On the last day of November 1936, the Bulgarian newspaper *Dyga* featured a spread on *Pyrviyaty bylgarski trik-filmy "Pakostnitsi"* (The first Bulgarian animated film "Villains"), to be produced by the end of the year. The subtitle underscored the most important novelties that should immediately attract the attention of public to this initiative: "a fly as the Bulgarian Mickey Mouse, an authentic film about ordinary life in the Bulgarian countryside, 24 pictures per minute, physicians who will give theatre to the countryside."[1] The young but already famous cinematographer, film director and actor, Vasil Bakyrdzhiev, in cooperation with young cartoonist Stoyan Venev, sought to make their film, aimed at educating ordinary Bulgarians about the dangerous role of flies as carriers of diseases, as authentic as possible. Bakyrdzhiev and Venev planned to demonstrate how disobedience to hygienic rules contributed to the contamination of various milieus within rural life, from field work to the private yard of every house in the village. This attempt[2] represents a testimony to how the reverberation of the global call for eradicating flies and the intention to be aligned with local peculiarities produced incredible palimpsestic intertextuality among health films, mainly aimed at teaching children, new immigrants and the working-class basic hygiene skills.[3]

The eradication of flies was one of the earliest health campaigns, based upon editing the initial series of animated moving pictures from Great Britain, *The Fly Pest*, by F. Persy Smith (1911). The campaign operated through fear and aversion: It depicted in detail the process of flies laying eggs as an intrusion into daily life or even the desecration of a saint. For example, in the film, a fly sits on a baby's mouth, on the leaflets a fly turns into a giant that bites off the head of a small child. Precisely, this moment was reproduced in the Bulgarian *Pakostnitsi*, in which poultry and livestock have lost their heads. But along with this horror, the filmmakers sought to make the common fly, one of the millions that whizz through the air, sitting on our food and transmitting disease, "a main character of their film."

Surviving sketches from the film feature a married fly couple, in which the wife convinces a not very trusting spouse about some plans she has hatched;

DOI: 10.4324/9781003272267-8

at the same time, a bacterium clearly appears behind the fly-wife. This schematic representation leaves no doubt regarding the similarity with the bacterium in the verse-book *More beasts for worse children* (Hilaire Belloc 1897), illustrated by Basil Temple Blackwood and translated into more than ten languages by the end of the 1920s.[4] The motif of family relations among flies and, even more, their "tragic love story" connects *Pakostnitsi* with another famous but lost health film, *Jinks*, from the studio Bray Production, commissioned in 1919 by the *National Tuberculosis Association*. The catalog of the films offered by the Red Cross for Eastern European countries provides the following description:

> It starts with a picture representing Jinks "not feeling well – no pep." He is indignant at his wife's suggestion to see a doctor and leaves for the factory, where his troubles still follow him. He does his work badly and is dismissed by his employer with the remark that "This is a factory not a hospital." Feeling very low spirited he tries to ensure his life but is met with a curt refusal by the office of the Insurance Company and they remark that "They do not insure wrecks." He then decides that his wife is right and he ought to see a doctor, which he does. One feature of the amusing examination is the catching of a microbe in a net by the doctor upon Jink's sneezing and showing it to him through a microscope. Terrified at this sight our friend rushes home and throws himself into bed only to dream of Microbeville and particularly of "Mike Robe" who has a plan of his (Jink's) lungs representing and ideal bungalow "No fresh air, no exercise, etc." Meeting a "lady" Mike Robe shows this plan to her and asks her to marry him. They enter an empty den, the marriage bureau, and quickly emerge followed by a long line of little microbes. They start out for Jink's lungs but to their disgust on arrival they find that he has awakened out of his dream, which has made so strong an impression on him that he immediately changes his mode of life and follows the rules of hygiene which he had previously neglected.[5]

The Fly Pest and *Jinks*, two extremes of using cartoons in health propaganda, the first suggesting horror and the latter parodying germs as infantile people, reflect the dynamic and controversial narrative about the visualization of carriers of disease, which had become an inseparable part of the discursive practices around bacteriology and medicine since the late nineteenth century. For Martina King, "encoding a variety of meanings, the living microbe reflects the paradoxes of modernism itself and likewise contributes to its paradoxical signature."[6] The very first steps toward visualizing germs were taken between 1880 and 1900 in Great Britain, Germany and France. They aimed at connecting the fledgling combat against germs with inter-country contests and calls for increasing national security[7] and even at proposing early models for a regime of global health security.[8] "[A] reciprocal normative identification of germs with political enemies or stigmatized human beings"[9] contributed to the role of anthropomorphism as one of the main vehicles for visualizing germs. Another driving force was the rapid expansion in direct-to-consumer advertising for sanitary products such as soap, disinfectant or toothpaste.[10] The equation "bacteria are like their carriers" determined two modes for presenting germs, whether frightening monsters or strange freaks, or a combination of both modes. This division was reinforced by the struggle among experts over educational films, who faced the education-entertainment dichotomy[11] or the contest between danger vs. delight as the possible outcomes of seeing health films.[12]

The question, "What role does imagination play in situating the potential danger of germs if, particularly for children, the germ character mirrors the very activities they themselves partake in?"[13] led to one of the central questions concerning health propaganda, namely, "How to find the balance between the call to present germs as a part of our everyday life but along with it as an outstanding threat?" A major part of the efforts to visualize germs started with the intention to make the invisible visible led to their familiarization; even the process of visualizing germs in illustrations for professional and public sources, or within pre-cinematic forms of visualization, was a process of familiarization per se. The appearance of cinematography and its photogénie or defamiliarization, giving viewers the opportunity to see ordinary things as if for the first time,[14] were immediately employed within the rapidly developing field of health propaganda. The specificity of health films, in comparison with other mediums of health propaganda, was that "A disease can function remarkably like a story: by knitting diverse people and places into reciprocal, if inequal, relationships."[15] Experiencing disease and treatments against disease emerged as a new line of social division, and films tried to present this line as independent of the individual's social status. This intention to avoid the issue of class was extremely important for early health films, which addressed diverse audiences. Attributing the role of the central villain to disease seemed to be a promising device for negating the role of social class.

The Fly Pest and *Jinks* exaggerated the role of carriers of diseases in the daily life of humans through oscillation between anthropocentrism and anthropomorphism in picturing germs and their victims, namely, ordinary people. This double effect, aligned with cinematic representation, was disseminated during the interwar period and defined by Béla Balázs as "the fullest account of the interrelationship between the face of man and the face of things, [a model] in which film gives face to human and non-human entities alike."[16] Despite different approaches to picturing the carriers of infection, *The Fly Pest* and *Jinks* embodied a new, cinematic, sensitivity to the expressions of emotions and utilized close-ups as the central and most significant cinematic tool.[17] In these films, the carriers of infection took on the position of independent agents, able to influence through visualization, as well as through new approaches for describing diseases, their courses and strategies to prevent them. Often, they were imbued with super strength and were compared with powerful forces. In one of his earliest articles for one of the first issues of the monthly journal of the Red Cross, Driml wrote: "There are still people in China who believe that diseases are spread by bad spirits, and the Red Cross has done a lot to explain to Chinese youth that impurity should be considered such an evil spirit. And in our environment, we have the same 'bad spirits' that bring disease, and these evil spirits are different insects: mosquitoes, flies, and lice."[18]

The Fly Pest and *Jinks* were purchased by the Red Cross for dissemination in Eastern European countries at the end of 1920.[19] They were often shown one after the other in meetings with children, representing one of the possible solutions to the dilemma of danger vs. delight. *Jinks* was normally the last film among the four or five films included in the program of each of the performances.[20] It was the most attractive, accompanied by the explosions of laughter, according to the reports of those who witnessed the performance of health films for children and who confirmed "the incredible reception of the film": "when the light in the hall is switched on again, a unanimous wish comes from the children's mouths: One more time!!!"[21] In 1922, *Podmladak Crvnog Krsta*, the Yugoslav branch of the Junior Red Cross, organized the competition among the schoolchildren for the best poster based upon the lectures targeted with informing about tuberculosis that included the demonstration of *Jinks* accompanied by the lecture of school physicians.[22]

Despite the positive reception of U.S. films aimed at disseminating knowledge about hygienic skills in struggling against the carriers of infection, since the early 1920s, health propagandists in Eastern European countries themselves sought to implement various strategies, including the production of health films targeted at involving people from different social groups in the eradication campaigns. *The Fly Pest* and *Jinks* played multiple roles in these attempts. Furthermore, these attempts to develop strategies for health propaganda campaigns contributed to the transnational level of health film production – mostly for children or social groups equalized with children. Even the description of *Pakostnitsi* and the surviving sketches point to exaggeration, the main cinematic strategy of U.S. films, as well as to a metauniverse reality in which carriers of disease behave as humans, not just in dreams but in reality. The work on the film was presented by the *cartoon* of Venev, who, in a very friendly manner, communicates with the fly and simultaneously draws her. This direct communication between the creator of the film and the fly points directly to the ability of films to present the world of carriers of disease as previously not only invisible or parallel but also unnoticed or even neglected.

Film, as a medium for visualizing this world and attracting the attention of the audience to its threats, started to become a part of the scenario that mixed rational explanation for disease (lack of hygiene) and the concept of *magical contagion*, a spell cast by evil forces that could be removed through the rite of purification. Presenting the story of infection and the struggle against it as aligned with the frames of magical contagion highlights the call for external intervention and places the main protagonists, those weak and sick, on the verge of objectification. Jinks needs to sleep and to listen to his subconscious, to tune in to positive changes and a healthy lifestyle. This specific culmination makes it possible to think about the presentation of unhealthy habits as unnatural and acquired in a dysfunctional environment. In *Pakostnitsi*, people from countryside recognize the terror of flies, who behave as invaders, along with the call for the physician to act as a noble knight that saves lives. The Bulgarian animation was not the first example of introducing magical contagion into the plot of films about hygienic skills and objectifying the target audience.

At the end of the 1920s, the Croatian artist Petar Papp and writer Milan Marjanović produced several animated films for the School of Public Health, which in one way or another reproduced the idea of magical contagion. Like *Pakostnitsi*, these films did not survive, but it is possible to explore them through descriptions and the various parts of the plots. *Komarac a njegov razvoj* (The mosquito and his development, 1929) mixed themes from *The Fly Pest* and *Jinks* in a way compatible with *Pakostnitsi* but attacked yet other dangerous insect, the mosquito, along with the disease seen as the most dangerous, especially in the south of the Balkans, malaria.[23] The scene of the nightmare from *Jinks* was transformed into the simultaneous coexistence of two worlds, human and mosquito, which demonstrated the threat to humans from dangerous insects during sleep.

More than 100 draft images of mosquitoes as part of a jazz band[24] give off the impression of presenting unsafe insects as sophisticated musicians who play and flirt and who perceive a sleeping person as a comfortable stage for nighttime entertainment. The thoroughness with which the figures of the mosquitoes were depicted, with a special focus on their emotions, their communication among them through eye contact and gestures and the obvious relation between psychological character and music instruments are a reminiscent echo of *commedia dell'arte*, one of the strong influences of Italian theater on Croatian theatrical culture and a favorite cultural context for the animated films by Lotte Reiniger (see Figure 5.1).[25]

Reiniger was one of the idols for many Eastern European artists and filmmakers, along with the *Institut für Kulturforschung* (Institute for Cultural Research), to which Reiniger was affiliated during the interwar period. The independent structure, which had not only achieved success in the field of filmmaking and the history of contemporary art, but had also managed to create several film genres and supported the idea that "those cultural institutions are not only a way to receive subsidies, but also a strategy for the development of real art,"[26] was seen as a sign of hope for people in Eastern Europe. In *Komarac*, as in other animated films produced in the same year, 1929, it is easy to recognize the influence of Reiniger's visual style, which mixed puppetry, drawn figures and silhouettes divided into pieces for creating the animation. While the figures of the mosquitoes and their movements were drawn, the figure of the sleeping man was created as a moving silhouette (see Figure 5.2).

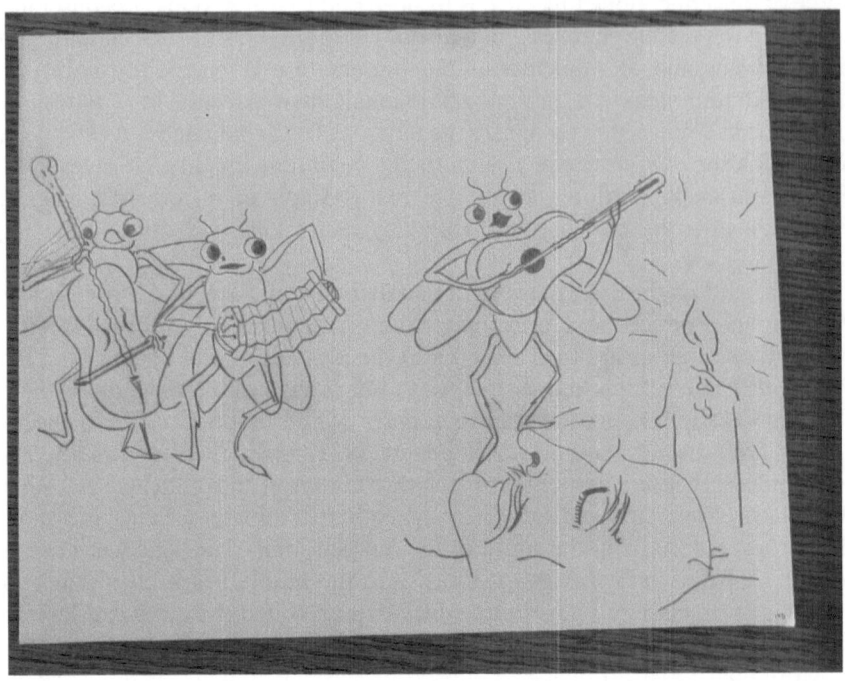

Figure 5.1 Echo of *commedia dell'arte* in the characters of mosquitoes in *Komarac* (Mosquitos, 1929).

Source: Kinoteka HAD.

It is reasonable to assume that *Komarac* became well known to Bulgarian filmmakers through their communication with Yugoslav colleagues within the *Jugoslovensko-Bugarsko filmsko društvo* (Yugoslav-Bulgarian Film Union) established in the early 1930s.[27] Both Croatian and Bulgarian attempts to create animated films were pioneering efforts not only within the health film movement but also with regard to the history of national film generally and adapting new Western trends in making animated films. But not only the visual method was a matter of adaptation.

Martin u nebo Martin iz neba (Martin goes to heaven and back, 1929) describes the story of careless Martin, who, only after reaching heaven and observing the ideal organization of the paradise countryside, learns about the secrets of sustainable farming, including the hygienic rules concerning care for poultry and livestock. Martin is so impressed by this new knowledge that he makes the decision to return and enlighten his still "backward" neighbors as well as to correct his own approach to rural labor.[28] *Martin u nebo Martin iz neba* can be easily interpreted as an inversion of another health film, *Peter and the Moon Man* commissioned by the Health and Cleanliness Council in 1929 for British audiences. Peter, a young boy, meets a man who has arrived

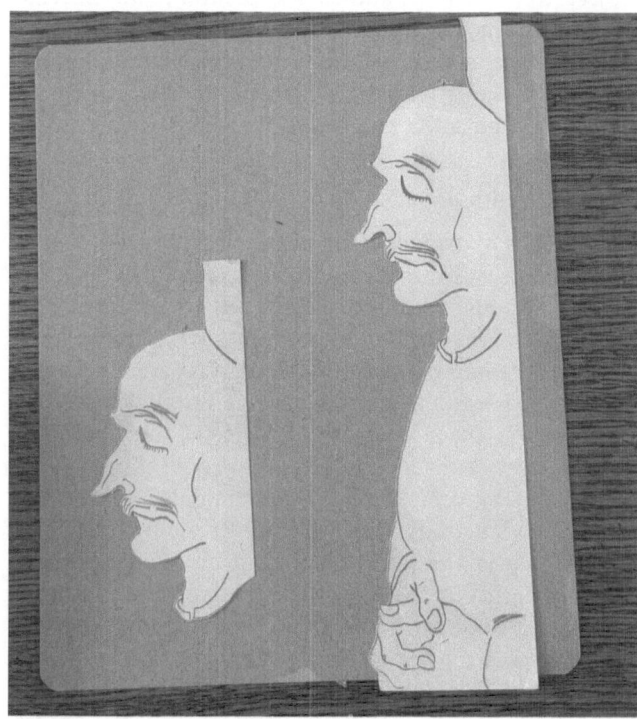

Figure 5.2 Following Reiniger's visual style in *Komarac* (Mosquitos, 1929).
Source: Kinoteka HAD.

from the Moon and invites him to tea. During this visit, the Moon Man learns the rules of hygiene and buys cleaning equipment, with which he returns to the Moon, which, over time, begins to glow brighter due to the fact that it was properly cleaned.[29] The difference in the identities of *Martin u nebo Martin iz neba* and *Peter and the Moon Man* attributed to target audiences (to follow good examples even though they seem to be unrealistic and relevant only to paradise and to be at the vanguard of the global and even interplanetary movement for higher hygienic standards) stresses the role of moral contagion for changing the plots: Only through experiencing death and travel to heaven would a man from the Croatian countryside be able to learn hygienic skills.

Magical contagion created a very powerful "account for the deliberate and continued visual alignment of disliked archetypes – the devil, the insect, the military enemy and the monster – with germs."[30] It shaped a specific genre of health propaganda, health fairy tales, which addressed children or those target groups whose perception and thinking were seen as child-like, namely, the rural population, and aimed at promoting hygienic skills and habits as indispensable to survival and progress, individually and collectively. Rick Altman has underscored that "genres appear as agents of a quite specific and effective ideological project: to control the audience's reaction to any specific film by providing the context in which that film must be interpreted."[31] One of the main contexts for the production and reception of health fairy tales in the genre of magical contagion was the unique role of puppet theater in Eastern Europe for developing health propaganda and health films in particular.

Puppet theater as a vehicle of health propaganda

The limited access to health films by people living in the periphery was one of the main reasons for developing and disseminating alternative mediums for propagating hygienic skills. Although the Red Cross tried to introduce traveling cinemas in regions where permanent cinematographs were unavailable, such as the majority of the Balkan states, in the mid-1920s, rural areas were not involved in systematic health propaganda. For instance, in Czechoslovakia in 1922, the first year of its operation, the mobile unit of the Red Cross organized 780 local presentations that were attended by 330,000 people (but only in Bohemia,[32] while Moravia and Slovakia became destinations for traveling health films only after 1925). In Yugoslavia, the practice of the traveling cinematograph was developed only in the late 1920s,[33] but mobile health film performances were introduced earlier, in the early 1920s, and remained the only option in Slovenia, Croatia and some parts of Serbia.[34] In Bulgaria, the systematic screenings of health films to the populations of the periphery started in the early 1940s.[35]

The process of instantiating microbes, infectious diseases and their carriers (insects) as a collective symbol was a part of shaping the global order of health security,[36] and ***collective participation in health propaganda*** was one of the central expectations from the side of international organizations such as the Rockefeller Foundation or the Red Cross. In his report on the first years of the Junior Red Cross in Czechoslovakia, Walter S. Gard, the first national director of the Junior Red Cross, described with great enthusiasm how 70,000 children took part in the Health Game in Prague.[37] Another expectation from the side of international organizations was achieving ***long-term effects of health education***. In the reports prepared by local physicians, or those responsible for local branches of the Red Cross, the recollections of events held among young participants were often cited as one of the main criteria for success. The physician, Libuše Rubelová-Berdanková, described her cooperation with the mobile educational film service organized by the Red Cross in Strážnici as a service in the name of *evangelium zdraví* (the gospel of health), one that should be regularized.[38] She illustrated her report with pictures drawn by children after several weeks of attending films in order to demonstrate how well they remembered the content and their emotions. Health propaganda was supposed to become not only ubiquitous and regular, but also ***interactive – involving the rising generations not only in consumption but also in production***. One of the earliest publications in Czechoslovak periodicals was a set of collective plays, for instance, *Hold vlajce* (Tribute to our flag) that should accompany the water play of children and connect the learning of hygienic skills with the acceptance of the symbols of new Czechoslovak state.[39] In 1945, a special issue of *Design*, dedicated to arts education policy, directly emphasized the phenomenon of collective creation as one of the central features of contemporary healthy childhood provided by the activities of the Junior Red Cross.[40]

One of the very earliest forms of collective, regular and interactive participation included various public activities such as the Days of the Red Cross for youth and children. These activities were disseminated in Eastern Europe,[41] along with others aimed at involving young people in a healthier lifestyle within the *Sokol* movement. But high numbers of participants were not the only expectation from such activities – the collective experience of struggle against disease should generate descriptive schemes shared by different social groups and cohorts, the functional purpose of any collective symbol.[42] This desirable outcome led to introducing various periodicals for youth and children aimed at disseminating "proper" discursive practices and achieving their sustainable reproduction. The Czechoslovak Red Cross started publishing *Měsíčník dorostu Červeného kříže* (Monthly magazine of the Red Cross for youth) in 1920, and in Yugoslavia, several magazines, including *Sokolska prosveta* (Enlightenment with *Sokol*), *Narodni napredak: list za unapređenje sela* (People's Progress: A Journal for the advancement of the countryside) and *Sokolska prosveta na sele* (*Sokol* enlightenment in the countryside), were established under the patronage of the *Sokol* movement. In Bulgaria, the special weekly newspaper *Zdravna prosveta* (Health education) started publishing special texts addressing schoolteachers, seen as the main agents for disseminating information among children and youth.

Because the activities and the periodicals directly depended on literacy, or, rather, the institution that ensured literacy (school), the lack of adequate literacy was seen as a possible limitation to collective participation. In the Rockefeller Foundation report of 1919, George E. Vincent describes "the naïve and straight performance" prepared for the Commission Américaine de Préservation contre la Tuberculose and written by Henri de Gressigny, which involved thousands of children of different ages and levels of literacy across France in the goal "to approach the unapproachable." The two-paragraph description of the puppet play and its performance was accompanied by a photograph of laughing children of different ages, watching the performance.[43] This example of "good practice" with regard to collective participation became one of the driving forces of the intensive institutionalization of puppet theater across Eastern Europe. Another factor was the exceptional role of puppet theaters for the promotion of national, "authentic" texts, as well as visual culture, as a part of shaping the collective identity of newly established nations.[44] As in Germany, Spain, Italy or Great Britain, in the nineteenth century, in interwar Eastern Europe, puppet performances were active agents in shaping the shared cultural codes that united nations. Both driving forces determined two interrelated means for the institutionalization of puppet theater: First, supporting amateur theaters, especially those established by schools or local districts, and second, establishing theaters and other professional bodies such as publishing houses for disseminating plays or even small manufacturing firms for producing puppets and decorations.

The *Sokol* movement intensified the interconnection between the development of puppet theater and nation-building within the multilevel, inter-country cooperation initiated in the mid-1920s aimed at preserving and advancing traditional Slavic puppet theater. *Sokol*'s periodicals were full of detailed articles aimed at sharing and disseminating puppet theater experiences: Advice on how to create puppet models, how to organize events to accompany performances, especially lectures on health, the "proper" education of children, childhood and psychology, including the perception of performances, were regular features in each of the issues of *Sokolska prosveta.* The associations of puppet theater masters constituted a subdivision of local branches of the *Sokol* movement. Another impact of *Sokol* included reinforcing the interrelation between health films and puppet theater as the main vehicles for health propaganda. The same activists of the *Sokol* movement often organized showings of health films and also created and disseminated puppet plays that used the plots of these films. This interrelation between films and amateur puppet theater was linked to the development of professional theaters.

Establishing the first puppet theater in Zagreb in 1920 was accompanied by the premiere of the first Croatian puppet play *Petrica Kerempuh i spametni osel* (Petrica Kerempuh and the clever donkey) by Velimir Deželić Jr., one of the founders of the theater.[45] The theater adapted the texts that became the classical legacy of national literature, such as August Šenoa's *Postolar i vrag* (The shoemaker and the devil) or fairy tales by Ivana Brlić-Mažuranić. Soon, it became common practice for the Croatian *Sokol* movement to organize short regional tours, not only to perform the plays but also to share the experience of how to prepare and perform.[46] The intention to advance national literature for children was directly reflected in the style and approaches to health-related puppet plays. Two main strategies for using puppet shows to realize the aims of health propaganda were introduced by Eastern European authors. While the Czechoslovak health puppet theater produced specific plays that simultaneously shaped collective identity and educated audiences about health skills, in Yugoslavia, both professional and amateur theaters adapted classical popular plays by adding some motifs about health and disease. For instance, in Slovenia, the folk play *Jurček dvorni zdravnik* (Jurček, the courtyard doctor) included information about diseases in order to educate children about their symptoms and prevention.[47] Both sets of plays reproduced magical contagion as the main plot for explaining the threat of disease and ways to prevent it. It is notable that the majority of the puppet characters discussed in *Sokol*'s periodicals were "bad" and "good" wizards – the main figures of the fairy tales based upon magical contagion.

Very early forms of puppet plays were presented in the Czechoslovak periodicals for children and named *Zdravotnické táčky,*[48] short, rhythmized stories of not more than 300 words. The production of *Zdravotnické táčky* was one of the earliest projects by Driml aimed at disseminating among children and youth the competencies regarding healthy nutrition, hygienic skills and the prevention of disease. From the very beginning, Driml followed the trend shared among European, and especially Eastern European, puppet theaters with their focus on the figures of Kasperl, Polichinelle, Kašpárek, Punch or Gaspar. These figures were not the main protagonists but rather the main supporting characters, very often the narrators, who link everything together and speak of morality and truth. Each of more than 20 short stories presented as conversations between Kašpárek and the children was accompanied by illustrations drawn in different styles. Even in these early attempts to create an interactive space for educational communication, Kašpárek utilized all the features of the spokes character,[49] especially because they included advertisements for toothpaste and soap in the plays. This double effect of the progressive Kašpárek would be fixed later in the films.

The very first *Zdravotnické táčky* were illustrated by Josef Lada, who, at the same time, started illustrating *Osudy dobrého vojáka Švejka* (The good soldier Švejk). Some later parts were illustrated in the style of shadow theater. But the main portion of these short stories, as well as the plays, was illustrated by Karel Štapfer, painter, illustrator and head stage designer of the National Theater in Prague, famous for his love of detail and multiple forms of visual metaphors. Štapfer was also a devoted propagandist of puppet theater. This early experience of visualization was continued in the production of puppets and theatrical decorations in different styles, which only reinforced the networking among enthusiasts of puppet theater as a medium of health propaganda – not only within Czechoslovakia but beyond. Between 1922 and 1928, Driml wrote more than 30 plays aimed at disseminating hygienic skills, healthy nutrition, vaccination readiness and information about diseases and ways to prevent them. Several plays were translated by Yugoslav enthusiasts of puppet theater culture.

For the Czechs, writing and disseminating health puppet plays started to become a strategy for improving international and national reception, as well as for winning the long-term competition between the German and the Czech traditions of puppet theater. Driml posited his writing as the continuation of the long-term tradition of Czech puppet performance as an agent of national revival.[50] The unprecedented role of the Czechoslovak puppet theater movement across Eastern Europe achieved its apex at the end of the 1920s. After organizing the nationwide and international exhibition of puppet theater in 1928, the *Masarykův lidovýchovný ústav* (Masaryk Institute of People's Education) established the *Svaz slovanských loutkářů* (the Union of Slav Puppeteers), and one year later, with the entry of Germany, Austria, France and the Soviet Union, it was transformed into the International Union of Puppeteers.[51] At the same time, the Czech tradition continued in a complicated relationship with the German tradition of marionette theater and its central figure Franz von Pocci, deeply rooted in Central European popular culture. For those Czech patriots like Driml, the influence of the German tradition was embraced as justification for culture war. This contest was only reinforced during the interwar period. Marie Jirásková and Pavel Jirásek have underscored that recruiting puppet theaters for the aim of enlightening the people led to the replacement of traditional Czech theater by more professional approaches, directly influenced by the tradition of Franz von Pocci.[52]

Mladen Širola, the director of the first puppet theater in Zagreb, explicitly described the relationship between German and Czech puppet theater traditions in terms of competition: "The good example [of using puppet theatre for the aims of enlightenment] by Czechs came on the heels of the Germans in developing puppet-theatre culture, including writing special plays aimed at educating children and adults."[53] Širola underscored the role of Czech propagandists of puppet theater for dissemination throughout the Balkans, stressing the outstanding role of Czech "colonists who loved puppet theatre from the bottom of their hearts."[54] But at the same time, he included more plays written by German authors in the list of plays recommended for the purposes of health propaganda and school puppet theaters. An even greater commitment to the German tradition was presented in Slovenia, where the first puppet theater production in Ljubljana was an adaptation of one of the plays by Franz von Pocci, *Die Zaubergeige* (*Čarobne gosli* in Slovenian). The contest between the Czech and the German traditions of puppet theater reinforced nationalistic motifs, especially in the competition for international reception. The direct attack against the German tradition of puppet theater and approaches to depicting germs became a driving force that ensured the national and international acceptance of one of the very first health puppet plays written by Driml, *Bacilínek*.

Notes

1 The first Bulgarian animated film "Villains," *Dyga* 30.11.1936, 170, p. 6.
2 The film did not survive, and, moreover, there is no information on whether the film was finished and screened or if the project was not completed; more in Nadezhda Marinchevska (2001) *Bylgarsko animacionno kino 1915–1995* [Bulgarian animation between 1915 and 1995], Sofia: Kolibri.
3 Bill Marsh (2010) Visual Education in the United States and the 'Fly Pest' Campaign of 1910, *Historical Journal of Film, Radio and Television*, 30, 1, 21–36, p. 31.
4 Hilaire Belloc (1897) *More Beasts (For Worse Children)*, London: Duckworth and Co.
5 The League of Red Cross Societies Geneva Switzerland (1921) *Conditions concernant le prêt des films par la Ligue des societies de la Croix-Rouge* [Prerequisites for loaning films by the League of Red Cross Societies], EMVZ, box 106 SNA.
6 Martina King (2013) Anarchist and Aphrodite: On the literary history of germs. In Thomas Rütten and Martina King (eds), *Contagionism and Contagious Diseases: Medicine and Literature 1880–1933*, Berlin: De Gruyeter, 101–130, p. 106.
7 Paul Weindling (2007) Ansteckungsherde. Die deutsche Bakereiologie als wissenschaftlicher Rassismus 1890–1920 [The sources of infection: German bacteriology as scientific racism in the 1890s and 1920s] in Philipp Sarasin, Silvia Berger,

Marianne Hänseler, and Myriam Spörri (eds), *Bakteriologie und Moderne. Studien zur Biopolitik des Unsichtbaren 1870–1920* [Bacteriology and moderne. The studies of biopolotics concerning invisible in the 1870s and 1920s], Frankfurt am Main: Suhrkamp, 2007, 354–374.

8 The idea of bacteria as "enemies of mankind" offered by Robert Koch was quickly disseminated throughout the world and became central to national and trans-national discourses of public health; more in Josep L. Barona (2019) *Health policies in interwar Europe: A transnational Perspective,* London: Routledge.

9 King Ibid.

10 James F. Stark & Catherine Stones (2019) Constructing Representations of Germs in the Twentieth Century, *Cultural and Social History,* 16 3, 287–314, p. 289.

11 Marsh. Visual Education in the United States.

12 Catherine Stones, James Stark, Sophie Rutter and Colin Macduff (2020) The visual representation of germs: a typology of popular germ depictions, *Visual Communication,* doi.org/10.1177/1470357219896055.

13 Ibid.

14 Laura Marcus (2003) How newness enters the world: the birth of cinema and the origins of man, in Julian Murphet and Lydia Rainford *Literature and Visual technologies Writing after cinema,* London: Palgrave Macmillan, 29–48, p. 32.

15 Miriam Posner (2011) Communicating disease: tuberculosis, narrative, and social order in Thomas Edison's Red Cross seal films, in Devin Orgeron, Marsha Orgeron and Dan Streible, *Learning with the Lights Off: Educational Film in the United States,* Oxford: Oxford University Press, 90–106.

16 Marcus How newness enters the world p. 35.

17 Ibid.

18 Karel Driml (1921) Náš společný nepřítel [Our common enemy], *Měsíčník dorostu Červeného kříže,* 1, 4, p. 8.

19 The League of Red Cross Societies *Conditions concernant le pret des films.*

20 Spoločnost Československoho Červeného Kríža [The Red Cross] (1926), Soznam filmov pre deti [List of the films for children], Fond of Košická župa 1923–1928, II. ZV, box 522.

21 Děti a zdravotně výchovná jednotka Čs.Červeného kříže [Children and the mobile unit of Czechoslovak Red Cross], *Měsíčník dorostu Červeného kříže* [Monthly magazine of the Red Cross for youth], 1923, 3, 7, p. 4.

22 Zdravstevni odsjek za Hrvatsku Slavoniju i Medjimurje i Zagreb [The Department of public health at Slavonia, Međimurje and Zagreb] (1922) Gradskom školskom nadvornišstvu [The letter to the Department of education] Arhiv Jugoslavije Ministarstvo socijalne politike i narodnog zdravlje Kraljevine Yugoslavie Broj fond 39, Broj fasikle 2.

23 Ibid. p. 47.

24 Komarac (1929) The sketches for the film. Kinoteka of the State Archives of Croatia, Fond of Skola za narodnog zdravja, box 1.

25 Whitney Grace (2017) *Lotte Reiniger Pioneer of film animation,* Jefferson, Horth Carolina: McFarland & Company, p. 185.

26 Franta Kocourek (1929) Institut für Kulturforschung [Institute for cultural research], *Nová svoboda,* 6 24, 375–377, p. 375.

27 Sokolska prosveta, 1934, IV 3–4 p. 150.

28 Vjekoslav Majcen (1995) *Filmska djelatnost škole narodnog zdravlja "Andrija Štampar": (1926–1960)* [Film activities of the "School of Public Health Andrija Štampar" 1926–1969], Zagreb: Hrvatski državni arhiv, pp. 46, 107.

29 'A National Encyclopedia of Educational Films and 16 mm Apparatus Available in Great Britain' (1935), pp. 160, 236.

30 Stones et al. (2020) The visual representation of germs.

31 Rick Altman (1984) Semantic/syntactic approach to film genre, *Cinema Journal,* 23 3, pp. 6–18.
32 Děti a zdravotně výchovná jednotka [Children and health education unit] (1923) p. 4.
33 Karl Kaser (2018) *Hollywood auf dem Balkan. Die visuelle Moderne an der europäischen Peripherie (1900–1970)* [Hollywood on Balkans. Visual Modernity in European Periphery (1900–1970)], Wien, Köln, Weimar: Böhlau, pp. 226–227.
34 Andrija Štampar (1925) *Socijalna medicina. Uz saradnju jugoslovenskih socijalnih lekara* [Social medicine: From the experience of Yugoslav physicians], First volume, Zagreb: Institut za socijalnu medicinu, pp. 281–282.
35 D. Orachovats (1942) Pismo do gospodin Lange Glaven sekretar' na Bylgaro-germanskoto druzhestvo [Letter to the Lange, chief-secretary of the Bulgaraina-German society], Sofiya 21.03.1942, CDA Fond Bylgarsko druzhestvo Cherven krst 156 207.
36 King ibid.
37 Walter S. Gard (1921) Playing a great game Junior Red Cross news, March, 101–103.
38 Vzpomínky dětí na zdravotně-výchovnou jednotku [The memories of children about the health education unit meeting], *Měsíčník dorostu Červeného kříže* (1925), 5 p. 59.
39 Jaroslav Sojka (1996) *Komenšti* [The successors of Jan Komenius], Brno, 3.
40 Junior Red Cross (1945), Design, 47:3, p. 19.
41 The national subdivisions of the Junior Red Cross were established in Czechoslovakia and Yugoslavia between 1921 and 1922.
42 King.
43 The Rockefeller Foundation, A review for 1919 Public health and Medical education in many lands, pp. 25–26.
44 Antonina Bogner-Šaban, Dalibor Foretić, Livija Kroflin, and Abdulah Seferović (1997) *Hrvatsko lutkarstvo* [Croatian puppet theatre], Hrvatski centrum Unima, p. 9. Remarkable that the heyday of puppet theatres including health puppet plays fell on the first decades of the existence of the German Democratic Republic. In 1967 the documentary that presented the history of socialist puppet theatre in health propaganda got the special prize of the International Festival of Red Cross and health films.
45 This play was adapted by Karel Driml in 1924 and retold as a story of survival by a good but naïve king, through a donkey, from unhealthy habits: *Král Asinus* Choceň: Loutkář.
46 Sa zbora župskih prosvetara [News from the meeting of local educators] (1934), *Sokolska Prosveta,* IV 5, p. 218.
47 Ibid., p. 219.
48 *Táčky* has two interrelated meanings. The first is a friendly conversation or discussion, for example, sitting in a peaceful neighborhood. The second denotes a small cart on one wheel often associated with amateur mobile puppet theatre. Notably, Karel Driml, who wrote the majority of health puppet plays, was presented not as the author but the "driver" of these stories.
49 Stones et all The visual representation of germs.
50 Karel Driml (1927) Zdravotní výchova loutkovým divadlem. (Proč jsem je angažoval?) [Puppet theatre for health education. Why have I engaged?] Česká osvěta [Czech enlightenment], 2, 3.
51 Marie Jirásková and Pavel Jirásek (2011) *Loutka a moderna: vizualita českého loutkového rodinného divadla, spolkového divadla a uměleckých scén v první polovině 20. století jako osobitý odraz avantgardních a modernistických snah českých výtvarných umělců* [Puppet and modernity: the visuality of Czech puppet family

theater, amateur's theater and art scenes in the first half of the 20th century as a distinctive reflection of the avant-garde and modernist efforts of Czech visual artists], Řevnice: Arbor Vitae, p. 301.

52 Ibid.
53 Mladen Širola (1927) *Marionetsko kazalište: u službi zdravstvenog prosvjećivanja* [Puppet theatre in serving the mission of health enlightenment], Zagreb: Tisak Jugoslovenske štampe p. 7.
54 Ibid p. 6.

6 *Bacilínek* (1922) on the stage of the national and global orders of health security

Bacilínek: The inception of the magical contagion genre in health propaganda

Bacilínek, a four-act play, was written by Driml in 1922 for the purposes of health education and specifically as a part of the campaign against tuberculosis. In the first act, Jedibaba (literally "poisoning woman" and a paraphrase with "ježibaba," a popular female villain in the Czech fairytales), who is the *mastičkářka* (medicaster), "an earthly companion of the devil, a faithful hell helper," motivates Beelzebub, the devil, to create Bacilinek, the bacillus of tuberculosis, as an insurmountable barrier to human progress:

> I will create strange small animals,
> They will be smaller than a dot
> They will gnaw people's lungs
> Like worms eating rotten mushrooms
> They will destroy joints and bones
> I will endow them with a special power of invisibility

Along with Bacilínek, Beelzebub creates the Fly, "the giant monster with wolf paws and chicken eyes that transfers bacilli from the sick to the healthy."

In the next act of the play, this pair of hell fiends arrives in the town Hloupá Lhota (literally "stupid" Lhota),[1] where Bacilínek observes the future paradise for his large family, the house of the shoemaker Emanuel Dratvička:

> Full of dirt, full of stench
> There is not a drop of air here
> Smells exceptionally like alcohol

Bacilínek sees Dratvička, who prefers to be treated by Jedibaba instead of going to the physician, as a perfect candidate for being infected by tuberculosis and becoming a good carrier of disease. Dratvička's wife is already sick, and we learn about her existence, disease and death at the beginning of the last act from the words of Dratvička. We also meet his four children, who

DOI: 10.4324/9781003272267-9

must sleep on the floor because their father spends all the money for *kořalka* (distillate) and tobacco as well as some "medicaments" from Jedibaba.

Along with Bacilínek, the narrator Kašpárek arrives at Dratvička's house and asks him to provide accommodation during the performances of his theater in Hloupá Lhota. Even just a short conversation with Dratvička and his friend Škrhola[2] persuades Kašpárek not only of their "backwardness" and myriad of unhealthy habits but also their distrust of public health as a legacy of previous times. Škrhola shares his unpleasant memories and his skepticism regarding physicians:

Once upon a time there was a doctor
All he did was write prescriptions
strange figures, hooks, badges
for those "gentlemen" from the pharmacy

Kašpárek promises these two that he will spend a vacation as the student of "a really good doctor," who has already discovered the bacillus and methods of treating tuberculosis. In the following act of the play, he travels to Berlin, to meet Robert Koch. Koch has given Kašpárek the task of cleaning a laboratory full of test tubes with bacteria and viruses, forbidding him to open them. Left alone to clean, Kašpárek is faced with the germs, Death and Beelzebub, who demands he release the germs from the test tubes, alternating temptation and threat in order to force Kašpárek's hand. But Kašpárek copes with his fears and does not release the germs. Koch, who is impressed by the brave behavior of Kašpárek, goes with him to Hloupá Lhota to treat Dratvička, his family and the entire community.

The final act of the play presents the struggle between Kašpárek and Koch on the one side and the dark strengths of Jedibaba and Beelzebub on the other. Although his confidence in the methods of Jedibaba is undermined (because they did not help his wife), Dratvička continues to question the benefits of the advice given by doctors and Kašpárek. Tired of the verbal skirmish between them, Dratvička posits a riddle, and the correct answer should prove the legitimacy of the argument either for continuing to drink *kořalka* or for following the advice of Koch and Kašpárek. Dratvička asks, "What is covered with skin, has one hoof, a long tongue, and a black face?" While Jedibaba relies on the assistance of Beelzebub, who tells her that it is him, Kašpárek, who understands Dratvička, provides the correct answer: It is a shoe. As a man of his word, Dratvička promises:

Glory, glory, three times glory
That's a funny head
I'll listen to his advice now

The fact that it is not a proper medical argument but rather personal trust in Kašpárek is decisive in favor of health only reinforces the motif of magical contagion and cleansing, just with the help of common sense and reason. Dratvička starts practicing physical exercises, stops drinking distillates and even joins *Sokol*. These metamorphoses lead to the suicides of Bacilínek, his fiancée Bacilinka and Jedibaba.

While the play's plot adapts a great deal from *Jinks*,[3] in terms of class and gender relations, *Bacilínek* can be significantly distinguished from *Jinks*. The main protagonist of *Jinks* belongs to an upper working class and lives in the city, while the inhabitants of Hloupá Lhota are lower-middle class and live in a small town on the verge of settlement. Remarkably, for Kašpárek to win over the attention of Dratvička at the beginning of their communication, he pretends that he accepts him as not a master of *boty* (shoes) but as a *professor of botany*. Undoubtedly, this respect, stemming from the wordplay, helps him lend some credentials to Kašpárek. Jinks's wife thinks progressively and plays a central role in the first steps toward reeducating her husband, but the wife of Dratvička remains invisible and inaudible. This gender-based imbalance, typical of many other plays by Driml, can be seen as one of the legacies of the puppet theater tradition introduced by Matěj Kopecký, in whose plays male characters and male views are predominant.

In the plays by Kopecký, female characters are passive, mostly presented by their social roles: Wives, servants, daughters or princesses, without names. Similarly, the three female characters of *Bacilínek* can be hardly recognized as central to the narration. The audience does not pay attention to the name of Dratvička's wife. Addressing the male audience reflects the vision of the target group of health propaganda, as well as viewing men as the central agents of nation-building. In this way, the plays by Driml reflect not only the aims of health education but also the mission to unite people around particular symbols and practices – reproducing the long-term tradition of Czech nation-building as predominantly masculine. It further reverberates with the predominance of the boyhood adventure genre, central to European literature for children, including the literature of Eastern Europe.[4] A definition of masculinity that combined "sportsmanship," chivalry and patriotism, which was advanced within imperialist metanarratives, took on new features, including the acquisition of hygienic rules as a means to become the master of one's own fate. In *Bacilínek*, Dratvička's engagement with *Sokol* can be read as a very early approximation of exploiting the boy's adventure genre in the late plays and films by Driml, whose male protagonists eventually become younger – teenagers.

With some variation and adaptation, *Bacilínek* continued to be performed until the end of the 1960s. Since the late 1920s, it was accompanied by a short lecture about the treatment of tuberculosis prepared by Driml.[5] Published first in 1922, the *Bacilínek* text was issued in 1925 and 1929, and then in 1950 – every time with a new cover. Two of the most remarkable covers were created by Karel Štapfer in 1928 and Vojtěch Cinybulk in 1950. Štapfer directly used visual matches with *The Fly Pest* and *Jinks* and very probably also with the recent British animation, *Giro the germ*, produced by Newhall Films for the

Health and Cleanliness Council in 1927; the chain of flying bacillus is very similar to the horde of the Giro germs in the British animation. Cinybulk, who engaged in the puppet-theater movement during the interwar period and was one of the artists who continued this tradition after 1945, styled the cover in a minimalistic manner. Both covers present Bacilínek as a wild creature, between an ape and a human that looks savage enough "to inspire disgust and consistent denial,"[6] one of the main aims of visualizing bacillus. Aligned with the logic of magical contagion, the invasion of such "wild" enemies of humanity should be stopped using the weapons of civilization, medical intervention and hygiene. Furthermore, its rejection brings it down to the level of "wild" bacteria.

Bacilínek became emblematic of Czechoslovak health propaganda in the early 1920s, and the images of its performances illustrated the great role of puppet theater in the success of public health campaigns.[7] Between the 1920s and the 1950s, under the recommendation of the Red Cross, *Bacilínek* was translated into Serbian (including Braille for the purposes of educating people with serious visual impairments), Dutch and German, as well as Japanese and Chinese.[8] Explaining the play's success in a much larger community than children in interwar Czechoslovakia inclines us to focus on its messages and cultural codes, which not only ensured the positive reception of *Bacilínek* but also made it a text "that pushed the boundaries of genre and texts that cross cultures"[9] in health propaganda and health films for children in particular. *Bacilínek* attacks two interrelated German canons: (1) visualizing bacillus as dangerous but beautiful creations; and (2) questioning the positive role of medicine in puppet plays, to root magical contagion and physicians as those "good wizards" as a central motif in health-related plays of films.

The cultural war between *Bacilínek* and anti-scientism

In the correspondence between Driml and Jindřich Veselý,[10] there is an unpublished translation of *Les Nègres et les Marionnettes* (The Negroes and the puppet-show, 1839),[11] one of the famous lyrical poems by Pierre-Jean de Béranger.[12] In his characteristic sarcastic and accusatory manner, Béranger compares the audiences of puppet theaters with slaves; the puppetry, similar to that arranged by the captain of a slave ship, calms them down and even prevents death from melancholy. The sequence of provocative comparisons among the characters in traditional puppet theater, like Polichinelle or Kašpárek, the devil and the police officer, points to the temptation of a collective identity, which "leaves us as slaves of the king's manipulation."

In contrast to the original, Driml does not use "us" – instead, he uses the definition *poddaní* (subjects of the king). What motivated Driml to translate and send this remarkable text, which combines anti-monarchic stances and negative attitudes toward popular culture, including puppet theater, is not clear. Undoubtedly, Driml could apply this critical view against one of his main competitors, the German aristocrat Franz von Pocci, one of the most influential confidants of King Ludwig the First of Bavaria. Von Pocci's public activities could easily be compared with the position of Driml, who was slated to lead the Subdivision of Propaganda of the Ministry of Health and Physical Culture, but he died before obtaining this position.[13] The belligerent tone of the play points to interpreting *Bacilínek* as the deconstruction of Pocci's view on medicine in favor of an uncritically positive acceptance of public health, one of the main missions for the public activities of medical experts in interwar Eastern Europe.

Von Pocci's attention to the public role of medicine and the ambiguous impact of medical assistance reflected the transformation of medicine as a semi-institution in the first part of the nineteenth century to a highly institutionalized instrument of surveillance since the last third of the nineteenth century. Von Pocci belonged to the pre-modern tradition of medicine when "diseases were not generally thought of as discrete entities,"[14] but medicine and its main representative, the physician, had already started to become a powerful influencer. The increasing trend to rely on medical progress that could defeat disease irritated von Pocci and relegated him to the edge of anti-scientism. With his characteristic skepticism, von Pocci presented in his plays a whole series of physicians and biologists whose ethics were questionable not only because they abused their knowledge for the sake of enrichment and power, but also because they committed open villainy.

Der Zaubergarten's cast of characters includes the bizarre botany professor, Kräutlmayer, who may be easily interpreted as a chief herbalist more interested in taking care of his plants than the people surrounding him. In *Casperl als Turner*, there are two propagandists of a healthy lifestyle, the medical adviser Fiberer, and the fitness instructor Barrenreck, who risk the lives of their patients. Professor Gerstenzucker (literally, "barley sugar"[15]) in *Schimpanse der Darwinaffe*,[16] who hires Casperl[17] to pretend to be his already dead chimpanzee to maintain the attractivity of Darwinian ideas, wins out over even the experienced scammers from the mayor's office. And a keen butterfly gatherer, Doctor Fleischmann (literally "man of flesh"), in *Hänsl und Grethel oder Der Menschenfresser* (Hansel and Gretel, or the maneater),[18] a *Naturforscher* (natural scientist) who lives with Katharine, the only surviving (not eaten) girl, who is also the housekeeper. Fleischmann not only feeds Hansel, Gretel and Casperl unhealthy food, such as small dumplings, to make them plumper but also intends to dissect Casperl in order to discover the reasons behind his strange anatomy.[19]

But the most consistent critical reflection of the changes in the public position of medicine is achieved in *Doctor Sassafras oder Doctor, Tod und Teufel* (Doctor Sassafras, or the doctor, death and the devil). The scenes in *Bacilínek* key for understanding the social responsibility of the physician should be read as directly interrogating this play. *Doctor Sassafras* was extremely popular among German-speaking Czech viewers in the nineteenth century and was even published in Czech translation in 1918 in *Frant. hrabě Pocci, klasik loutkových her* (Franz von Pocci, the classic of puppet plays), a collection of the plays by von Pocci. It was selected by the leaders of the Czechoslovak puppet-theater movement Jan Bartoš, Jaroslav Hloušek and Karel Kobrle, who defined this play as "delicately poetic but intertwined with hilarious scenes."[20] Moreover, other Eastern European puppet theaters performed *Doctor Sassafras.* In the Croatian translation, *Doktor Medikuš* (Dr. Medicus) was recommended as one of the most relevant plays for educating youth about the role of public health.[21] Posing *Bacilínek* as a direct negation of von Pocci's view on medicine, Driml continued the cultural war between the Czechs and the Germans for acceptance at the international level. His main argument involved opposing the progressive view coined in *Bacilínek* to von Pocci's skepticism, seen as "backward" and abusive of the attractiveness of puppet theater.

From the very beginning, Sassafras is presented as a talented practitioner who applies a wide range of all possible methods, depending on the needs of the patients, even those that were seen as mutually opposed, such as allopathy and homeopathy. Casperl who is sincerely attached to his master is the main servant of the physician who often worries about his master because he works too hard. This connection is reproduced in *Bacilínek* through the respectful trust of Kašpárek for Professor Koch and the readiness to serve him. But as in other Diml plays, Kašpárek represents a servant not of a particular master (as in Pocci's plays) but rather a servant of progress.[22]

Due to his outstanding success, Sassafras is often dubbed the second Hypocrite or Paracelsus. But von Pocci names this character after a small tree, the sassafras, brought to Europe from the United States. Sassafras had become one of the main components in European homeopathy, symbolizing wealth and financial gain, the values that are the top priorities of Sassafras. Having gained his reputation by treating ordinary people, Sassafras is now interested only in rich patients who can provide him with a more respected and luxurious life. While Casperl must substitute for his master, treating poor farmers, Sassafras is pulled into a dependent relationship with the vastly rich baron, Steinreich, who is healthy and whose heart pains emanate from his heartlessness toward others. In contrast, the joint efforts of Koch and Kašpárek, aimed at eradicating tuberculosis in Lhota, are diametrically opposed to the arrangement of characters in von Pocci's play.

Notwithstanding the contest between the German and the Czech traditions of puppet theater in health propaganda, Driml reproduces in *Bacilínek* all the patriotic tropes concerning the figure of Robert Koch, introduced by German bacteriology at the end of the nineteenth century. Koch, who accepted Kašpárek's invitation to help the inhabitants of "stupid" Lhota represents the "Father of Bacilli," a crusader fighting enemies in faraway lands who became one of the symbols of the German revival.[23] The very idea that the human body and the nation's boundaries are a matter of applied hygiene is re-produced in *Bacilínek*, through equalizing the "backwardness" of particular inhabitants and an entire location, the town of Lhota.[24] This uncritically positive attitude toward Koch[25] is based upon Driml's own view on progress as an unconditional good.

The key antagonist of progress is attributed to Beelzebub, who creates Bacilínek specifically to interrupt progress. Jedibaba, who seduces those who already suffer from disease through her poisoning potions, is an additional driving force of this "un-natural selection." The motifs of social Darwinism in explaining infectious diseases are reinforced by the monist view on the origin of bacillus,[26] which Driml also attributes to Beelzebub. Beelzebub directly equalizes humans and bacteria as originating from the same "dirty" substance when he responds to Jedibaba's doubts about his ability to create Bacilínek:

> God created man out of clay
> to worship God forever
> Why doesn't the devil create bacilli out of clay?

In complete correspondence with the views of the most famous monists in bacteriology, Ernest Haeckel and his successor Wilhelm Bölsche, Beelzebub describes the appearance of bacillus as an act of transforming an unanimated world into an animated one:

> Dragon eye, fox hair
> Clay from the grave, Yaga's saliva
> Dust and dirt from under the nails[27]

Driml often exaggerated the power of evil wizards by attributing to them such outsized Darwinism as a key source of magical contagion. For instance, in another play, *Špindimůra* (literally "dirty nightmare"), an evil sorceress, intends to cover weak people who do not follow hygienic rules with dirt, in order to transform them into a dirty substance. The idea of spontaneously emerging bacteria, which connects the unanimated and animated worlds, echoes in one of the final scenes, in which Bacilínek proposes hand and heart to Bacilinka:Ba

> cilínek: But let's look - my love, Bacilinka, goldilocks. I kiss your hand - bent to the ground in the dust.
> Bacilinka: My Knights - Bacilín,
> Have you found another house yet?
> I don't want to live any longer in the dust
> You have to get a seat for us!

Attributing sex to bacillus and even particular visual characteristics such as hair color is reminiscent of the famous comparison of the first bacillus with Adam and Aphrodite, made by Wilhelm Bölsche,[28] one of the pioneers in visualizing bacteriology for the public and for professionals. The comparison of bacteria Bacilinka with Aphrodite, born from sea foam, is easily associated with metaphysical Darwinism. And the intentional appearance of bacteria Bacilínek, who, like other live entities and Adam, must struggle for survival, reflects the indispensable role of social Darwinism in the history of visualizing bacteria and other carriers of infectious diseases.[29] This overlapping of two different Darwinisms only reinforces the role of bacteriology as a new secular religion that brings together natural science and a creation myth.[30] Driml exaggerates this effect by labeling this view as an indispensable part of the evil forces that should be defeated by powerful wizards – physicians.

The physicians in both plays achieve enormous power over disease. Sassafras makes a deal with the devil to prevent blackmail from Death, which demands Sassafras give him (in the play Death is *Herr Knochmeyer*) half of the patients, including the richest ones. This bargain permits Sassafras to cure the most hopeless. The doctor captures death by placing Death in a devil's chair, from which Death cannot escape. Koch achieves his power over carriers of diseases by capturing them in test tubes. His laboratory represents the triumph of reason over disease. At times, Kašpárek finds Death in the laboratory too – but without a scythe, which makes Death helpless. Both Casperl and Kašpárek face direct threats from the side of Death by being present where Death has been captured – but these scenes have mutually opposite meanings.

Von Pocci demonstrates the meaninglessness of the attempts to triumph over Death, the natural end of a natural process. Moreover, one of the monologues by Death, about the equality of people facing mortality, is key for understanding the changes in the behavior of the main characters, who ultimately reject their ambitions in favor of justice even at the price of their life. But Kašpárek intends to snatch people from the clutches of death. In contrast to von Pocci's play, in *Bacilínek*, only one patient, the invisible wife of Dratvička, dies – in favor of launching his move toward a healthy life. In both plays, the image of the collective patient is directly associated with less educated and "simple" people who are often presented in von Pocci's plays through the figure of Bayern, and in the Czech tradition by the character of Škrhola. Casperl names the usual group of poor patients who try to approach Sassafras *Rudel* (the horde). The scene depicting the treatment of a farmer who has eaten dumplings and asks for relief from his stomach pains most likely coincides visually with the scene in Driml's play depicting the meeting between Kašpárek and Škrhola.

In his usual manner, asking questions rather than answering them, von Pocci constantly doubts the existence of boundaries between the worlds, which are considered to be parallel and uncrossable. In *Doctor Sassafras*, the difference between the world of the living and the world of the dead is decisive. The culmination of each of the acts, the decision making made by Sassafras, Steinreich and his secretary, a young man with a kind heart and noble motives, takes place in a cemetery. For these characters, the boundary between life and death is uncrossable but not so for Casperl, who considers the boundaries between social classes much more unapproachable than the option to cross the line between death and life. In *Bacilínek*, it is not a violation of the natural law that creates a metauniverse reality but rather it explains something on the verge of inexplicability, namely, the origin of germs, as a part of the magical contagion plot.

Driml uses the story as a source of memes decisive for the purposes of propaganda: Bacillus are those wild creatures who make thoughtless people sick – and block them in their ability to move ahead; contamination occurs because there exist enemies of humans; healing is a contra-action regarding contamination that requires the presence of external forces, physicians and medicine. *Bacilínek* takes on the predispositions for a story to become a meme: Audiences of different cultural backgrounds recognize it as relevant, and the play is repeated through action and behavior. The story of infectious diseases and their successful treatment as magical contagion continued "to justify itself through an ongoing process of replication,"[31] not only in the puppet-theater movement in Eastern Europe but also in several film projects targeted at child audiences in Great Britain and the United States.

Notes

1 *Lhota* is a popular name for Czech villages in different regions.
2 Škrhola is a character from traditional Czech marionette theater, who represents the behavior of a village "primitive.".
3 Undoubtedly, Driml got a chance not only to watch *The Fly Pest* and *Jinks* during his U.S. scholarship in 1920 but also to be trained in how to use films and puppet shows for the aims of health propaganda. Moreover, Driml had the opportunity to observe the enormous success of *Jinks* among young viewers in different parts of Czechoslovakia. Měsíčník dorostu Červeného kříže [Monthly magazine of the Red Cross for youth], Vzpomínky na pana Broučka [Memories about pan Brouček], Dorost Čs. Červeného kříže obecné školy v Knyku [Youth of the Red Cross of the secondary school in Knyk] (1924) 4, 5, p. 67.
4 Robyn McCallum (2018) *Screen adaptation and the Politics of childhood,* London: Palgrave, p. 41.
5 Karel Driml (1928) Propagace a boj proti tuberkulose na podkladě statistik a evidence [Propagation and the struggle against tuberculosis on the grounds of statistic data and evidences], *Věstník Masarykovy ligy proti tuberkulózy,* IX, 8.
6 Jan Malík (1950) *Bacilínek* IV. Výdaní Umění lidu Moderní loutková scéna, 6, 1.
7 Karel Driml, (1923) "Puppet Plays Teach Health to Czechoslovak Children," *The Nation's Health* 7/6, 464–465, p. 464.
8 More about various adaptations can be found in the publication: Object of the Month: Bacilínek https://muzeum.nlk.cz/2021/01/predmet-mesice-leden-2021.
9 Robyn McCallum (2018) *Screen adaptation and the Politics of childhood,* Palgrave, p. 22.
10 Jindřich Veselý (1855–1939) was the patriarch of Czech puppet theater, who historically connected several generations of Eastern European puppeteers and remained an icon of the puppet theatre movement. He supported using puppet theatre in health propaganda, and remained to be one of the most referential people for Karel Driml. František Černý (1985) "Jindřich Veselý" *Československý loutkář* [Czechoslovak Puppeteer], Vol. 12. Stanislav Cífka, Cífka, (1986) *Jindřich Veselý, tvůrce moderního českého loutkářství* [Jindřich Veselý, Creator of Modern Czech Puppetry], České Budějovice: Jihočeské nakladatelství.
11 Karel Driml, Otroci i loutky Fond Veselý Jindřich undated document *LA PNP.*
12 Œuvres complètes de Béranger, H. Fournier, 1839, 2 (p. 320–321), the translation into English: William Young (1850) *Beranger: Two hundred of his lyrical poems,* New York: Georg P.Putnam, p. 249.

13 In the early 1950s, *Bacilínek* started to be criticized for its lack of a complex approach to the risk factors of diseases and for a simplistic, or even vulgar, misuse of the effects of puppet theatre: Vlasta Brychlová Potřebujeme loutkové hry [We call for puppet plays] *Lidové noviny* 20.08.1950, p. 7.

14 Rachel Kahn (2019) *Best Common Enemies: Disease Campaigns in America,* Oxford: Oxford University Press, p. 24.

15 A hint of foreign (French or English) origins, countries where barley sugar sweets were typical, and at the same time, the lollipop, sweet to sugary, unnatural.

16 Franz von Pocci (2010) Lustiges Komödienbüchlein [Funny little book of comedies], Vol. 5,. Edition Monacensia, Allitera Verlag.

17 Instead of the more common spelling "Kasperl," Pocci used "Casperl".

18 Franz von Pocci (2008) Lustiges Komödienbüchlein [Funny little book of comedies], Vol. 3, Edition Monacensia, Allitera Verlag.

19 The echo of these educated villains reverberates in crime and mystery fiction. Multiple villains in the stories about Sherlock Holmes, including Professor Moriarty or Stapleton, or in *Dr. Hannibal Lecter* by Thomas Harris, can obviously be seen as successors of Dr. Fleischmann.

20 Jan Bartoš, Jaroslav Hloušek and Karel Kobrle (1918) *Frant. hrabě Pocci, klasik loutkových her* [Franz von Pocci: The classic of puppet plays], Chocneň: Čeněk J. Mojžíš, p. 17.

21 Širola *Marionetsko kazalište* pp. 42–43.

22 Richard Rus (1924) Kašpárek ve službách pokroku: loutkářská příručka s Kašpárkovými besídkami pro sokolské a lidovýchovné malé i velké pracovníky [Kašpárek in the service of progress: a puppet guidance with Kašpárek's plays for small and big educators in Sokol and people's initiatives], Pardubici: Vzdělání lidů.

23 Christoph Gradmann (2014) Exoticism, Bacteriology and staging of the dangerous in Thomas Rütten and Martina King (eds.) *Contagionism and Contagious Diseases: Medicine and Literature 1880–1933,* Berlin, Boston: De Gruyter, p. 65, 69.

24 Ibid. p. 73.

25 Notably, the character of Koch was replaced by Driml in the 1929 edition prepared by Veselý, after the death of Driml.

26 Universal or metaphysical Darwinism or monism are based upon the idea of a common source of the origin of the animated world.

27 It is remarkable that in the latest socialist version, published in 1950, only the description of the nutrient medium for bacillus survived while the explanation of their "divine" origin disappeared.

28 Wilhelm Bölsche (1903) *Vom Bazillus zum Affenmenschen. Naturwissenschaftliche Plaudereien* [From the bacillus to the ape-man. Scientific conversations], Leipzig: Diederichs, p. 106.

29 King pp. 122–123.

30 King p. 125.

31 Jack Zipes (2012) *The Irresistible Fairy Tale: The Cultural and Social History of a Genre,* Princeton: Princeton University Press, p. 67.

7 Health films for children

Between cultural reciprocity and popular scientism

Western health animation for children in the service of social and biological awareness

"A germ becomes the film star 'Giro' to act the villain" was the slogan for promoting the first film in a series of adventures about gangs of germs and their leader Giro started in 1927:

> "Giro," a germ, is the latest screen star. He is the villain of the piece, and he will make his first appearance in a film to-day at King George's Hall, ... on behalf of the National Baby Week celebration ... the first scene is in a dustbin, and Giro who emerges from his lodgings there, hails a fly as a taxi, and visits the house of Mr. and Mrs. Grimy.[1]

One of the most popular animated interwar series in Great Britain narrates the adventures of Giro, not a germ of a particular infection but the personification of the collective image of a germ. Giro embodies multiple signs of "savage" behavior, such as "primitive" language, mostly non-verbal communication, and dancing "wild" dances, reminiscent of apes or even stereotypes of African people.

For creating the characters in the first film of the series, the rotoscope technique, tracing live-action footage into cartoon drawing, was used, not only adding realism, including the portrayal of germs,[2] but also providing all the predispositions to make Giro one of the spokes-characters in interwar animation and to introduce the mission of social advertising to health films for children. Bars of soap, brushes, baths and showers represented the main opponents of Giro, and British children were invited to play this enthralling game. The consistent interactive nature of the series was reinforced by multiple practices of retelling and revision. The authors of the films introduced visual matches between Giro and the most popular films and genres to reinforce the image of the villain. For instance, in the final film, *Giro Fast and Loose* (1935), there are visible motifs from contemporary gangster movies and from James Whale's Frankenstein (1931).[3]

DOI: 10.4324/9781003272267-10

Along with developing the image of germs as villains, the series *Giro the Germ* introduces multiple analogies between disobedience to hygienic rules and other forms of asocial or even criminal behavior. Pejorative names for these characters only emphasize these analogies. For instance, the family with which Giro stays in Episode 1 has the surname Grimy, and in Episode 2, the boy who does not wash himself regularly has the surname Grubby. In the final episode, the accomplice of Giro the Germ, Slacky the Sloucher, releases Giro from the "jail" of hygienic rules. Magical contagion remains the motor for narration in each of the episodes but in contrast to *Bacilínek*, or other films produced in Eastern Europe, not the physician or public health but soap, electricity and hot water help to defeat germs.

The genre's variability and the multiple development of the characters that maintained the audience's attention and formed memes of perception of hygiene rules can be connected with different motifs. Such motifs varied from the ultraliberal intention to replace professional healthcare with the self-discipline of ordinary people[4] to using *Giro* episode screenings during local epidemics of disease, such as scarlet fever.[5] *Giro* started to be included in various actions that addressed children and adults in different parts of the United Kingdom. Notably, in the events organized with the participation of the Red Cross, the *Giro* episodes achieved the status of the *Fly Pest* and were shown together with *Jinks*.[6] And the episode *Giro and His Enemies* (1935), in which the germ and his gang invade the town of Healthiville, can easily be seen as a reversion or even a parody of the *Fly Pest*, but with a substantive change at the end of the film – all-out victory over microbes by the Soap Army.

The biological awareness among the child audience shaped by the series was meant to be instrumental – the series explains the mechanisms of contamination but not the disease itself. Furthermore, the series systematically translated the idea of sharing responsibility among citizens for achieving hygienic standards to ensure a secure life. Each citizen could be either on the side of hygiene and progress or against it, together with the germs. Cleanliness was presented as a public good, and germs as public enemies. Another popular animation, the U.S. *Goodbye, Mr. Germ* (1940 by Edgar Ulmer), presents germs as public enemies too, but specifically with regard to another public good, the elimination of tuberculosis. The main protagonist of the film, the father of two young children and a professor of bacteriology, claims that "Tuberculosis, ancient misery, should disappear," and the entire film embeds the desirable skills and competencies regarding tuberculosis and its prevention in the history of the progressive struggle in the name of future generations: "When we will grow up, our children will not have tuberculosis," is the very last phrase said by the daughter to her mother.

In contrast to *Giro the germ*, which constructs the world of germs as mostly external and something that must be accepted as coexisting with humans forever, Ulmer puts the world of germs inside the human body and tells the story of their invasion of private, mostly family, life as the main threat of disease. His film maintains an emphatically individualistic view relevant to the target audience – middle-class children. From the very first moments, Ulmer takes the children – both the characters and the viewers – away from the outside world, led by a thunderstorm outside the window, to the armchair of a wise father, who is ready to share a new, entertaining and instructive story. The safety and calm of family life is the main motif used for persuading audiences of the necessity to become aligned with assessment and treatment aimed at eradicating tuberculosis, the disease that "destroys happy families." While the general message of Ulmer's film is similar to other health films about bacillus for children, "What is bad for people is good for germs and vice versa," *Goodbye, Mr. Germ* accompanies this message with a complex explanation aimed at significantly improving the biological awareness of children.

The film is constructed as a multiplicity of stories within one, central narration: The regular evening ritual of telling fairy tales to children. The son asks about the image of tuberculosis germs, and his father decides to tell the children the dramatic story of struggle against this horrible disease. He offers his children an imagination of what it would be like if germs could talk – "while they could breathe and move like we, humans." The professor in the story knows the language of germs like Dr. Dolittle knows the language of animals; the action of the film is then transferred to a fairy laboratory in the clinic of the protagonist of a series of children's novels, *The Story of Doctor Dolittle* (1920 –1948 by Hugh Lofting). This reference to the popular book and its 1928 film adaptation stresses the power of the professor as a mani-festation of medical progress; he can manage animals or the animated world. In his laboratory, the professor is surrounded by animals: A cat walks on his table, a monkey and rabbit are waiting for their favorite treat, and he com-municates with Mr. Germ as one of his pets or, rather, even a trophy taken from the lungs of one of the patients, in the same friendly manner. Meanwhile, the professor starts to observe Mr. Germ through a microscope, simultaneously making a call. At that very moment, Ulmer interrupts the atmosphere of security with a close-up of a skull on the table near the microscope, accompanied by disturbing music.

Making Mr. Germ a part of the animation emphasizes the difference between him as a dangerous pet, not similar, or only pretending to be similar, to other animals. Mr. Germ is depicted as a middle-aged man with a sedate gait, in a cylinder hat, with only his pointed ears protruding from the brim of the hat indicating that he is not entirely human. The more detailed and psychologically complex character of Mr. Germ, in contrast to the majority of previous visualizations of germs in health propaganda, including *Bacilínek* or *Giro the germ*, aims to underscore the role of personal struggle with the main psychological barriers to proper treatment against tuberculosis, namely, overconfidence and lack of attention to alarming symptoms. Multiple examples of such behavior are integrated into the film: A woman who is infected by tuberculosis does not limit her communication with her young nephew about whom she cares, and when he becomes a young adult, he eschews healthy habits and provokes the aggravation of his disease, transmitted from his aunt. Mr. Germ distinguishes himself by outstanding self-confidence: "I love to talk about myself," he says at the beginning of the film. But during a conversation with the professor, this confidence fades and at the very end, the headphones through which he communicates put him down, he dies and the headphones put his hat on his stomach – a final ironic touch to the picture of the miserableness of the bacillus. But what sends him to lockdown?

The dialogue between the professor and Mr. Germ is a history of struggle against tuberculosis that interconnects emotional metaphors of the disease and scientific explanations regarding its specifics through flashbacks. The film presents tuberculosis step-by-step from the contamination through describing the various reactions of organisms to the disease, followed by assessment and treatment. The moment of contamination is first presented as an act of irresponsible behavior by those who do not pay attention to the symptoms. But for Mr. Germ, it is the act of occupation of the lungs, which he describes through the slogan, "Lungland Lots and lots for sale." Dancing bacillus look much more organized than Giro's gang, as an army rather than a tribe or a family, as Mr. Germ describes them. The process through which the tubercle appears, a round capsule with germs inside, as a result of the attempts by the body to protect itself against the dissemination of bacillus, is described by Mr. Germ as "like imprisoning ordinary thieves." The professor "translates" the jargon of Mr. Germ into scientific language, adding to the image of the tubercle as a prison of bacillus an enlarged image from an anatomy textbook. In the same manner of exchanging scientific explanations provided by the professor and the simplistic notes by Dr. Germ, the film explores diagnostic procedures, tests and x-rays.

Along with providing sufficient scientific explanation, the film cultivates fear of the disease. A rare example in which the film focuses on the metaphoric description is the crisis in the development of the disease; the appearance of blood in a cough is presented as an act of sabotage by bacillus, who explode the blood vessels. Another emotionally powerful moment is featured when the professor shows the lung x-ray of a young girl who suffers from tuberculosis, and Mr. Germ starts brushing his beard smugly and smiles. The monkey near the professor immediately hides; this performance is dreadful for her. The tone with which Mr. Germ describes his victims reflects in the manner with which the Professor communicates with Mr. Germ: Polite in a formal way but full of attempts to insult and to demonstrate to Mr. Germ what a weak creature he has become. Along with presenting Mr. Germ as a sophisticated manipulator, the film stresses the multiple gaps in his competencies – he regularly repeats his questions and obviously does not fully understand scientific explanations. Because of the mission to cultivate fear of the disease and its sophisticated carriers, Ulmer opts for a consistent masculine narrative in which there is no place for active women – the young and pretty wife of the professor appears only at the end to offer her family tea and biscuits and to listen to a short report about the professor's story from her daughter.

Giro the Germ and *Goodbye, Mr. Germ* presents two extremes in addressing the task of shaping social and biological awareness through health films as "stories with a 'cleanliness' moral in an attractive way and tell the germ theory in a form which makes it sufficiently intelligible to young children."[7] A British cartoon series puts forward the idea of shared responsibility and presents hygienic skills as a part of responsible citizenship. The film by Ulmer, like some of the most successful U.S. health films for children released earlier, relies on individual superiority due to enhanced medical competencies. The different strategies employed in the two films relied on different cultures of childhood and expectations from children. Moreover, the films presented different, widely circulated strategies, and children in many countries experienced different approaches to conscious acceptance of hygienic rules as one of the foundations for behavior. The films made in Eastern Europe can be easily interpreted as an attempt to combine different strategies for shaping social and biological awareness and for furthering the mission to foster national identity.

Kašpárek kouzelníkem: Our children deserve more care than royalty!

Health propaganda for children in interwar Czechoslovakia was saturated with a motif concerning the creation of a new state and its salvation against enemies, including infectious diseases and their carriers. The imagined dispute between a flea and a louse about who is more important ends with the victory of the louse, who, unlike the flea, carries deadly diseases such as typhoid. But the whole story culminates in a moral message about hygienic rules as an indispensable part of statehood:

> Youth, you hear the truth:
> Soap, brush, warm water,
> Kerosene and washing soda
> They saved the Czech Empire.[8]

Children were seen as the royalty of this new empire. This view was easily adopted for producing two Czechoslovak health films for children made one year before celebrating the first decade of Czechoslovak statehood. This fact should be seen as decisive for interpreting the syntax and semantics of these two films. Along with *Kašpárek kouzelníkem* (Kašpárek the magician), aimed at propagating milk as the ground for healthy nutrition for children, and *Kašpárek a Budulínek* (Kašpárek and Budulínek), targeted at oral hygiene, the same team of filmmakers set out to bring the most popular fairy tales to film, *O popelce* (Cinderella) and *Perníková chalúpka* (Hansel and Gretel).[9] Like health fairy tales, these films fix particular behavior as desirable or not for growing children. One of the central motifs concerned the role of proper balanced nutrition as a prerequisite for healthy physical development.

Along with guidance for teachers featured in *Vyučování výživě a stravování školní mládeže* (Teaching nutrition and eating to school children, 1924),

Driml dedicated several puppet plays to the mission of instilling proper habits of healthy nutrition. *Zázračný encián* (Miraculous gentian) was written "for children who dawdle at meals and with their parents" in cooperation with Otakar Teyschl, a famous pediatrician. The aim of the play was "to shape the interdependence between healthy nutrition and outdoor activities." Máňa and Jenda (or Jeník) are children who are spoiled by their mother. It is only through the cooperation of their father and the doctor, who describes a magic remedy from a magic herb, which the children must collect on their own on the hillside, that the children have a chance to become reeducated. Echoes of the story about Hansel and Gretel capture the attention of a child audience. Instead of encountering a witch, these siblings meet two young, poor shepherd children, Ferda and Lojza, who reveal the doctor's plan to the hungry spoiled Máňa and Jenda. The mocking tone of the poor children, who do not suffer from a lack of appetite, but quite the opposite, does not prevent their desire to help Máňa and Jenda and to share with them a simple lunch made up of bread and milk. Notably, one of the sarcastic jokes includes naming the town where Máňa and Jenda live *Rozmazlená Lhota* (literally "spoiled" Lhota), in contrast to *Hloupa Lhota* ("stupid" Lhota) in *Bacilínek*. The artificial worries of the mother and her over-medicalized approach are diametrically opposed to the naturalness and authenticity of ordinary children, who represent the future of the new state, through acquiring new healthy habits. Máňa and Jenda emancipate themselves from the negative influence of the "backward" parents – namely, the mother. This general motif was reproduced in other plays and health films targeted at children.

In the film *Kašpárek kouzelníkem*, this motif is reinforced by dividing the narration into two parts: (1) a fairy tale in which the king and the whole royal court are treated with ordinary milk and remedied; and (2) a documentary part that presents the various actions aimed at supplying children with milk. The film had not survived but negatives and photographs provide a very plausible resemblance of the film plot with another play by Driml, *Princezna Bledule* (Pale Princess, 1925). The play tells the story of a struggle for influence upon one royal family through their eating habits. The cunning and nosy chef, Vařečkini, convinces the entire royal court to eat exclusively meat, which transforms all the butchers into rich people who share their capital with the chef. Only two people, the astrologist and Kašpárek, understand the probable health damage, but they realize that they cannot explain it directly to the people because of their obvious limits in understanding.

The skeptical and pessimistic view on fairy-tale nobility is reinforced through a scene featuring a medical examination of the princess by pseudo-doctors whose inconsistency is exposed by Kašpárek, who also pretends to be a doctor. The astrologist and Kašpárek enact a prediction that tells the princess to eat more fresh vegetables and to marry out of heartfelt inclination. At the end of the play, the audience learns that the chef is marrying a vegetable saleswoman who is about to become the richest woman because of the changed fashion in nutrition. In *Kašpárek kouzelníkem*, the astrologist plays an important role, and the chef represents one of the negative characters, according to his appeal in the photographs. The presence of a large retinue can be interpreted as a possible reproduction of the skeptical view on the limited abilities of people to develop proper biological awareness. Obviously, the child audience achieves these competencies through opposing their common sense to the limits of former ruling social groups. The film ends with a depiction of the collective activities of children, who purchase milk or directly drink this magic product at school.

It remains unknown whether the film reproduces the sad story of Kašpárek and his enforced unhealthy nutrition in childhood that Driml attributed to this most important narrator of health fairy tales in his very first *Zdravotnické táčky*. Undoubtedly, the majority of children who had watched *Kašpárek kouzelníkem* were familiar with this part of the fairy biography of their favorite character, stolen by a "Gypsy" circus, and forced to drink *kořálka* and to eat badly so as to remain lilliput, according to the idea of the circus chef. In his early plays (until the mid-1920s), Kašpárek often underscores his small size as a source of limits or even impairment. Generally, his early image balances between a disabled person and a "freak." While *Kašpárek kouzelníkem* exploits this tradition, the following health film for children significantly revises the image of Kašpárek.

Kašpárek a Budulínek: A health film to save future generations and national manufacturers

If parents can send their grown children into the world with healthy teeth, they can easily say that they have brought them 32 protectors and helpers. Healthy teeth are not only protection of the body against diseases but also helpers in the struggle for life and existence. Healthy teeth recommend a person better than an elegant business card. For a girl, a nice tooth actually means part of a dowry, because it gives her beauty. Even in shops, offices and factories where contact with customers is important, employees who make a pleasant impression tend to have priority. A person with defective teeth will find it difficult to compete.[10]

This passage from an interwar lecture by Driml, directed at parents, reproduces the main message of two American films, *Tommy Tucker's tooth* (1922) and *Clara cleans her teeth* (1927), commissioned by Kansas City dentist, Thomas B. McCrum, which garnered the attention of the Laugh-O-Gram studio, Disney.

Tommy Tucker's tooth starts out as a lecture for young children in kindergarten, about older children whose successful coming of age directly depends on the health of their teeth. Two boys, Tommy Tucker and Jimmie Jones, have totally different approaches to caring for their health. While Tommy cleans his teeth regularly and properly, Jimmie thinks that such behavior is only for girls. They get mutually opposed feedback from the side of the adult world. If Tommy is praised by doctors and gets his first job because he takes pride in himself and would do so in the job, Jimmy comes under fire from the side of male experts, namely, the physician and the potential employer, who says that the dentist is the best friend of young men. Being wise enough, Jimmie accepts the advice and finally gets the same good start as his peer Tommy.

The story of reeducating Jimmie is accompanied by multiple analogies aimed at explaining to children the reasons for toothaches and ways to prevent them. Disney effectively introduces elements of animation for demonstrating the decay of the tooth due to improper care. The caries bacteria, "acid demons," destroy the tooth. As the tooth decays, the number of "demons" increases until they stumble upon an alarm – a nerve that painfully signals the need to go to the dentist. Multiple analogies with everyday life, such as preserving meals in a cold, not warm, place, the necessity to darn the hole in a stocking until it is small. Analogies accompany direct instructions concerning the procedure for cleaning teeth. While the film only lasts ten minutes, it can be seen as comprehensive guidance that orchestrates the acquisition of biological awareness as a part of responsible coming of age aligned with the individualistic ideal of the U.S. middle class. The fact that film continued to be screened in the United States, Canada and Great Britain until the end of the 1940s provides evidence of its efficacy.

Another piece of evidence demonstrating the demand for such educational films includes the production five years later of *Clara cleans her teeth*. The film addresses girls and the main threat to them is the risk of being excluded from the company of their peers and even becoming a subject of bullying. Clara is a pretty girl who attracts the attention of boys. One day, on the playground, she is involved in the activities of her peers but when they have a snack break, they realize that Clara cannot eat biscuits without putting them in milk because her long improperly treated teeth hurt her. All the children, except one boy, stop playing with Clara, but when her parents offer her the opportunity to go to the dentist and resolve these issues, she rejects it. Late at night, she dreams and, in her nightmare, a toothbrush, a glass of water and toothpaste cannot persuade Clara to clean her teeth. Then her teeth abandon her. Clara wakes up in horror and tells her mother that she is ready to visit the dentist. After treatment, Clara is again accepted by her peers, especially the boy that she obviously likes. The film was purchased by the Dental Board of the United Kingdom, among nine other films aimed at improving oral hygiene among British children.[11] It was widely circulated throughout Europe, together with *Tommy Tucker's tooth*, until the end of the 1930s.

During his stay in the United States, Driml paid special attention to approaches for promoting dental hygiene for children and youth. He published *Zubní profilaxe ve Spojných státech amerických* [Dental prevention for the youth in the United States] as one of his outputs of his Rockefeller Fellowship. Healthy teeth had started to be seen as one of the main predispositions for proper development since the end of the nineteenth century and easily became a priority in health propaganda, due to the reverberation of political and commercial interests. If experts in many countries recognized oral hygiene as the main condition for proper nutrition, those who produced toothpaste and other dental hygiene items were interested in their mass consumption. Interwar Czechoslovakia was no exception.

The Austrian *Kalodont* and the German *Odol* were the leaders in sales of dental hygiene products in the Czech lands before 1918 and throughout the first years of independent Czechoslovakia. The toothpaste *Thymolin* started to be produced in 1899 by the *Spolek československých zoubních lékařů* (Union of Czechoslovak Stomatologists), The Union had ambitions to achieve a kind of monopoly, and the campaign for healthy teeth for future generations of Czechoslovaks represented a main strategy to realize this goal. "Not advertisement but propaganda should become our ally," shared Viktor Hájek, the commercial chief of *Thymolin*, in his memoirs about the interwar triumph of the Czech producer.[12] Driml was recruited by *Thymolin* as the designer of the advertising campaign, and since the mid-1920s, the Czech Junior Red Cross organized the annual Weeks for Healthy Teeth in direct cooperation with *Thymolin*. Children received kits with toothpaste and toothbrush free of charge and also participated in various activities. Multiple leaflets were disseminated among dentists, and guidance for parents, youth and physicians was published.

In many respects, this campaign reproduced the success of British policies aimed at improving the state of teeth among children and young people – including special performances. First, the puppet play *Budulínka bolí zoubek* (Budulínek has a toothache) appeared in amateur puppet theaters. Budulínek suffers from a toothache but does not want to be treated – because it is too uncomfortable. The very first replicas explain health issues by the fact that Budulínek is an only child and therefore very spoiled by his mother and grandmother. The women are accustomed to motivating the child to behave with candies, but the toothache is stronger, and Budulínek is demotivated. Additionally, he is afraid of doctors and dentists in particular. The dentist kills the tooth with arsenic and promises Budilínek a painless end to the treatment the following day.

In the night before his visit to the dentist, in his dream, Budulínek observes Zubovrt (literally "tooth hole-borer") and Kazizub (literally "spoiler of the tooth"), two bacteria, in the play a father and a son, in an attack against Zoubek. They aim to make a big black hole for the large family of bacteria in Budulínek's mouth. But their plans are not implemented because of Kašpárek, who rescues Budulínek with a sword, a toothbrush and a magic weapon, toothpaste. Shaking with fear, the bacteria flee, and the rescued tooth thanks Kašpárek for making him again a "panna" – a virgin.[13] In this way, the obvious motif of presenting a lack of hygienic skills as a lapse of virtue emerges. In the early morning, after awakening, Bodulínek not only immediately cleans his teeth but also rejects the candies offered by his mother – because he wants to keep his teeth "strong as oaks." This analogy situates him back in the world of men, in which not virginity but strength and resistance to diseases are valued.

In 1927, the play was adapted for film. *Kašpárek a Budulínek* significantly rewrote the story. Budulínek becomes older – while in the play, he is not older than six or seven years old, in the film we observe a younger teen who is not interested in candies but in good entertainment. Despite his toothache, Budulínek intends to attend a puppet performance, and his impression is so strong that he forgets about his toothache. But his father, a shoemaker, does not. Without his father's permission, but with the support of his mother. Budulínek attends the performance. This part of the film documents in detail the practice of traveling puppet theater: The performance takes place in an ale house in which one section is separated from the tables for adults. The film's viewers experience double pleasure by observing the performance, the story about the struggle of Kašpárek against two devils, as well as the emotional response in young viewers, mostly boys. Like in the plays aimed at forming proper healthy habits regarding nutrition, *Kašpárek a Budulínek* introduces children from "simple" social groups as the protagonists of progress. Full of emotions, Budulínek comes back and shares his impressions with two boys, apprentices of his father who are unable to attend the performance because they are banned from doing so by their master but who obviously share the affectation by Budulínek. Then Budulínek goes to sleep and observes one more time the same performance, but with his direct participation as a victim of the two devils, performed by young boys. Kašpárek presumably performed the role of one of the young actors playing the apprentices of Budulínek's father, who expels the devils from the boy's life (see Figures 7.1 and 7.2).

It is difficult to judge whether the film was accompanied by a medical explanation because the second part did not survive. It is reasonable to

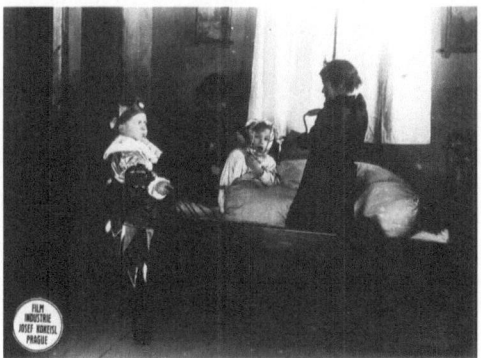

Figure 7.1 Magical contagion: the attack of bacteria in *Kašpárek a Budulínek* (1927).

Source: NFA, ©OOA-S, Prague 2021.

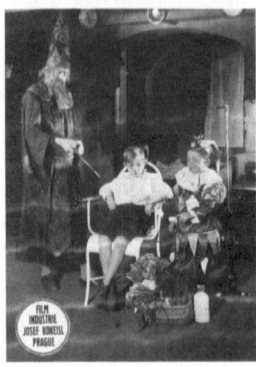

Figure 7.2 Magical contagion: the miracle of healthy nutrition in *Kašpárek a Budulínek (1927)*.

Source: NFA, ©OOA-S, Prague 2021.

assume that the play and the film addressed social awareness more than the medical competence and practical skills relevant to oral hygiene. Notably, in a review of the fairy tales by Kokeisl, in cooperation with Driml, *Kašpárek a Budulínek* was named an "educational fairy tale," *while Kašpárek kouzelníkem* was labeled as propagandist.[14] One year after releasing the film, Driml prepared a special lecture aimed at providing further biological awareness. *Milá mládeži!* (My dear youth!) was presented as a special edition in the celebration of the tenth anniversary of Czechoslovakia. Both the film and its accompanying lecture adapted many of the methodological techniques used in Disney films. In the lecture, the function of teeth was presented as a kind of manual labor, depicting teeth as an instrument. The lecture started with an image of a saw and the Czech proverb: "A saw with blunt and broken teeth does not cut."

The novelty of Driml's approach included an analogy between coming of age and an increased need for healthy teeth. In his lecture, he focuses on the replacement of primary teeth by permanent teeth as a process in which success directly depends on systematic and proper oral hygiene. Multiple analogies between the growth of teeth and the typical activities of boys, such as lining up to measure growth during physical education lessons or comparing teeth among the members of a scout team, or eating damaging foods, are compared to lifting weights regularly for muscle training. These analogies embedded the texts of the campaign within the idea of male maturation, a central motif in the play and the film.

The film could be seen as a coming-of-age story for several male characters: Budilínek, Kašpárek, and probably his father, whose character resembles Dratvička from *Bacilínek* – violent and obviously not an adherent of a healthy lifestyle at the beginning of the film. At the beginning of the play and the film, Budulínek's whim has a direct connotation with the behavior of a young girl: His father describes his behavior using the expression "natahoval moldánky" what means to sulk and be capricious, normally associated with female behavior. He then experiences collective activities, such as attending puppet theater, sharing his experience with peers and struggling together with them against devils. The transformation of Kašpárek in the peer of Budulínek is another significant sign that focuses on developing identity as a main mechanism for acquiring hygienic skills. While there is no information about the destiny of the film after 1945, the play continued to be performed even in the 1950s as a part of the regular activities of local public health boards.[15]

The campaign, including the film, achieved considerable success in advancing the *Thymolin* brand on the national market. In cooperation with the Junior Red Cross, the special packing of *Thymolin*, with images of Kašpárek and Budulínek, was produced for dissemination among children who were the members of the Junior Red Cross for 2.5 crowns instead of 4 crowns. Along with its national success, *Kašpárek a Budulínek* became a role model for Croatian filmmakers to propagate personal hygiene routines, which they did through a fairy tale about meeting water spirits who teach capricious children these rules but in a strict manner.

Campek nevaljalac: The indisputable values of personal cleanliness in controversial times of political pollution

Campek nevaljalac (The rascal Champek, 1929) tells the story of a boy who does not follow the request of his not pedagogically gifted parents to wash himself. Neither the father nor the mother are able to persuade him to wash his face and hands, or to clean his teeth. He defies not only his parents, but also even the lord of water, who requires the boy to observe personal hygiene. In fact, the wizard captures and imprisons the boy for not practicing personal hygiene. Instead of accepting his fate, the boy escapes with the help of cunning – while the wizard shows him how to wash, the boy abandons the dungeon. On the way home, he meets a younger version of the wizard – a boy wizard, who, despite the same demands to learn how to wash, is more friendly. The young wizard worries more about the unhappy parents who believe that they have lost their only son. But their happiness after finding the prodigal son does not last long at all – the father harshly punishes his son, and Campek escapes again, only to meet the lord of the water and become mortally ill after taking a sip of the lake's water. Only the young wizard is able to rescue the disobedient boy by asking the older wizard for help. The father begs for the same, and Campek is resuscitated from the dead. Only after this experience does the boy begin to wash himself with great enthusiasm.

The double meaning of definition *nevaljalac* in the film's title, both "dwarf-like" and naughty, exaggerates the motif of coming of age or becoming full-sized and obedient. As in the Czechoslovak films, not parents but peers are the protagonists of new healthy habits who help disobedient boys to accept the rules that regulate the behavior of responsible adults. Remarkably, *Campek nevaljalac* reproduces the same class and gender dimensions of family life as in *Kašpárek a Budulínek*: A middle-class family with a working father and a stay-at-home mother who has many opportunities to spoil her child. Another supplementary motif in both films is the fact that the main protagonist is an only child, which can easily be interpreted as one of the main reasons the child is so spoiled.

The film was screened in conjunction with a course on home and school hygiene organized by the Junior Red Cross in Yugoslavia, in operation since 1927. Along with a campaign aimed at teaching the rural population personal hygiene, including the rules for establishing toilets and systems of disinfection, this film, as a part of systematic health propaganda, bore the same message as a campaign among the rural population that relied on the slogan *Tko znade – i tko hoće može se sačuvati od griže!* (Those who know – and who want – can save themselves from worry!). It further reproduced analogies well-known from the cartoon series *Giro the germ*: The equalization of irresponsible people with the carriers of diseases, criminalizing fleas, and objectifying the target groups of propaganda.[16] The "pro-man" focus of health propaganda was a common trait for both campaigns among school youth and the rural population.

Men and boys remain the only protagonists, and the masculine component of the film is only reinforced by the fact that in a room in the house, there is a portrait of an obviously official person, very probably the tsar Alexander the First (see Figure 7.3). With the exception of the tsar's face on the portrait, viewers have no idea how the characters of the film look, because *Campek nevaljalac* was produced using the technique of a shadow play. This artistic decision shaped the feeling of benevolent paternalism from the side of authorities, as well as the idea of uniting all citizens around the figure of the

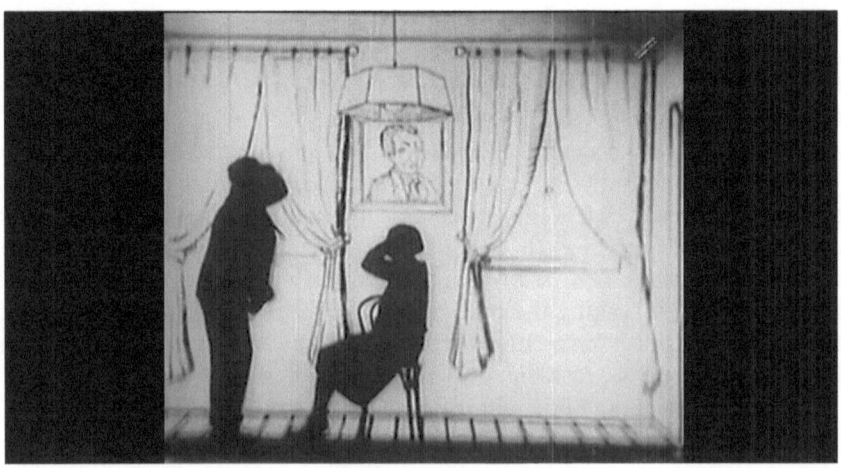

Figure 7.3 Benevolent paternalism vs parental helplessness in *Campek nevaljalac* (The rascal Champek, 1929).

Source: Kinoteka HAD.

tsar, and values such as obedience to hygienic rules. This approach could be seen as an attempt to avoid any personalization through ethnicity within a campaign aimed at rallying people together around the mission of public health, one of the strategies of the School of Public Health, under the pressure of centrifugal political processes surrounding Yugoslav statehood. The attempts by the School and its leaders, including Štampar, to connect Yugoslavism and the public good of promoting people's health, had seen negative consequences for the public acceptance of the School since the late 1920s.[17] If the nationalistic pathos of Czechoslovak health films for children required many details for translating the message "When you care about your health, you save your country," then the eight minutes of screen time, the laconic but expressive dynamics among the movements of all five characters (four men and the immovable portrait of a representative of the highest power of the tsar) was enough for *Campek nevaljalac* to broadcast the same message.

Notes

1 Westminster Gazette –Tuesday 05.07.1927, p. 7.
2 Jez Stewart (2021) The Story of British Animation London The British Film Institute 55–56.
3 Ibid.
4 Mr. Cash looks forward to workless doctors Derby *Daily Telegraph* - Wednesday 18.06.1930, p. 3.
5 *South Yorkshire Times and Mexborough & Swinton Times* – Friday 19.10.1934, p. 12.
6 *Rugby Advertiser* – Friday 15 November 1929 p. 4.
7 Muir, W. A. Green, George H. Buchan, G. F. (1938) *Health and cleanliness: a textbook for teachers,* London: Health and Cleanliness Council.
8 Karel Driml (1922) Zdravotnické táčky *Měsíčník dorostu Červeného kříže,* 5 13, p. 9.
9 Steffen Retzlaff (2017) Der tschechoslowakische Märchenspielfilm (1920–1989) in Ute Dettmar, Claudia Maria Pecher and Ron Schlesinger (eds) *Märchen im Medienwechsel: Zur Geschichte und Gegenwart des Märchenfilms,* Stuttgart: J.B. Metzler Verlag, pp. 229–250.
10 Viktor Hájek (1967) Jak jsem reklamu dělal [How I made advertisement] Part 2 6 *Propogace,* pp. 132–133.
11 *Belfast News-Letter* - Monday 29.02.1932.
12 Viktor Hájek (1967) Jak jsem reklamu dělal [How I made advertisement], Part 1 *Propogace* 5, pp. 105–107.
13 The motif of virginity is one of the most prevalent in the plays by Driml. For instance, in the play *Čarodějka Špindimůra* (literally witch named "dirty" and "nightmare"), there is obvious word play on the verge of the normative and the pejorative in the Czech language. The word *pindík* or *pinďour*, meaning penis, adds more "dirty" motives to the play, aimed at convincing children to clean their rooms. Kašpárek, who won over the witch *Špindimůra* with soap and hygienic rules, says that "his mission is to make Czech land tidy and beautiful as a virgin." Karel Driml (1927) *Čarodějka Špindimůra* Choceň: Loutkář p. 10.
14 Filmová industrie – Josef Kokeisl (1927) Zpravodaj Zemského Svazu kinematografů v Čechách,[Newsletter of the Union of filmmakers in Bohemia], 7, p. 10.

15 Takové jsou: Sestry z Okresního ústavu národního zdraví v Holešové [Such are: Nurses from the District Institute of Public Health in Holešov] (1956) *Zdravotnická pracovnice. Časopis pro střední a nižší zdravotnické pracovníky* [Journal for middle and lower level healthcare professionals], 6, p. 20.
16 The draft of the leaflet Škola narodnog zdravija u Zagrebu NDH 1940 3/517.
17 Željko Dugac (2005) Protiv bolesti i neznanja: Rockefellerova nadacija v međuratnoj Yugoslaviji [Against disease and ignorance: The Rochofeller Foundation in interwar Yugoslavia], Zagreb: Srednja Europa, pp. 134–135.

Part 3

Men and women in the focus of health films

8   Health films as *Bildungsroman* for teaching men

The options and limits of health films for men in the late 1910s

In autumn 1920, the Czechoslovak Ministry of Defense organized a massive public campaign among military men in Eastern Slovakia, aimed at preventing the dissemination of venereal diseases. The campaign employed a wide range of strategies to inform the men about diseases and to motivate them to seek medical attention at the first sign of illness. This campaign featured lectures and health film screenings, including the American *The End of the Road* (1919), the French *On doit le dire* (It must be said, 1918) and the German *Es werde Licht* (It will be light, 1917). The campaign was supported by local branches of the Sokol movement, in making its argument in favor of an immediate call for help in case of infection more persuasive through adding the rhetoric of prostitution as an enemy of the nation. The films and lectures were presented for most of soldiers and officers in "the most polluted places," such as Prešov, Košice and Turčiansky Martin.[1] According to the reports of regimental physicians, the output was not impressive; even after finishing the campaign, they continued to register more than 1,000 new cases of sexually transmitted diseases among military men every month until the end of 1921. The main reason for this incidence was the rupture between the aims of the propaganda and the limited access to medical treatment, especially a lack of physicians and hospital beds. But clearly, the instructions and motivations translated by the films made during the Great War were insufficient for the post-war audience.

In *The End of the road*, *On doit le dire* and *Es werde Licht*, the audience could easily recognize the very strong motif of male immaturity as one of the central reasons for becoming infected and transmitting venereal diseases to the innocent – wives and children. In these and other films produced in the late 1910s and targeted with disseminating information about venereal diseases, the focus on men can be only partially explained by the main target audience of these films, military men of different countries who faced the same issue – the risk of infection through the unsafe sexual intercourse.[2] *Bildungsroman* for men as a genre of health propaganda had been introduced by the campaigns aimed at preventing venereal diseases in the last third of the nineteenth century in different Western countries.[3] Coming of age ideally

DOI: 10.4324/9781003272267-12

dovetailed with the task of combining moral lessons and clinical instruction, one of the main predispositions for effective health propaganda.[4] The new experience of being infected, treated for disease and healed should be seen from two interrelated positions, new emotions and new knowledge, which would make men more responsible, more farsighted and more thoughtful, or, in short, more mature. Along with the changing role of fiction films, as a more important medium for disseminating information,[5] World War I reinforced the *Bildungsroman* as one of the most suitable genres for these purposes.

The films were a part of the campaigns that employed persuasion rather than punishment as a more promising strategy to prevent venereal diseases.[6] Film producers were inclined to mix the frames of single-focus or dual-focus narratives for achieving the best possible result in motivating men toward disease prevention. On the one hand, a tale about two men with identical social profiles, who develop in mutually opposite ways – healthy and responsible vs. unhealthy and irresponsible – in response to the same situation of being infected, can be easily interpreted as the characteristic opposition between the orderly forces of civilized life and those who would challenge order and civilization.[7] In the French *On doit le dire*, the role of civilized and progressive behavior was attributed to Matthieu, a French soldier, while Mattéo, an Italian soldier, destroyed himself and his family by ignoring the signs of syphilis. A responsible physician and a childish artist were the main protagonists of *Es werde Licht*. And in the American film, the cockered Pauk Horton and the selfless Doctor Bell present the most extreme opposition of irresponsible patient vs. good physician, who struggle to court the same young woman.

Typical of dual-focus narratives, "the textual progression depends on an omniscient and omnipotent narrator,"[8] in this case, performed by the figure of the physician, whose comments help the audience to recognize fateful decisions as right or wrong. For instance, the opening scene of *On doit le dire* is a public lecture about syphilis, given by a prominent physician, and in *The End of the Road*, the physician is the demiurge whose acts regulate the behavior of others against the chaos introduced into the lives of the characters by the disease. The image of the physician as a quasi-parental figure, who takes on the role of mentor and senior friend for the young man "in trouble," remained the most memorable legacy of this cohort of films within the next generations of health films addressing the prevention of venereal diseases in the interwar period.

On the other hand, the main characters are presented as choosing one way or another to behave after being infected, typical of the single-focus narrative and its particular emphasis on independence and emancipation.[9] Since the middle of the 1910s, the rationalization of the response to the risk of venereal diseases started to be promoted as exemplary and mature behavior for men, instead of feeling guilty and sinful.[10] Through accepting or rejecting treatment, the protagonists either usurped control or permitted the disease to usurp control over their lives. The films showed young adult men, which reverberated with the trend to limit the role of parents in sex education for their children, an idea that began to compete with the more traditional opposition of responsible and irresponsible parents in the very first films against sexually transmitted diseases.[11] But coming of age, one of the central motifs connected with the single-focus narrative, is presented in these films exceptionally as a form of success in practicing self-control, through following the rules aligned with the moral obligation to be healthy, reinforced by war rhetoric. Fear and shame,[12] emotions that should be overcome by the pro-tagonists of war films, did not offer a sufficient range of feelings for achieving psychological plausibility in depicting men's coming of age after the war.

The oversimplicity of feelings reverberated with the univocality of moral prescriptions. The expectations from the men who were at risk of being infected were formulated in terms of binary oppositions: Instead of "pseudo-medicine" (either self-treatment with "folk" drugs or visiting unreliable physicians) "real" mature men should be treated by proper physicians affiliated with the public health system that would prescribe proper medicine; not to postpone treatment but to obediently follow the results of a medical examination; and, finally, to be responsible for not spreading disease to other, innocent, people such as spouses or children. The univocal opposition of mature to childish behavior linked self-responsibility with obedience to a certain order. This approach, stemming from the call for preventing military men in the situation of war, was not aligned with interwar social and political trends.

Along with uncontrolled prostitution in the aftermath of World War I, the interwar struggle against venereal diseases faced new challenges due to the massive restructuring of gender relations, which mostly connected venereal diseases with issues such as infant mortality and birth rates. Prioritizing demographic policy as the main realm within which the majority of health issues started to be interpreted redefined the reliance on men's health as one of the main preconditions for achieving the purposes of this policy.[13] If in war-period films, the physician, usually a regimental officer, was a central figure in surviving and ensuring coming of age, interwar health propaganda and films in particular, began to reflect the intensive institutionalization of public health and relevant fields, including health and life insurance, which replaced the character of the physician in providing a feeling of sustainability and hope.[14] The multiple internal contradictions in approaches to gender compelled interwar filmmakers to revise the genre of the health *Bildungsroman* in favor of reconstructing the complex relationship between community and public health institutions as the main context for the successful struggle against venereal diseases and men's coming of age.

The interwar social order reflected the juxtaposition of the pre-war hier-archical division of gender roles and the multiple challenges to women's access to political rights articulated by the war.[15] But not only the struggle for political rights delineated the gender-based inequality of the time. The unambiguous division into "valuable" and "non-valuable" women gave way to mutually competing interpretations of the diversity of female identities. The task to combine the roles of the "modern woman," who wants to live her own life, and the "mother," who gives life,[16] introduced new challenges as much for women as for those who reflected these trends in cultural, political and social life. Furthermore, the growth of public critical reflections reinforced the activities of those who continued to promote an intolerant attitude toward prostitution. Within the realm of public health, women continued to be seen as a problem more than a solution, which explained the tendency to attribute blame to Romani, Jewish and Hungarian women for venereal disease, and in Bulgaria or Yugoslavia –to Jewish, Romani and Turkish women.

In Eastern Europe, the struggle against venereal disease manifested in boundary work between "civilized" and "non-civilized" people, ethnic groups and even countries. In 1922, Doctor Meška, the chief physician in Košice, resented the apparently offensive comparison of Slovak seasonal workers to African migrants, typical of the French press, which had accused migrants as the main carriers of syphilis.[17] Meška underscored the role of medical examinations, established by Czechoslovak authorities as an effective measure aimed at preventing the risk of disease transmission by Czechoslovak migrants and turned the discussion in the opposite direction, toward the number of those infected during their stay in France or Germany. Along with understanding the impossibility of stopping migration, Meška relied on education and international efforts to inform people about venereal diseases and how to avoid the risk of transmission. While such measures were not introduced with regard to Western Europe, a control point on the border between Czechoslovakia and Hungary was established, since the flow of infected people emanated from there.[18] Moreover, experts stressed the lack of beds in hospitals especially for women who were not prior patients,[19] which damaged the international image of Czechoslovakia. The systematic emphasis on Europeanness in public discourses regarding venereal diseases could thus be seen as a defense against such a derogatory view.

A three-page instruction booklet on venereal disease for school graduates in Bohemia informed students about endemic syphilis as a disease transmitted not through sexual intercourse but due to insufficient hygienic conditions such as the common use of the same dish and "typical of not-cultural people (Balkan peninsula, Russia) while in the Czech lands remained a rarity."[20] The highly intolerant critics of the ban on brothels introduced by Czechoslovak authorities with the *Zákon o potírání pohlavních nemocí* (Law on Combating Sexual Diseases 1922) embraced a multilevel racialized view on prostitution and women of the periphery in particular:

> The removal of brothels and, therefore, the previously operating official controls carried out earlier that regularly removed at least the most virulent forms of sexually transmitted diseases, as well as the introduction of "Western" methods of treating sexually transmitted diseases, are useless with regard to the low cultural level of certain layers of the population, which differ in their truly oriental indifference to health. Sexually

transmitted diseases caused by soldiers after the war, together with the physical and mental filthiness of Gypsies, from whom secret prostitutes are mostly recruited, only aggravated the current and quite desolate state of the rural population ... There is no promises of any tendency towards regression.[21]

Notably, in practice, numerous medical examinations of Romani women did not confirm these fears and prejudices. For instance, according to the reports of local physicians, among fourteen detainees, "twelve gypsies and two workers," only one was infected; the rest were healthy.[22] Another district reported that among 28 cases of mostly "Gypsy" women and waitresses, only three cases were positive but "among military men many more cases were indicated, and officers should be seen as the main carriers of disease."[23] Another issue was the fissure between the enforcement of the measures introduced by law and the multiple organizational gaps that prevented the application of such measures in cases of actual infection. For instance, local authorities complained that a "Gypsy woman who was detained and who was diagnosed with a dangerous venereal disease was sent to the local hospital but, because of the lack of a bed, was released."[24]

Along with criminalizing prostitution, the public discourses of interwar Europe and North America started to highlight the satisfaction of sexual needs as a manifestation of healthy behavior.[25] Harmonious sexual relationships began to be promoted by health films. Marital life represented the most secure form of providing this basic need, predominantly for men. In interwar Eastern Europe, not being treated in the case of sexually transmitted infection was presented as a crime against one's own people, family and conscience: "[T]o bring, knowingly or unknowingly, illness into the family is not only condemnable from the point of view of hygiene and morality but should be considered a crime."[26] Public campaigns mainly addressed men, who were warned about the need for timely treatment before marriage. In 1935, the weekly Bulgarian newspaper, *Narod i prosveta* (People and education), launched a public campaign aimed at disseminating information about venereal diseases, especially syphilis. One of the first articles explained in detail the disastrous consequences of untreated syphilis, especially for men's health. Male infertility, sexual neurasthenia and chronic prostatitis are just some of the items on the list of the consequences mentioned in the article.

Interwar politics concerning venereal disease extended the responsibility of physicians to the proper sex education of future generations. In contrast to the first cohort of health films against venereal diseases, these films minimized the role of parents in educating their children about sex and its shadowy sides, including risky sexual intercourse. If *The End of the Road* depicted the opposing approaches of the mothers of the two main female protagonists to sex education, later, this function started to be attributed to public health institutions. The interwar discursive practices around sex education and venereal diseases not only complicated the division of women into "valuable" and "dangerous" but also questioned the boundaries between public and private life in combating venereal disease, reinforcing the class-based differences in health propaganda. The question, "Should middle and upper classes have more rights to privacy within the campaigns against venereal diseases than workers?" reverberated with the question "Who in terms of class and social status should be the protagonists of health propaganda and health films in particular?"

In his play, *Reigen: Komödie in zehn Dialogen* (The circle: A comedy in ten dialogues, 1897), Austrian physician and writer Arthur Schnitzler univocally blamed the upper classes for irresponsible and corruptive practices that hampered the efficient prevention of sexually transmitted diseases. While during the war, the pro-socialist and class-based view was relegated to the margins of discursive practices, after the war, connecting the issues of prostitution, venereal disease and multiple forms of inequality came to be in demand more and more. Schnitzler not only introduced the theme of class-based explanations for prostitution and the limits in controlling venereal diseases,[27] but also systematically deconstructed the dual-focus narrative typical of health propaganda. In his play, the idea of achieving equilibrium was turned inside out – venereal diseases were disseminated in a circle, from one pair of occasional lovers to another, a motif conditioned by the constant reproduction of class distinction. This multilevel negation of pro-state and pro-hierarchical health propaganda ensured the long life of Schnitzler's play, adapted more than twenty times and which continues to be performed nowadays.

The play was clearly a cultural context used by Jenő Janovics, a famous Hungarian theater and film director who produced *Világrém* (Menace, 1920), one of the first postwar attempts to promote new discursive practices concerning venereal diseases. Janovics tells the story of a stellar theatrical couple, in which the husband of a famous opera singer cheats on his wife with another actress and contracts syphilis from her.[28] Instead of seeking treatment, he tries to keep his illness a secret, endangering the lives of his wife and children. The husband's best friend and part-time physician saves the family: He offers the latest treatment for syphilis and conducts a kind of shock therapy in its focus, subjecting the unfaithful spouse to all sorts of irreversible consequences of syphilis, inviting his unlucky friend to his clinic.

Janovics built the narration around opposing the figures of the physician and the actress (who is secretly a prostitute) as symbols of good and evil in the life of protagonists. For these purposes, the film director effectively used the nightmares of the main protagonists for revealing to viewers the true emotions and affects in the process of making a "proper" or "improper" moral choice. These scenes were directly connected with various operas, which only reinforced the expressive manner of narration.

Along with multiple novelties in artistic devices, the promotion of *Világrém* can be seen as a know-how of health propaganda: The famous physician and successful researcher with an international reputation, Constantin Levaditi, who offered treatment for syphilis with bismuth, prepared a lecture that preceded the movie. The film gained international acceptance and was shown in Paris in 1921.[29] *Világrém* can this be seen as a transition between the earliest cohort of films aimed at struggling against venereal diseases and the interwar films that were relevant to the new context.[30]

After World War I, the task of producing new films adapted to the needs and contexts of civilian life elevated the subject-object dichotomy of health films. The questions important for the genre coherence, such as "To what degree are the characters free in their actions, and who establishes the limits?" mirrored in such practicalities: "What does timely treatment entail?"; "How to involve innocent victims in treatment?"; "What violations of privacy are acceptable in the case of sexually transmitted and other diseases?"; and many other issues that called for new strategies aimed at motivating people to be treated not only in the case of infection but also to engage in preventive measures such as pre-marital counseling and medical examination.

Multi-focus narration in *Il était une fois trois amis* and *Damaged lives*

In her classification of interwar health films against venereal diseases, Anita Gertiser classifies *Falsche Scham* (False shame 1925/1926 by Rudolf Bierbach), *Il était une fois trois amis* (Once upon a time there were three friends, 1927 by Jean Benoît-Lévy and Marie Epstein), and *Damaged lives* (1933 by Edgar Ulmer) under the same subcategory, as focusing on the psychology of the characters and their sufferings.[31] Interpreting these films from the point of view of *Bildungsroman* for men, and the development of this genre within health film production, leads to the assumption that the latter two films deliberately challenge the main moral messages of *Falsche Scham*.

Falsche Scham works on transforming the previous generation of films created to combat venereal diseases, extending the audience to include young men and boys. However, the main set of genre devices used for achieving this purpose very much resembles the previous generation of health *Bildungsroman* for men: The formula includes rationalizing the situation and understanding emotions for better self-control. Five different situations are connected through the figure of the physician, who offers very different advice for each situation and presents a variety of options to gain timely information, including visiting hygiene exhibitions and viewing health films. Shame is seen as an obstacle to the intention to receive proper treatment, a sentiment that should be eradi-cated. For Benoît-Lévy and Epstein, as well as for Ulmer, shame is not a matter of eliminating or oppressing a focus on the social origins of shame in the face of venereal diseases and its impact on the destiny of men and their families. The culmination of both films includes impressive scenes of catharsis that transform shame into the energy to overcome disease.

In contrast to previous cohorts of health *Bildungsroman*, both films question the necessity of becoming an adult – at the beginning of the films, viewers observe the pure, unadulterated joy of life. The three friends and their fiancées spend their time dancing, eating delicious food, drinking good champagne and loving each other. Mary Louise Roberts explains this "frenzied hedonism" of the postwar years in France as a kind of emotional response to "a sudden and dramatic metamorphosis" of post-war social life.[32] According to Vignaux, *Il était une fois trois amis* develops the idea that only those humans or nations who do not have a history remain entirely happy – but people (and nations) are destined to become adults.[33] This paradox works for *Damaged lives* too.

In *Damaged lives*, Donald and Joan are born with a silver spoon in their mouth: They are rich and, moreover, not spoiled by an upper-middle-class mode of life. Ulmer consistently shapes the image of Donald as a playful, emotionally open young man, friendly with people of different social classes. Joan is not only pretty but also open hearted and spontaneous. Donald's charisma stems from his *joie de vivre* and his relationship with Joan is one of the most important sites for experiencing this joy. Like the lives of the three French friends in *Il était une fois trois amis*, their happiness is suddenly ended by pregnancy and the revelation of the fact that they are infected with venereal disease. This spousal crisis is resolved in a very dramatic way – Joan tries to kill herself and then Donald, but he prevents her from doing so. Ulmer introduces different visual analogies for demonstrating the discomfort of growing up and accepting responsibility in the last part of the film, when both have learned that they are infected. Visually, Donald and Joan are either "compressed" by their circumstances – for example, in a cramped car or sitting on the floor with their backs against a narrow sofa, or they appear ready to lose their balance and fall due to shock. Asking "How to take responsibility but not to lose playfulness and spontaneity?" *Damaged lives* redefines the idea of maturity and challenges many of the cliches concerning coming of age used in earlier health films. Notably, both films actively use the metaphor of managing one's own life through comparing it with driving a car – in the first part of *Il était une fois trois amis*, Georges and Charles go to Jacques's farm and have a lot of fun by teaching their fiancées how to drive. Then Charles is informed about the complications on the birth of his child while he is repairing the car. In *Damaged lives*, Joan drives a car to get married and Bill, the friend of Donald and Joan, takes them totally destroyed back to the car after they learn that they have syphilis.

A not entirely positive view on coming of age permeates the films to produce a much more sophisticated morality regarding the differing abilities of people to cope with the challenges of coming of age, including such experiences as having a venereal disease. If the morality of previous films stemmed from imbuing the identity of viewers with a positive character that could be easily interpreted as symbolic violence, the moral messages of *Il était une fois trois amis* and *Damaged lives* are open to audience interpretation. According to Altman, recognizing a transformed version of a familiar situation[34] in unfamiliar material opens new options for following and mapping the narration, and these films offer neither dual-focus or single-focus narratives nor a mixture of both; instead, there is a multi-focus narrative about becoming an adult that requires more interpretative energy from audiences, "more efforts and more courage to go out of the frontiers of more comfortable narrative strategies."[35]

Both films depart from the tradition of opposing two characters in dual-focus narration and from the focus on the fate of one protagonist in single-focus narration. The French film tells the story of three friends and their relationship, and the American film focuses on a couple and their relationship with their immediate environment. The characters of three different men, the driver Charles, the bank officer Georges and the farmer Jacques, do not satisfy the need for personal identification with one of the film's exemplary characters typical of a single-focus narrative.[36] Instead their friendship is the engine of the storytelling, coping with illness and saving their community. Georges, a bank clerk, demonstrates the most rational behavior among the three friends and makes a decision concerning pre-marital examination and seeking treatment for syphilis, but he remains on the margins of the narration and does not provoke an emotional tie with his story from the side of the audience.

Like Georges, Jacques has been infected through occasional sexual intercourse and steadfastly refuses to accept this fact as the main cause of the death of his newborn children. In opposition of the approaches by Georges and Jacques toward treatment, it is easy to recognize the vicissitudes of destiny of Matthieu and Mattéo from *On doit le dire*. Instead of blaming Jacques, *Il était une fois trois amis* introduces viewers to a dramatic scene depicting the birth and death of Jacques's son, full of emotion, including the catharsis of Jacques, which eliminates any options to blame him as a non-innocent man. Moreover, when the physician offers Jacques treatment, without informing his wife about the infidelity, Jacques refuses and explains his readiness to share the information with her by referring to their mutual love and trust.

Like earlier films, *Il était une fois trois amis* traces "the moral careers" of characters "who are corrupted by temptation and face the consequences of their dubious decisions,"[37] but finally the film leaves the viewer with the idea that it is never too late to start treatment. Despite the motto of the film, "There are no shameful diseases; there are shameful patients," the motif of "become stigmatized only to suffer shame and a damaged reputation" is replaced by empathy for the characters and the shared joy of their success in treating the disease. Benoît-Lévy and Epstein invite viewers to become virtual members of this imagined community by following the destinies of the main protagonists. The fact that the film's casting was familiar to the audiences of the health films by Benoît-Lévy and Epstein, who had already recruited the actors in previous films, only reinforced this interactive effect.[38]

Damaged lives avoids any binary oppositions between characters, even in the case of Joan, the respectable wife and Elise, the society girl who has infected Donald; they are opposed not due to morality but to social status. Moreover, Ulmer blurs the line between righteous and non-righteous women, attributing to Elise and Joan a similarity in emotional responses to the information about their illness, including suicide attempts. Ulmer focuses primarily on the vulnerability of girls like Elise, and instead of presenting her as the enemy of happy family life, the film's director translates a very strong message about how unlucky it is to be poor but pretty. Elise seduces Donald not because of money, lust, or ambition but because of loneliness and the need for emotional acceptance. She is doomed to be manipulated by those men "who cannot maintain sufficient control over their primal urges"[39] and that does not make her happier or wealthier.

Her shame and inability to say directly that she has been infected only reinforces this feeling of vulnerability. Donald, who was unable to stop Elise, survives along with his wife, which gives them hope. In contrast to the pre-determined unhappy fate of Elise, Donald and Joan have their chance at happiness. Donald, who makes all the possible mistakes known from early films, including being treated by a charlatan, refusing to accept the truth about the disease and infecting his own wife, nevertheless receives a chance at recovery, gaining dignity and preserving love. The absence of a clear division of the characters into those worthy of public approval or deserving of censure reverberates with the central role of medical institutions and the community as decisive for coping with the disease.

Il était une fois trois amis and *Damaged lives* attach the story of combating syphilis to a particular social group, the petty bourgeoisie in the periphery and the upper-middle class in the city, respectively, in order to achieve the most representative group for the films' mass audiences. This choice is determined by the intention of the film directors to address not only potential victims of disease but also the broader society because the "moral crux ... is fearing ostracism and stigmatization people could fail to pursue proper treatment."[40] While the French film insistently promotes the positive role of a small community made up of three families in a provincial town, the American film puts forward the emancipation of an infected spousal pair from the pressure of friends and relatives as decisive for overcoming the internal barriers to coping with the disease. Both films reference the threats of large cities but do not emphasize the opposition of city vs. nature or city vs. small town as central for telling the story.[41] At the moment of leaving the hospital, Joan envisages, one by one, each of her relatives and friends who will be horrified by what happened, and, in reality, it becomes more painful – when Laura, her best friend and the wife of Billi, Donald's best friend, forbids Joan to touch their little son, whom Joan loves. She recovers from this emotional pressure at the moment she staves off the suicide attempt of suicide, when she must answer the call of her pregnant friend, Marie, who asks for Joan's help because she has eaten too many pickles, which she believes could damage her unborn baby. In comparison with the risks that Joan has experienced, these ridiculous worries make Joan and Donald laugh, which reflects their ability to emancipate themselves from the ridiculous reactions of their community.

The characters' emotions, mostly despair and hope, set the rhythm of the narrative in both films. Benoît-Lévy and Epstein connect emotions with temporality – the film is built around multiple flashbacks that not only depict memories of the protagonists but also bring a repressed past with its unresolved problems to the present. These two timelines, "an anachronistic time of the past, normative because it seeks to regulate through treating the disease, and the present time where the reality of a continuously changing community is embodied,"[42] questions the ability of men to manage their lives and health without the assistance of institutions and community. The film alternates a transformation from hope to despair and back again, along with the moves of the protagonists to and from the farm of Jacques's parents, which symbolizes security and sustainability, as well as the fragility of its power in the face of the threat of disease.

The growth of uncertainty and despair is expressed in Ulmer's film through the successive "collapse" of the space surrounding the main characters. If at the beginning of the film, Donald and Joan move around the city and even from city to city, by the time of their diagnosis, their space is portrayed by a piece of the floor near the sofa in the living room, on which they find themselves after preventing a suicide attempt. Ulmer makes full use of the music to highlight the catharsis of the main characters – which accompanies only the scene of the suicide attempt, and which sets the viewer up for a happy outcome to this dramatic situation.

Both films delineate the internally contradicted interconnection between public and private spaces concerning disease and its treatment. Public health institutions help but they also intervene with private life and inevitably damage it. The opposition of public to private rearranges the gender-based inequality – while public space belongs to men and is managed by physicians, private space tends to be associated with wives and mothers. The protection of privacy is one of the central values of both films, even though they apply completely different strategies for promoting it. In *Il était une fois trois amis*, the audience is allowed to observe the public space and the community space, but the private, family life of the characters remains behind the scenes. Family life is shown just twice in short-time sequences with close-ups of the parental families of the heroes: Charles's parents, destroyed by the disease of the father, and Jacques's mother, who places a baby's cap back into the dresser with tears in her eyes after the death of another newborn. The audience does not observe the spousal life of the main heroes – the viewers must rely on the words of three friends, normally full of emotions when they share the details of their family life with each other. *Damaged Lives* puts married life under the loupe – fixing viewers' sympathies for both young people, introducing some elements of comedy to reduce the drama, and emphasizing the impact of disease on destroying the mutual trust created solely in intimacy.

The instructive parts of both films reverberate with the predominance of recognition and empathy, which should stimulate reflection and doubt. The French film focuses on the physiological response of an organism to contamination and the destructive power of disease, along with a treatment made up of a mixture of three different substances – palladium, arsenic and mercury. *Il était une fois trois amis* depicts the process as a part of a lecture for medical students and includes elements of animation that show the infection as an invasion by treponemas while the treatment is portrayed as purification from the infection and its carriers. This lecture is followed by a long dialogue between the physician and Charles, which connects abstract knowledge with a typical case of the disease.

Charles suffers from hereditary syphilis and, until the moment his child is born, he does not know about this fact. Charles learns firsthand how early intervention into hereditary syphilis is organized from the female patients he observes in the counseling center where the physician has taken him. Charles enters the waiting room, full of mothers with babies, and with suspicion asks the accompanying physician if these children are ill. The reply comes from one of the mothers, who shares that she had noticed the "bad blood" of the child in time and turned to the right place. Later in the film, this experience plays a decisive role in the remedial process of Jacques, with whom Charles shares his positive experience. In *Damaged lives*, the instructive part is relatively short and includes several cases of being infected and not treated in a timely manner. Doctor Leonard, a friend of Donald's father, focuses his efforts on helping Donald accept responsibility through the realization of all the possible risks, but not to lose faith in the greatness of life. This very personal approach reverberates with the informal support from the side of the multiple patients who help Donald when Joan faints.

The performances in both films aimed to involve women, even though censorship and public opinion were not totally aligned with this intention. *Damaged lives* was banned in New York for four years after its release,[43] and the Canadian audience was segregated by gender: Women and men attended the film showing on alternate days. *Damaged lives* was supplemented by 29-minute reels, each different for men and women, in which Dr. Gordon Bates, General Director of the Canadian Social Hygiene Council and clinical supervisor for the film, appeared and gave a lecture accompanied by images of the more horrendous effects of venereal diseases.[44] The affectation of the European public by *Damaged lives* did not exclude some tensions with censorship issues, even in Great Britain and France: "[S]o subtly and cleverly has this objective been achieved ... the entertainment value of the picture allowed to suffer, impart a telling sympathy into lesser roles."[45] *Il était une fois trois amis* was criticized for lacking Christian morality. The film had to receive special permission for being shown to young women.[46]

Along with transforming the role of women and introducing multi-focus narration, *Il était une fois trois amis* and *Damaged lives* illuminated the gender-based imbalance in politics and practices against venereal diseases formed during the period of the Great War. Vignaux has stressed the impossibility of solving the contradictions and further has highlighted the Manichaeism in the position of women in health films, to whom exceptionally conservative ideals were attributed.[47] The strictly defined limits of women's activities regarding their own health gained unprecedented importance in the health propaganda of interwar Eastern Europe. The Czech health film *Osudná chvíle* (Fortuitous moment, 1935) resolved these contradictions by narrating the story of the story of Ladislav Dvořák, a decent man, but en-tangled in his own fears, and his selfless fiancée Marta, as a male-female double *Bildungsroman*. Also, only Ladislav gained knowledge about the threats of venereal disease – while Marta has come of age through experi-encing devotion, patience and forgiveness.

Osudná chvíle as a health *Bildungsroman* for men

Eric Schaefer underscores the role of the titles of the films targeted with venereal diseases as having "succinctly summed up their lessons about damaged goods and lives, reflected bourgeois ideology, as well as capitalist demands for a productive citizenry,"[48] but the title of the first health film that included sound produced in Czechoslovakia, *Osudná chvíle*, focused the attention of the audience on the question: What is the moment of decline for those infected and their relatives, the moment they realize the necessity to be treated (or vice versa) and are able to meet the proper people ready to help? Another title, *Hra náhody* (Play of fate) directly pointed to the fact that anyone can contract a venereal disease and "lose" their fate. Two medical experts, Hynek Fügner and Karel Hübschmann, who wrote the screenplay in cooperation with Josef Kokeisl, echoed the doubts of Donald, a protagonist in *Damaged lives*, who refuses to believe that "it" has happened to him. As conceived by the filmmakers, Ladislav has a lot of similarities with the character of Donald but because of the long tradition in national literature, he could not be wealthy by birth. The young man is the best clerk at the bank, and the play of chance brings him to the boss's daughter, the discreet beauty Marta, who falls in love with Ladislav. By framing the tale around ardor, ambition and the desire for risk as qualities that can serve both well and poorly for men, *Osudná chvíle* indirectly but consistently normalizes the ex-perience of venereal disease for men but not for women. A comparison of the draft script[49] and the final version of the film indicates the range of ap-proaches recruited by the authors for translating this message to the audience.

The filmmakers brought together foreign films targeted at venereal diseases and male-female double *Bildungsroman*, quite a popular genre introduced to the Czech public by such female authors as Sofie Podlipská and Anna Srbová, alias Věnceslava Lužická,[50] who efficiently adapted this genre "congenial to the woman novelist who wishes to emphasize the way in which a society that rigidly differentiates between male and female gender roles"[51] to the aims of the Czech revival. *Osudná chvíle* reproduces the tripartite structure of double *Bildungsroman*, which consists of an introductory part that presents the idyllic period of spending time full of happiness and shared joys together, followed by separation, often through the escape of the man and the uncertainty of the woman, who awaits his return and reunion for achieving previous harmony.[52]

The first, idyllic part of the film presents the protagonists during their shared entertainment. For Ladislav, it is an introduction to the joys of the higher society to which he would belong after marriage with Marta. Together with Marta and her father, he visits the hippodrome, and this pleasure in observation is obviously opposed to more dangerous ways of spending one's free time, than seeing off freedom in a nightclub in the company of a spoiled friend in the next part of the film. In the draft of the scenario, the couple in love is spending their holidays at a ski resort in the Tatras, which only reinforces the impression of an ideal and near-wild life for Ladislav and Marta. Notably, Marta's father, when asked if they are going to the mountains in Switzerland, replies that there are wonderful places in their native land. Then, the former and older schoolmate of Ladislav, Reich, invites him to a night club, and the separation between Ladislav and Marta begins. Ladislav distances himself not only from his fiancée but also from his own mother, who hopelessly awaits her son. In the club, Ladislav meets Mimi – a temptress beauty, in the script a dancer, and in the film, a singer, who starts flirting with Ladislav. Reich not only fixates his attention on these nonverbal signals but also leaves Ladislav and Mimi alone. According to Goodman, a man's sexuality often operates as a driver of separation in the *Bildungsroman*, and the scenario draft describes how Ladislav gazes at the dance pole through his glass of wine and observes the figure of Mimi wearing only a veil and bending seductively in the glass.[53]

In the draft script, Ladislav does not offer an account of what is happening, due to excessive drinking, but in the film, he is instead under the psychological pressure of his friend and Mimi. The seduction scene in Mimi's boudoir is absent in the draft but is shown in detail in the film. Mimi seduces Ladislav for the sake of her lover – who makes a living by blackmailing his girlfriend's lovers. But Ladislav, instead of the expected fright, begins to fight, and, as it appears to him, kills the blackmailer. Horrified by what he has done, he flees to Belgrade, where, after a while, he realizes that he has been infected with gonorrhea. First, he tries to treat himself with "magic tea," which he has read about in the local newspaper (see Figure 8.1). But after unsuccessful attempts and another outburst of rage, now against a teapot with a "medicinal drink," Ladislav accidentally meets a Czech physician, a specialist in venereal diseases. In the draft, Jiří Materna is a former schoolmate of Ladislav who now works in Belgrade – in the film, he is an older man who represents a quasi-father figure for the young man (see Figure 8.2).

While Ladislav corrects his deed, Marta devotedly looks after his mother and waits for her lover. Ladislav is not only recovering from gonorrhea but also realizes that he did not commit the murder. It is noteworthy that in the draft, he remains unsure of whether he committed murder until he arrives home. The physician informs him about the death of his mother and gives him money for a ticket to Prague. After visiting his mother's grave, he returns to his home, where Marta is waiting for him, and who, in response to Ladislav's attempt to confess and apologize, says that she does not want to

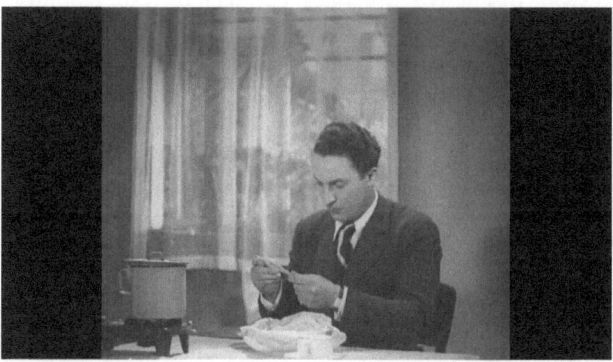

Figure 8.1 "Magic tea" and desperation of the protagonist in *Osudná chvíle* (Fortuitous moment, 1935).

Source: NFA.

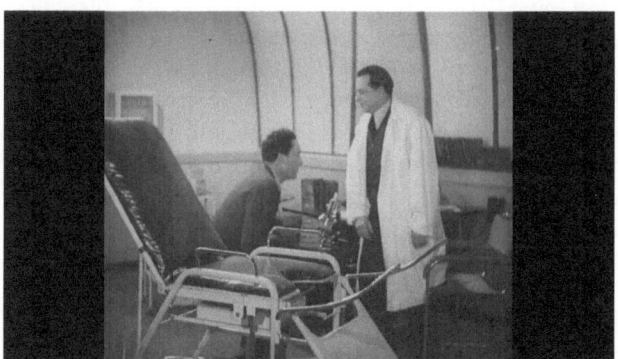

Figure 8.2 A quasi-father figure for the young man in *Osudná chvíle* (Fortuitous moment, 1935).

Source: NFA.

spoil the wonderful day. The father gladly accepts Ladislav, in whose place he had to accept Reich, and informs him that his friend suffers from an inconceivable disease, as a result of which he is paralyzed. The film ends in the garden of the villa, where Ladislav, Marta, their two children, and Marta's father enjoy another wonderful day. The very final slogan of the film is "Healthy family – healthy child – healthy nation."

The film does not deviate from the main discursive practices of the public campaign against venereal diseases that started in the middle of the 1920s that mainly addressed young men coming of age.[54] In a way very compatible not only with American and German campaigns but also with the attempts of Czech physicians to disseminate information about sexual relationships and self-protection, the interwar discursive practices connected responsibility, freedom, and self-control:

> You have been brought up by your family and school so far, and you will soon achieve almost complete freedom when you continue your studies. This freedom can be very fatal to you if you do not control your sexual instinct, succumb to it, and become infected by the venereal diseases that can destroy the roots of your entire physical and mental development. That's why you need to be educated about sexually transmitted diseases that hardly any of you still have the right ideas about.[55]

In these instructions, young women were mentioned only once: "Extramarital intercourse, however, is just as dangerous for girls as it is for men who have sexually transmitted diseases. But to that is added: Social exclusion, the danger of getting pregnant, discarded parents, and finally, a desolate life ending in prostitution."[56] Since the early twentieth century, the fine line between prostitution and promiscuity was typical of moralizing rhetoric among Czech experts. In 1903, Otakar Rožánek (1862–1931), a physician from Podebrady, presented his review of the politics and practices aimed at eliminating prostitution in different countries, with a particular focus on sexual immorality as a driving force behind prostitution: "Prostitution is usually preceded by extramarital sexual intercourse allegedly for 'love', and, therefore, it is necessary to understand this circumstance in the fight against prostitution."[57] Interwar experts often stressed the social origin and economic uncertainty among the driving forces behind prostitution. Notwithstanding, it is difficult to accept the opinion that this benevolent paternalism stood in opposition to the more conservative criminalization of women who were seen as being of "easy virtue."[58] The character of Mimi, the "occasional prostitute" in *Osudná chvíle*, embodies the interrelation of these two views. If in the draft, her criminalization reaches its maximum – Mimi is in a conspiracy with her lover – in the film, it is visible that Mimi is under pressure and duress by her lover.

Mimi is opposed not only to "valuable women," namely, Marta and Ladislav's mother, but also to her lover – while he is forced to be treated against venereal diseases and placed into a clinic, the viewers do not learn anything about treatment for her. The factor uniting all the women in the film is their lack of familiarity about venereal diseases. While Marta's father is informed about Ladislav's escapades, his daughter is not. The view of women as limited in their ability to accept the fact of venereal disease and to be able to cope with it through "open eyes" had been widespread in the professional practices and public discourses of Czech physicians since the start of dissemination of sex education in the early twentieth century.

From the very beginning, sex education presented men as those who should learn how risky sexual intercourse could be. Meanwhile, women were divided into innocent victims of venereal diseases for whom it would be better not to know much and those "easy-virtue" women who were their main carriers and also did not need any information. This multiple division was enshrined in the conductive fiction and multiple manuals for men and women disseminated between the end of the nineteenth century and the early twentieth century.[59] The exception that only confirmed the general rule was the short tale *Pitva* (Autopsy), by Otakar Hanuš,[60] who tells the story of an affair between the young medical student Lola Holmová and the patient Jaroslav Goll, who has infected her with syphilis; upon the autopsy of his body, she realizes that her lover was a syphilitic. The story concludes with Lola's announcement to her professor that she is sick and should be treated. The fact that Lola has missed all visible symptoms of syphilis because of her sexual passion could be seen as one more testimony of the limited ability of women (even future physicians) to recognize the threat in a timely manner.

Anna Honzáková, the first woman to graduate from the Czech Faculty of Medicine and one of the leaders of the Czech women's suffrage movement, was not only a consistent and influential opponent to the legalization of abortions but also practiced uninformed treatment of venereal diseases among women.[61] One of the friends of Honzáková, Marie Šebová shares the following story:

How deeply she empathized with her patients is demonstrated by this case: one of my employees, a beautiful, cheerful, and healthy girl, became ill shortly after her marriage, and withered like a wilted flower. I turned to the nice Mrs. Dr. Honzáková with a confidential request for help. She discovered a dangerous venereal disease and dealt with this sensitive issue energetically, delicately, and without delay. She invited the young husband, the mother of the young woman, and their united efforts and purposeful treatment by an experienced doctor managed to heal the young woman without her knowing what she was affected by. After two years, she became the happy mother of a beautiful, healthy boy, and to this day, she does not know what she owes to the dead Dr. Honzáková.[62]

The documentary part of *Osudná chvíle* remains aligned with this tradition. The filmmakers had transformed the earlier strategy of stopping sex hygiene films midway through to offer live lectures[63] – such lectures had been incorporated into the film as a documentary part lasting more than thirty minutes. The character of Materna shares a detailed description of the step-by-step contamination of the male and female organisms by gonorrhea bacteria and uses the analogy of an invasion, similar to the animation in *Il était une fois trois amis*. Along with a detailed description of the disease by which Ladislav is infected, Materna describes two other venereal diseases, chancroid and syphilis, included in the Law about the Combat against Venereal Diseases. This description reproduces the information presented in the manual "Pohlavní zdravověda a sebeochrana" ("Sexual health knowledge and self-protection" by Vladislav Kurka, first published in 1911 within the *Biblioteka lékařských spisů populárních* or the Library of Medical Publications for the Public).

The documentary portion of the film compares data about sources of disease contamination in Czechoslovakia and France through labeling women who infect men, finishing with a bravura description of the successes of the Czechoslovak pharmaceutical industry in the manufacture of drugs for the treatment of sexually transmitted diseases. As in the fictional part, the documentary part mostly focuses on men and men's health – even though the spread of the disease is depicted in the female genitals, the documentary part does not specify the dissemination of venereal diseases among women.[64]

But it was not only long-time tradition that shaped gender-based inequality in sex education – the political initiatives of Czechoslovak authorities to move away from the Austria-Hungarian politics of regulationism to abolitionism regarding prostitution as a pillar of the struggle against venereal diseases were inconsistent and poorly organized, which led to the negative reception of these politics by key actors such as physicians and local authorities. The ban on brothels was critically accepted, even by many physicians who overtly considered this legal regulation inefficient and elusive:

> Unfortunately, it can be stated that the result of this humanitarian legislative act was that prostitutes continue to do their business, being free to rely on themselves. We had to issue new instructions for control, which we are guided by. Our officials and the public agree that the closure of brothels has not brought any positive results, which would either reduce sexually transmitted diseases or combat criminal prostitution.[65]

Along with depicting the consequences of these politics, the film replaces the focus on treatment for those already infected and reconstructs a kind of hierarchy in which the more innocent could be treated through a more respectable approach, like the one in which Ladislav receives treatment from a Czech physician, who is clearly involved in the process of civilizing another country, the Kingdom of Yugoslavia. Meanwhile, the derogatory procedures of detention and compulsory treatment would be applied to regular visitors of the night club. Reich, who has involved Ladislav in an immoral adventure, remains on the top of this hierarchy of male irresponsibility, being inconceivably sick.

The domestic reception of *Osudná chvíle* underscored the ambiguity of the film, which led to many unrealistic and psychologically implausible collisions, such as the overly naïve behavior of well-educated men like Ladislav.[66] But the instructive value of the film was not a matter of doubt and question. The film was one of the latest health films made in interwar Czechoslovakia and it is reasonable to accept it as a culmination of interwar health propaganda that brought together tradition and novelty and reflected one of the most typical features of Czech health films, namely, using the genre of double *Bildungsroman* for claiming the predominance of men in the struggle for the people's health within the intensive process of institutionalizing public health. What role did the double *Bildungsroman* play in health films – in Czechoslovakia and abroad?

Double *Bildungsroman* in Czech and international health film

The garden and the spring season that provide the backdrop for many of the romantic scenes of *Osudná chvíle* are important symbols for understanding the film's message, which promises viewers who would be treated for venereal disease in a timely manner a life in a prelapsarian mythic garden, where kindred souls merge into one – a happy family. During the interwar period, the utopian but attractive idea of "family as a biological, functioning unit, the human organism of man plus woman ... ideally to be complementary"[67] gained extraordinary popularity among various thinkers, with implications mainly for the eugenics movement. In interwar Czechoslovakia, as in other European countries, the complementarity of sex roles within the family was discussed at multiple levels of producing and disseminating biological knowledge, including fundamental guidance for future physicians[68] and for the public too.

These audible androgynous motifs are the core of the double *Bildungsroman* and its main idea of seeking and finding such a soul and being able to reinforce the mutual feelings necessary to rekindle lost harmony.[69] Furthermore, Roman Roda-Růžička, who performs the role of Ladislav, can easily be attributed to the androgenic type, with his refined posture, big eyes and sensitivity. The fact that he performs all the male protagonists in the health films made by Kokeisl leads to the consideration of the impact of *Bildungsroman* on Czech health films. The films made earlier, in 1928, practiced the same type of narration that focuses on the internally contradictory figure of a man, simultaneously the driver of change and a force for achieving equilibrium.

"If wives knew what widows knew, neither uninsured husbands nor neglected children would exist" was the last sentence the viewers of *V blouznění* (In delirium/When frost creeps into the nest, 1928) read. The plot, about an ideal middle-class family with two young children whose prosperity and serene life end because of the unexpected misfortune of the father and his short-sighted refusal to procure life insurance, is one of the earliest examples of using double *Bildungsroman* in health films. While Jan relies on his health and the ability to work, he has purchased a nice home for his family on credit. But when he receives an advertisement for life insurance with the rhetorical questions, "Who is sure about the future? Have you already insured your family?" and an offer to sign a life insurance contract, he only laughs and invites Julinka, his wife, to share in his skepticism.

On the following winter day, Jan, who works as a wood appraiser, is forced to return later than usual, due to a breakdown of the sled, and being caught in a blizzard, he loses his orientation, falls and seriously injures his leg. He is doomed to certain death in the snow, but devoted Julinka finds him with the help of a local hunter and brings him home. The cold develops into croupous pneumonia, and the father dies. The widow is unable to pay the mortgage, and viewers witness scenes of debt extortion, including the repossession of the sofa while the children sitting on it, and removing the widow's necklace and earrings directly from her neck and her ears. The apparent exaggeration of this scene is immediately followed by a scene in which the sick Jan wakes up and shares his nightmare with his wife. The physician caring for Jan informs him that thanks to being a non-smoker and not a heavy drinker, he has a chance to survive. The first thing Jan does after recovering is to sign a life insurance contract.

V blouznění was not a health film in terms of its main purpose, to propagate life insurance, but it was informed by the same ideological frames and participated in its rooting.[70] The film coined the gender model of health propaganda in interwar Czechoslovakia based upon attributing to men the role of those who become more mature because of experiencing health issues and coping with them; meanwhile, women were the objects of care, able to devote themselves to their men but not to make decisions and to become more experienced and equipped for future challenges. This distribution of the roles was only exacerbated by a traditional, bourgeois view on family life, with the man as the breadwinner and the woman as the keeper of the hearth. Along with his many obligations, Jan practices modern forms of parenting: He spends time with his children and helps his wife with the housework. Julinka is portrayed as a courageous but naive woman who relies on her man, and whose trust could not be betrayed. While Jan learns a great deal from his experience of disease, Julinka only learns that her husband is the only source of her wealthy life.

V blouznění employs a wide range of analogies typical of double *Bildungsroman*. The idyllic part takes place during the warmer months, and the scene of Jan playing with the children in the garden is the culmination of life as heaven on earth. Conversely, the separation and mortal threat occur in a fierce winter. The nest of swallows at the beginning and the end of the film symbolizes the natural beginning of the desire to protect one's offspring. At the foundations of the double *Bildungsroman*, the audience can easily discern the Adam and Eve story that "can properly be read as a single-focus account of the birth of desire, repeatedly retold within single-focus texts."[71] The sustainability beyond any vicissitudes of the protagonists' lives is one of the central attractions of this narrative: "Eden is still Eden, Man and Woman are still Man and Woman."[72] The health-related double *Bildungsroman* re-interprets the biblical story as the expulsion from paradise due to illness as a consequence of irresponsible behavior and the return to paradise as the result of timely treatment.

Using a motif typical of health propaganda, namely, obtaining true and important knowledge through dreaming, reverberates with the tale about coming of age through experiencing disease and coping with it not alone but by becoming a part of larger social institutions (such as insurance) that aim to protect people from various threats, including inevitable evils like diseases or executors. *V blouznění* opposes the univocally positive institution of life insurance (presented by the hand-written letter) to the bank and the court who deprive the widow and orphans of the latter in favor of a court decision.

The pro-state interest to involve people as much as possible in the insurance system is mirrored not only in the content of film but also in the performance. The premiere of the film took place on June 21, 1928 at the cinema *Passage*, the first in Prague aligned with professional standards, with an 800-seat hall and affiliated with governmental structures during the interwar period.[73] The film was welcomed by the representatives of several Ministries including the Ministry of Industry, Commerce, and Trade and the Ministry of Health and Physical Culture. Then, the film was purchased by *Svaz československých pojišťoven* (The Union of Czechoslovak Insurance Companies), which asked the screenwriters to prepare a puppet show based upon the film for dissemination in rural areas, where mobile film services were unavailable.[74]

The double health *Bildungsroman* introduced the opposition of human vs. community and man vs. woman as challenges that not only taught audiences to cooperate with public health representatives but also ensured easy-to-understand but gripping storytelling. *V blouznění* advances the role of life insurance as a preventive measure against false confidence in one's own solvency, as well as a warning about the limits of assistance from the side of community. Even the very storyline of *V blouznění* convincingly shows the transformation of interwar health *Bildungsroman* for men into a more sophisticated narration that included the opposition of male and female roles as one of the main devices for maintaining the interest of the audience and encouraging them to adopt the "proper" behavior of the protagonists.

Pramen lásky or *Láska kvete v každém věku* (The seed of love/Love blossoms at any age, 1929), another film produced by Kokeisl, with Roda-Růžička in the role of the main protagonist, doubled the frames of double health *Bildungsroman*. The plot consists of the stories of two couples: The older widow Eliška and her first love, Jiří Světlý, whom she had to abandon after marrying a wealthy business owner and whom she meets again after many years, and the younger Helenka, a niece of Eliška who falls in love with another, younger Jiří Světlý, a nephew of the older Světlý, who, after emigrating to the United States, changed his surname to Light. Juxtaposing the two histories of separation and reunification provides more opportunities for bringing together gender, class and cohort as the main drivers of behavior. The main action takes place in Poděbrady, in one of the Czech spas, which began to emerge in the interwar period; in fact, the film was commissioned by the company distributing mineral water from the Poděbrady springs. Eliška is surrounded by those who want to marry a rich widow – retrogrades who think only about profit and lead an unhealthy lifestyle. Being sensitive and healthy in nature, she is wary of this attention and prefers to spend time with her niece, who is infatuated with the young patriot. Helenka and young Světlý demonstrate all features of the new interwar elite: They play tennis, swim a lot, walk and discuss Czech history, while those who represent the former elite eat cakes even as they drink mineral water, imbibe in alcohol and prefer to sleep under the sun instead of swimming. The natural sexuality of the main protagonists is opposed to artificial flirtation, as is the authentic patriotism of the old and the young Světlý, with pretensions of old elites

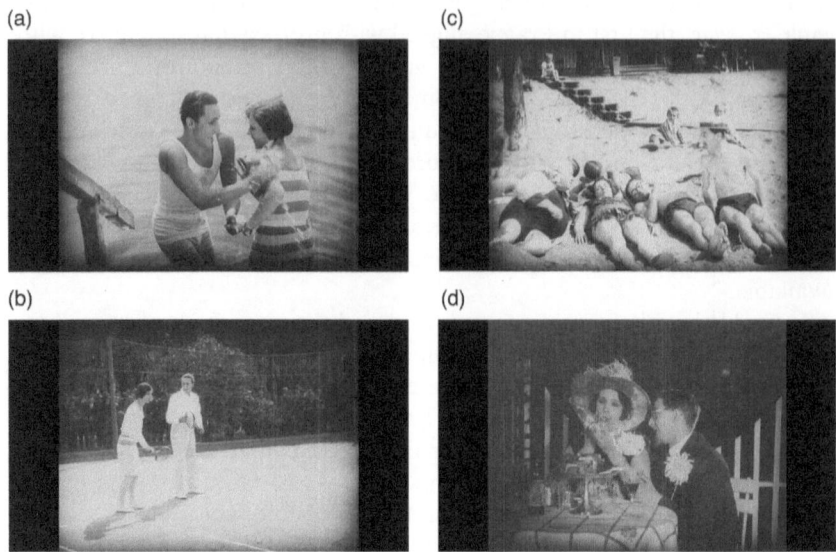

Figure 8.3 Opposition of new and old elites in *Pramen lásky* (The seed of love, 1929).
Source: NFA.

being patriots (see Figure 8.3a–d). These multiple dichotomies are reflected in the bodies of the characters: The progressives are thin and athletic, while the retrogrades are obese. Eliška's return to the bosom of the Czech nation is the main pedagogical message of the film, reinforcing the boundary between former and new elites who establish and promote the mutually interconnected norms of health, family life and leisure time.

In 1940, Edgar Ulmer made the exemplary double *Bildungsroman*, *They Do Come Back*, for the National Tuberculosis Association, interested in addressing various social groups seen as the most vulnerable and the least likely to be treated for tuberculosis in a timely manner. The target group for *They Do Come Back* would be young, working-class people class who needed to be motivated to undergo medical examinations and timely treatment. The story of two young lovers, Roy and Julia, consists of three parts: Their ideal life, including first, the enjoyment of healthy entertainment on the beach together; then, separation due to tuberculosis, which they both have con-tracted, and a long rehabilitation process, including vocational counseling and retraining for Roy; and finally, their reunion, not as an upper-working-class young couple but as a middle-class family with their own car and home. According to Altman, *Bildungsroman* often has a plot that results from a temporary imbalance between the two sides,[75] and Ulmer embodies this idea: The moment of disclosing the fact of disease comes when Roy, who, in a fit of joy, twists Julia around his shoulders, but is then forced to put the girl on the ground – because he loses his balance due to coughing and bleeding. The film connects finding balance through medicine and social rehabilitation – in which both Roy and Julia gain new economic and social stability, Roy – through mastering the profession of a drafter, and Julia – in the process of improving their housekeeping skills in accordance with the most modern ergonomic theories. At the very end of the film, the happy couple achieves their Eden – a small house with a nice garden to which Julia adds one more flower. The whole team of medical professionals who help to young pair to "come back" is easily associated with angels and presents public health as the perfect machinery of Eden on Earth. In the very final scene, viewers follow Roy and Julia, who are walking in the center of Philadelphia totally alone, like the first humans on Earth.

During the interwar period, when recasting gender roles became one of the predominant trends in high-brow and low-brow literature and film, health-related *Bildungsroman* reestablished gender-based hierarchies and recreated the feeling of stability – for those target groups considered in need of an unambiguous distribution of prescriptions to men and women, middle-class men or those aspiring to the middle class. The films produced by the School of Public Health brought forward another genre for achieving similar goal, to recruit the rural population into systematic actions aimed at preventing the dissemination of infectious diseases.

Notes

1 Presidium Československého vojenského ředitelství v Bratislavě [Central Committee of Czechoslovak Military Headquarters in Bratislava] Dopis Ministerstvu národní obrany [Letter to the Ministry of Defence] 18.11.1920 Fond EMVZ 97 SNA.
2 Susanne Michl (2014) Mapping the war: gender, health, and the medical profession in France and Germany, 1914–1918, Medicine, Conflict and Survival, 30:4, 276–294.
3 Alexandra M. Lord (2010) Condom Nation: The U.S. Government's Sex Education Campaign from World War I, The Johns Hopkins University Press, p. 12.
4 Eric Schaefer (2011) Exploitation as education in Devin Orgeron, Marsha Orgeron and Dan Streible (eds.) *Learning with the Lights Off: Educational Film in the United States* Oxford University Press, 316–337, p. 319.
5 Anja Laukötter (2021) *Sex – richtig! Körperpolitik und Gefühlerziehung im Kino des 20. Jahrhunderts* [Sex – right! Bodypolitics and education of feelings in the films of the twentieth century], Göttingen: Wallstein Verlag, p. 67.
6 Christian Bonah (2015) "A word from man to man". Interwar Venereal Disease Education Films for Military Audiences in France *Gesnerus* 72/1, 15–39, p. 18.
7 Rick Altman (2008) *A Theory of narrative,* Columbia: Columbia University Press, p. 104.
8 Ibid p.99.
9 Ibid p.105.
10 Lord, ibid.
11 Ibid., p. 31.
12 Laukötter, ibid., p. 45.
13 Virginie De Luca Barrusse and Catriona Dutreuilh (2009) Pro-Natalism and Hygienism in France, 1900–1940. The Example of the Fight against Venereal Disease, *Population* 64, 3, pp. 477–506.

14 Todd Wider (1990), in his article "The positive image of the physician in American Cinema during the 1930s," *Journal of Popular Film and Television* 17:4, pp.139–152, explains the rapid growth of positive images of physicians in popular American films by the tectonic changes in the interrelation between public health and the insurance system due to the economic crisis. It is reasonable to add the global trend of the intensive institutionalization of public health as one of the decisive driving forces in this trend.

15 Julia Roos (2010) *Weimar through the Lens of Gender: Prostitution Reform, Woman's Emancipation, and German Democracy, 1919–33* Ann Arbor, Mich.: University of Michigan.

16 Mary Louise Roberts (1994) *Civilization Without Sexes: Reconstructing Gender in Postwar France, 1917–1927*, Chicago: The Chicago University Press, pp. 120–121.

17 Aleš Meška (1922) Poznámka k boji proti pohlavním chorobám mezi našimi krajany v cizině [The remark to the struggle against venereal diseases among our compatriots abroad], *Dermatologie* 7. 9., pp. 2–4.

18 Okresný úřad v Turčianskom Sv. Martine [Local authority office, Turčiansky svatý Martin] 25.07.1925 Vlád. Nariadenie k zákonu o potieraní pohlavných nemoci. Prievodný výnos k nemu. Zriadenie venerického oddelenia a Wassermannovej stanice při žup. Nemocnici v Turč. Sv. Martine. [Governmental guidance on implementing the Law about the combat of venereal diseases. Supplementing information. The establishment of venreal subdepartment in Wassermann station at the district hospital in Turčiansky svatý Martin] Fond EMVZ 97 SNA.

19 Ibid.

20 Ministerstvo veřejného zdravotnictvi a tělesné výchovy (1923) [Ministry of health and physical culture] Poučení o pohlavních chorobách [The instruction about venereal diseases] Fond EMVZ 97 SNA.

21 Tekovský župan Zlaté Moravy [District Tekov, Zlata Morava] 10.06.1922 Policajný dohlaď nad prostitucí na Slovensku [Police surveillance over prostitution in Slovakia] Fond EMVZ 97 SNA.

22 Senica [District Senica] 19.01.1928Výročná zpráva o prevádzaní zákona o potieraní pohlavních nemocí [Annual report about implementing the Law on Combating Sexual Diseases] Fond EMVZ 97 SNA.

23 Okresný úřad v Turčianskom Sv. Martine [Local authority office, Turčiansky svatý Martin] 10.01. 1927 Výročná zpráva o prevádzaní zákona o potieraní pohlavných nemoci [Annual report about implementing the Law on Combating Sexual Diseases] Fond EMVZ 97 SNA.

24 Policejní ředitelství v Bratislave [Police Headquarters in Bratislava] 24.03.1922 Dopis Zdravotnímu oddělení města Bratislavy [The Letter to the Department of Public Health, Bratislava] Fond EMVZ 97 SNA.

25 The books, including Marie Carmichael Stopes (1918) *Married Love: a new contribution to the solution of sex difficulties,* London: A.C. Fifield and Th. H. Van De Velde (1928) *Ideal marriage: Its physiology and techniques,* London: William Heinemann, were enthusiastically accepted in many European countries.

26 Ivan Ivanov (1935) Brak i triper [Marriage and gonorrhea] *Narod i potomstvo* [People and offsprings] 01.02.1935.

27 Laura Otis (1995) The Language of Infection: Disease and Identity in Schnitzler's *Reigen, The Germanic Review: Literature, Culture, Theory,* 70:2, pp. 65–75.

28 Zsuzsa Bokor (2013) *Testtörténetek - A nemzet és a nemi betegségek medikalizálása a két világháború közötti Kolozsváron* [The History of bodies - The Medicalization of the Nation and Sexually Transmitted Diseases in Cluj-Napoca between the Two World Wars] Editura ISPMN, pp. 112–114.

29 Thierry Lefebvre (1995) Représentations cinématographiques de la syphilis entre les deux guerres: séropositivité, traitement et charlatanisme [Representations of

syphilis in the film between the two wars: seropositivity, treatment and charlatanism] *Revue d'histoire de la Pharmacie,* 83,306, pp. 267–278.

30 Delia Enyedi (2021) Janovics' Menace: inquiries into a duplicated silent film script *Studies in Eastern European Cinema,*12, 1, pp. 1–12.

31 Anita Gertiser (2013) *Falsche Scham: Strategien der Überzeugung in Aufklärungsfilmen zur Bekämpfung der Geschlechtskrankheiten 1915–1935* [False shame: The strategies of persuading and educating within the struggle against sexually transmitted diseases between 1915 and 1935] University of Zurich, Faculty of Arts P.26.

32 Roberts, ibid., pp. 1–5.

33 Valérie Vignaux (2007) *Jean Benoit-Lévy ou le corps comme utopie* [Jean Benoit-Lévy or the body as utopia] Paris: AFRHC p. 101.

34 Altman, ibid., p. 311.

35 Ibid., p. 291.

36 Ibid., p. 299.

37 Schaefer, ibid., p. 321.

38 Vignaux, ibid., pp. 99–100.

39 Noah Isenberg (2014) *Edgar G. Ulmer: A filmmaker at the margins,* California: University of California Press p. 47.

40 Ibid. p. 53.

41 More about the different approaches to construct and apply such dichotomies can be seen in Joël Danet (2015) Representation of Dangerous Sexuality in Interwar Non-Fiction Sex Hygiene Films: A Franco-German Comparison, *Gesnerus* 72/1, pp. 39–55.

42 Vignaux, p. 101.

43 Rare Edward G. Ulmer Unknown newspaper AMPAS Personal collection of Edgar Ulmer folder 62.

44 Films restored by the national archives of Canada Montreal 1993 62 Canadian Film Research AMPAS Personal collection of Edgar Ulmer folder 62.

45 Damaged lives coming to the Lido *West Middlesex Gazette* 25.11.1933.

46 Vignaux, ibid., p. 102.

47 Ibid.

48 Schaefer, ibid., p. 319.

49 Hynek Fügner and Karel Hübschmann (1934) *Osudná chvíle. Námět.* [Fortuitous Moment. Draft] Filmová industrie Josef Kokeisl [Film production by Josef Kokeisl] NFA.

50 Victoria Shmidt (2020) Female bildungsroman in Czech conduct periodicals: The inception of the genre, *History of Education & Children's Literature*, XV, 2, pp. 407–428.

51 Charlotte Goodman (1983) The Lost Brother, the Twin: Women Novelists and the Male-Female Double Bildungsroman *NOVEL: A Forum on Fiction* 17: 1 pp. 28–43 p. 30.

52 Ibid., p. 32.

53 Fügner and Hübschmann, ibid., p. 32.

54 Often in the texts about sex education the authors used *doba kvasu* – literally "time of fermentation".

55 Ministerstvo veřejného zdravotnictvi a tělesné výchovy (1923) [Ministry of health and physical culture] Poučení o pohlavních chorobách [The instruction about venereal diseases], Fond EMVZ 97 SNA.

56 Ibid.

57 Otakar Rožánek (1903) Pud pohlavní a prostituce vývoj a poruchy pudu pohlavního [Sexual instinct and prostitution: development of sexual disorders], Praha: Hejda a Tuček, p. 135.

58 Milan Hes (2017) *Dandy nezná lásky k ženě: Tragické příběhy českých dekadentů* [Dandy knows no love for women: tragic stories of Czech decadents], Prague: Epocha pp. 58–59.
59 For instance, in the Czech lands, along with the translation of German, French, and British manuals between the late 1900s and early 1910s such as Auguste Debay (1908) *Muž a žena v manželství* [Men and women in marriage] Praha: I.L. Kober, more than ten different popular books written by Czech physicians and aimed at teaching men and women sex appeared. The most popular were Otakar Rožánek (1906) *Choroby pohlavní u muže a ženy* [Venereal diseases of men and women], Prague: B.Kočí; Vladislav Kurka (1911) *Pohlavní zdravověda a sebeochrana* [Sexual health knowledge and selfprotection], Kladno: K. Stejskal; Karel Malý (1916) *Žena, její krása a život pohlavní (ženy sebeochrana a pohlavní zdravově*da) [Women, her beauty and sexual life: Self-protection and sexual health knowledge for women], Prague: Rudilf Storh. No one offered information about venereal diseases to women, even in the books that directly addressed them, including the manual by Malý. The exception was the translation of the manual *Die Ärztin im Hause* [The Doctor at home] by Jenny Springer (1911), made in 1925, in which an entire chapter was dedicated to sexually transmitted diseases.
60 Otakar Hanuš (1914) *Portréty milenek* [Portraits of mistresses], Královské Vinohrady: Přerod, pp. 92–102.
61 Honzáková was guided by class divisions and ascribed to women from lower social groups the ability to maintain responsibility and kindness, but not the ability to cope with the task of independently preventing certain diseases. Many of her feminist activities were submitted to the mission of nation-building; for instance, the right to vote was seen as central because of the reliance on Czech women's participation as a trigger for reaching a majority of pro-Czech politicians. And the fight for obtaining the right to higher education was connected with the competition with German women, who had tried to obtain the same rights. One of the latest refusals to accept Czech female students (before they were widely welcomed) was explored by the fact that German authorities did not want to allow the victory of Czech women, who would have received the opportunity to receive medical education before German women. More in Anna Honzáková (1936) Úsilí žen o vysokoškolském vzdělání [Women's efforts in higher education] PNR Fond Honzáková Anna, 1875–1940 Č.Inv. 93 22/76. *LA PNP.*
62 Marie Šobová (1945) Moje vzpomínky na MUDr. A.Honzákovou [My memories of MUDr. A.Honzáková] PNR Fond Honzáková Anna, 1875–1940, Č.inv. 134–135 22/76 p. 1 *LA PNP.*
63 Schaefer Exploitation as education p. 324.
64 The obvious oversight of women in sex education remains an issue that must be explored in order to trace the impact of interwar health education (including films) on later manifestations of health propaganda. The examples of gender-based inequality in sex education so common within interwar health propaganda can be seen clearly in late Soviet campaigns such as the short film *Gonorröa iseravimise ohtlikkus* (The danger in self-treatment of gonorrhea, 1986, Tallinfilm). The protagonist and the only character in the film is a young man, who, due to a promiscuous sexual life, becomes infected with gonorrhea, At the beginning, he self-medicates and fails, after which he turns to a venereal disease treatment dispensary - which takes care of him anonymously. Women in the film are not only shown as fragmented, but also remain associated primarily with the source of infection.
65 Župný úřad Zvolen [District authorities of Zvolen] 29.05.1923 Dopis Expositúre ministerstva verejného zdravotníctva a telesnej výchovy v Bratislave [The letter to the Ministry of Health and Physical Culture] Zatvorenie nevestincov [Closing brothels], Fond EMVZ 97 SNA.

66 Osudná chvíle 1935, *Film a diapositiv v osvětové práci a ve škole* 13 1 p. 4.
67 Jane Lewis and Barbara Brookes (1983) A Reassessment of the Work of the Peckham Health Centre 1926–1951, *Health and Society* 61, 2, 307–350, p. 329.
68 Jan Bělehrádek, Vladislav Růžička and Vladimír Bergauer, (1934) *Obecná biologie* [General Biology], Prague: Melantrich, pp. 19–20.
69 Goodman The Lost Brother p. 31.
70 *V blouznění* was filmed by the same team of filmmakers with Karel Driml and Josef Kokejsl at the head as four other Czechoslovak health films made by the tenth anniversary of Czechoslovakia between 1927 and 1928.
71 Altman, ibid., p. 131.
72 Ibid.
73 *Filmový kurýr* [Film courier] 01.09.1928, p. 12.
74 Miroslav Marvan and Josef Chaloupecký (1993) Dějiny pojišťovnictví v Československu [The history of insurance companies in Czechoslovakia] Volume 2: Dějiny pojišťovnictví v Československu (1918–1945), Bratislava: Alfa Konti, 206–207, p. 345.
75 Altman, ibid., p. 91.

9   Masculinity in health films for the rural population

The health education of peasants as a manifestation of progressive agrarianism

> The peasant is the best assistant if he feels that you are his best friend and that you wish him well. He does not trust us as a rule because he has traditionally developed that feeling towards the inteligentzia.[1] We should endeavor to overcome this feeling and make it become a thing of the past. There can be no progress in our rural districts if in our rural constructive plan the peasant takes no part; the family of the peasant is the basis and the unit for every constructive piece of work.[2]

This passage is from the 13-page letter by Andrija Štampar to Alice Masaryková that not only harshly criticized the approach of the Czechoslovak government to institutionalizing public health in the Eastern periphery but also presented the core of Štampar's own vision concerning the most reliable trajectories of health education, posed as "the most important thing that should occupy the first place, but it is also one of the most difficult as it requires a thorough study of the peasants, their life, their psychology and their needs."[3] In Štampar's conceptualization, physicians played a decisive role in connecting the progress of services, health education and involvement of the rural population:

> For this reason, one must study the conditions and environment of the peasants among whom he intends to work … . physicians due to their purely medical orientation show sometimes not only an unfriendly attitude towards socio-hygienic work, but also an attitude that may be directly harmful to public health.[4]

The roots of this belief in the primary role of the physician can be found in Štampar's early career period, when he took part in the measures aimed at stopping the cholera epidemic in 1913 in Nova Gradiška, a town near the border of Bosnia and Herzegovina. In his report about the spread of the infection and the obstacles to stopping the epidemic, Štampar outlined the

DOI: 10.4324/9781003272267-13

challenges to the sustainable development of public health that framed the main priorities for his conceptualization of social medicine for rural areas. At that point, he had achieved the position of one of the main experts on the issue of public health in rural areas, not only in his country but also at the global level.[5] A significant part of the report consisted of descriptions of the population's resistance to sanitary measures: "[A] family with four adults and numerous children used water from a polluted river, and a sign about the epidemic, which was supposed to hang on the house, was not found during the sanitary control."[6] Another problem was the uneven financial support for the efforts to stop the epidemic: "[T]he public physician who led the struggle against the epidemic for last three months did not get his salary at all."[7] The predominant position of the figure of the (male) physician reverberated with the very clear analogy between the rural population and weak and unintelligent women who "are mostly sick and more contagious like in the rest of the world."[8] This view was reinforced by the idea that infection came from the threatening East – Bosnia.

As a main cause of the epidemic, Štampar presented the fact that the local population utilized water from the Sava River, and in most villages, the river was not fenced off from sewage. In his opinion, sanitation would be the more important prerequisite for winning the fight against the epidemic, as opposed to medical treatment. Later, in criticizing school medicine in Slovakian rural areas, Štampar developed this argument by stressing the principle of connecting health education and the operation of health services through practicing mutual relevance: "[R]ural health care reform that focuses on medical aspects and neglects the need to take into account the social aspects of villagers' life, such as family budget, housing conditions, is helpless. What is the use of teaching children good hygiene at school if they return home with no proper latrine?!"[9] Notably, the sanitation of the water supply started to become a priority in the politics concerning the development of local public health,[10] as well as in the matter of health propaganda. One of the first projects undertaken by the School of Public Health was the production of two different films about sanitation in rural areas and the different approaches to repairing water supply systems that would align with hygienic rules.[11]

The reform led by Štampar dovetailed with global trends that sought to improve the accessibility of medical services and to involve working class and rural populations in new practices of preventing diseases and receiving timely treatment. In different regions, these global trends reverberated with the task of reinforcing the construction of nation-states and legitimizing their independence through claiming that care for people's health was an internationally shared priority. Along with Soviet Russia and Turkey, Yugoslavia was seen by global experts as a newcomer to the global system of public health after the Great War. Yugoslavia had introduced more "revolutionary and esoteric services" than even developed countries, making it an outstanding case of rapid progress in public health.[12] This stellar evaluation of Yugoslavia's success has often been attributed to the nature of Štampar's personality; it is thus reasonable to embed his strategy of educating the population (including the use of health films) into the wider contexts of interwar public health and the diversity of its institutionalization.

The adaptation of foreign initiatives aimed at improving public health and health education should be seen through the lenses of progressive agrarianism, the political platform that was not only shared by Štampar but also actively built and disseminated. Interwar agrarianism developed as the systematic negation of previous conceptualizations of rural life among urban minds,[13] in favor of the "articulation of a peasant [as] political subject."[14] One of the massive reforms in interwar Yugoslavia, "a fairly complete transfer of the land into peasant ownership,"[15] was a primary driving force that attributed to Yugoslav peasants and their political representatives a major role in uniting the nation. The call for giving agency to the peasant in encounters with modernity[16] determined the main pathway for the activities of the School of Public Health, including the empowerment of the rural population in light of the challenges facing the countryside, such as depopulation, lack of representation in public policymaking, and economic crisis.[17]

In an untitled text, the draft of a public speech written after 1925,[18] Štampar interpreted the approach of the brothers Antun and Stjepan Radić as *seljački pokret*, the ideology of human progress through the progress of the rural population. Štampar's main critique against the brothers came from their "relegating the idea of progress to the margins because of the predominance of the political struggle against centralism." Rudolf Herceg, who mostly engaged with enlightening activities for rural populations in the 1920s, was presented by Štampar as the real successor of progressive agrarianism. A promising future for progressive agrarianism was seen in its intercountry dissemination to places with economic, social and cultural similarities: Croatia, Slovakia and Ukraine. The films produced under the supervision of Štampar were a part of this ambitious task. The desirable political mobilization of the rural population to participate in nation-building inclined the ideologues of progressive agrarianism to present "their struggles as a microcosm of the struggles taking place in the wider nation."[19] Along with education, public health bridged the rural routines and the building of the nation. But progressive agrarianism not only reverberated with the priorities of interwar experts in public health, who were, like Marta Fraenkel, interested in bringing together medical and non-medical views on diseases and their prevention as a precondition for efficient health propaganda. Fraenkel, a German physician of Jewish origin, was one of the leaders of health education in Weimar Germany and the head of the exhibition at the Museum of Hygiene in Dresden between 1929 and 1933. Her responsibilities included the development of the concept of the exhibition and the entire range of work aimed at promoting the exhibition and presenting it to various audiences.[20] In response to Štampar's request, Fraenkel sent him a detailed critical analysis of the compilation of several films about public health in rural areas, produced by the School of Public Health for representative purposes. She shared the intention to use the films for educational purposes because "hygiene work, presented through its performance, must interest, captivate and convince."[21] She evaluated film as a generally excellent tool for propaganda but with a particular irony, she underscored the "noticeable reproach for insufficient detailing of what is shown, because of the understandable desire to avoid monotony."[22] This irony stemmed, obviously, from two interrelated positions.

On the one hand, Fraenkel was convinced by the different impressions that the films made among peasants and international experts, another target audience for the health films produced in Zagreb. On the other hand, she stressed that the films should explore and clarify what was an experiment, a model village, and what was reality, and how closely the desired model and the state of art resembled each other:

> If model villages are the nucleus of the hygienic movement, you need to provide expedient explanations such as maps or graphs with more detailed information concerning the scope of such centers, along with health schools and other relevant institutions, since for 95 percent of the medical audience the concept of hygiene is new and novel.[23]

Fraenkel highlighted the lack of information, such as more detailed plans of village houses and their redevelopment in accordance with the rules of hygiene, noting that such absence prevented positive reception by international audiences. In quite a delicate manner, she stressed that her opinion was the opinion of a medical expert, rather than non-medical experts who could provide other advice. She further developed this point in another critical remark: "For non-medical professionals, the connection between epidemics and unhygienic drinking water, perhaps even the connection between malaria and swamp areas, should be pointed out in a somewhat obvious way."[24]

Štampar answered immediately, informing Fraenkel about his readiness to polish the films according to her comments.[25] Indeed, the most disseminated films were complemented by more detailed information regarding the dissemination of the new practices and with a focus on a clearer connection between disease and lack of hygiene. In the second half of the 1930s, the films, along with the general approach to health education in rural areas, garnered overwhelmingly positive reception – one of the driving forces behind this success was not only progress in public health but also the embeddedness of the approach by Štampar and his colleagues in the most evident interwar trends for reforming public health.

The Dawson report, issued in the United Kingdom in 1920, was among one of the earliest initiatives that introduced the most comprehensive argumentation for a community medicine approach and relied on the solidarity of the people in favor of improving the health of the nation.[26] The British strategy, along with the approaches in other countries, helped to build an international model that was discussed at the global level. Štampar was certainly aware of these efforts and worked to modify these expectations concerning reform for the case of Yugoslavia. In his private correspondence,

Štampar mentioned several foreign approaches to organizing education for the rural population that seemed to be promising for rural areas in Eastern Europe. For instance, in correspondence with Masaryková, he mentioned that he planned to establish a school for rural women and men aligned with the model of the folk school offered by the Danish priest Nikolaj Frederik Severin Grundtvig in the first half of the nineteenth century. This choice was not coincidental.

Grundtvig's ideas reflected the process of emancipating Denmark from the Kingdom of Norway and transforming into an independent state; the mission of educating the adult population was embedded in the nation-building process.[27] Due to a lack of education, Danish farmers were limited in their participation in the civil engagement decisive for building the nation and an independent state; accordingly, folk education with a focus on the rural population should compensate this gap. Grundtvig asserted the necessity to enlighten not just individuals but entire communities, in order to foster collective identity and more efficient strategies of local cooperation. It is reasonable to assume that Štampar was affected not only by the methods offered by the Danish priest but also by the cultivation of the people's myth about Grundtvig as a builder of the Danish nation.[28] Like Grundtvig, Štampar brought forward the figure of the educator – in the case of health propaganda, the physician who would be responsible for shaping new national authenticity that did not interfere with the mission of progress. The eighth principle of the ten main principles of public health for the rural population offered by Štampar in 1926 was: "The physician is the teacher of the people."[29]

Another influential example stemmed from the Peckham Health Centre established in South London, whose employees, mainly educated as physicians, "give up their role as advisors on anything to do with health (for example, dietary, antenatal and infant care) and confine themselves to the role of 'therapeutic agents'."[30] It is unlikely that he shared the idea of separating prevention from conservative medicine, but the ideological foundations of the work of the British center concerning the role of family and care for the family, not just for individuals, but as a priority for public health, are very close to those of Štampar. The overt neo-Lamarckism in the stances of George Williamson and Innese Pearse, the Peckham Health Centre founders, was another shared ideological point – concerning the interrelation between public health and eugenics. The environment and its improvement seemed to be a more predominant explanation than inheritance. These stances inevitably led to an understanding of the family and the community as an organism, which attributed to them the position of agents of their own evolution. As with the ideology of the center, the orientation toward organicism also led Štampar's propaganda strategy toward a particular role for women, who complemented men and simply followed the men's choice to be healthy or not. This paradox of agency that was exclusively attributed to men was a predominant motif in the films produced by the School of Public Health for the rural population, namely, the unity of the efforts by physicians and the manhood of rural areas.

Representations of masculinity in *Dva brata: film o sušuci*

When a farmer is healthy, his economic situation improves; when a farmer is sick, he loses money and cannot work. The sanitation (*Gesundung*) of the village does not cost a lot of money, but the farmer must learn to improve his life by simple means.[31]

The above quote comes from the leaflet for the exhibition "Hygiene auf dem Lande" ("Hygiene in rural areas"), prepared by Andrija Štampar in 1931 under the request of Hermann Georg Otto Seiring, the director of the Zentralinstitut für Volksgesundheitspflege, Deutsches Hygiene-Museum in Dresden. This slogan reflects one of the main approaches developed by the School of Public Health to motivate the rural population to accept the practices and regulations of preventive medicine. Aimed at disseminating rules designed to stop the spread of tuberculosis, the film *Dva brata: film o sušuci* (Two brothers: A film about tuberculosis, 1931) embodies this approach through opposing the stories of two brothers, whose father died because of tuberculosis, and who both become sick, younger Ivan because he lacks basic knowledge about hygiene and older Pavel because of drinking and other habits of toxic masculinity. While Ivan and his wife Jaga have learned how to be healthy and wealthy, Pavel has drunk the last of what he has, losing his horse and his health, and subsequently dies (see Figures 9.1 and 9.2).

The story is set in "our Turopolje" and depicts the interrelation between two improper modes of behavior: Irresponsible and unfettered drinking (in contrast to the desire to earn a living) and a variety of unhealthy habits such as eating from the same plate, the whole family (including the infected) sleeping in the same bed, and cooking and sleeping in the same room. Narrated on behalf of a physician, the 40-minute film is divided into three parts that oppose the *Gesundung* of Ivan's house and family life to the

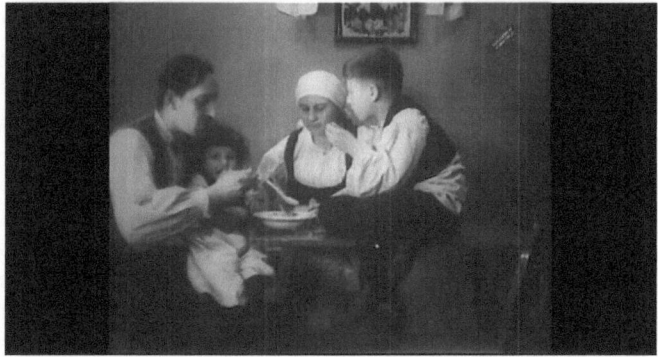

Figure 9.1 Ivan as a potential symbol of healthy masculinity in *Dva brata: film o sušuci* (Two brothers: A film about tuberculosis, 1931).

Source: Kinoteka, HAD.

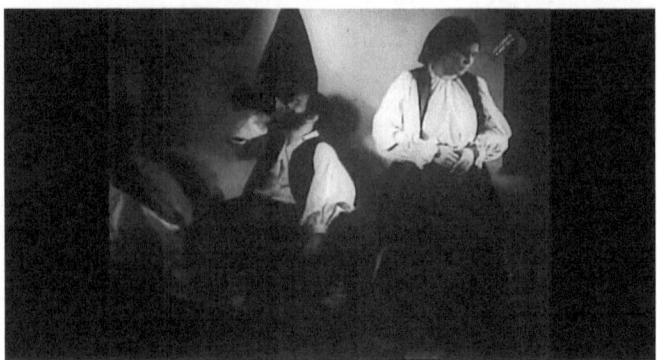

Figure 9.2 Pavel as a symbol of toxic masculinity in *Dva brata: film o sušuci* (Two
          brothers: A film about tuberculosis, 1931).

Source: Kinoteka, HAD.

disintegration of the drunken life of Pavel and his wife Mara, which occurs as
everything is destroyed, including Pavel's lungs. Each of the parts opens with
detailed introductory medical information and ends with a meeting between
the brothers. Such temporal sequencing creates a clear connection between
the tasks of informing audiences and motivating them to change their
behavior in line with new competencies and skills.

The first part opens with information on mortality in Yugoslavia and the
enormous role of tuberculosis, the cause of every fourth death. This information is represented by crosses in a cemetery, with every fourth one more
prominent than the three others. (These figures were an exaggeration – even
in the most problematic areas in 1930, the death rate from tuberculosis was
no more than 16 percent of all deaths.[32]) The main fear underlying the
massive campaign against tuberculosis had escalated in different regions of
Yugoslavia in the early 1930s – the public fear concerning the rapid spread of
the disease in a great number of infected households – and this fear directly
shapes the film plot.

The audience is invited to follow a typical day in the lives of Ivan and
Pavel. While Ivan works in field, Pavel spends the entire day at the local pub –
the *birtija* – where he drinks with a few other men. He returns home only to
attack his poor wife and to take money for another day in the *birtija*. Ivan, in
contrast to Pavel, not only likes working but also loves his family; the viewers
observe multiple toys that he has made for his sons, and another sign of love
is the children's anxious glances at their coughing father. Ivan does not want
to worry his family and only occasionally does Jaga disclose that Ivan has
hemorrhaged, but the following day, he continues his farmer's routine, and
after milking the cow, he goes to the field, where he loses consciousness. Pavel
finds his brother and instead of help, he offers him the alcoholic drink, *rakija*.
This moment is not only the culmination of Ivan's helplessness but also the

pinnacle of Mora's powerlessness. Mora seeks help from the nurse, but the nurse cannot convince Pavel to return from the pub to home. In contrast, Jaga and Ivan immediately receive all the attention of the nurse.

The second part mainly conveys instructive meaning: The nurse exerts much effort to improve housing conditions and to teach Ivan and his wife how to minimize the damaging effects of the disease for them, their children and other inhabitants of the village.[33] Ivan's condition deteriorates so much that he is forced to stay in bed and simply wait for improvement. This part of the film translates the expectations of public health services and their representatives, physicians and nurses, from the rural population. In his comprehensive guidance for coping with tuberculosis, Vladimir Ćepulić, the head of the *Institut za tubarkulozu u Zagrebu*, wrote: "Isolation remains the most effective measure in coping with tuberculosis and involves the removal of the patient from an unhygienic environment. An asocial patient must be forcibly admitted to a hospital."[34] The trust in and uncritical acceptance of public health officials and their superior knowledge culminates in the moment when the nurse stops Ivan from smoking – by taking the cigarette from his mouth.

If the nurse is the central figure for communication in the film, the role of the physician seems more modest – at least until the moment when Ivan's treatment is interrupted by Pavel, who decides to attend to his brother and to offer him alcohol as the best medicine against any disease. Pavel finds Ivan reading a chapter in *Narodna čitanka o zdravljiu* (The people's health reader), aimed at reviewing the diseases of the respiratory tract, including tuberculosis. While Ivan is lying in his room, Pavel very obstinately offers him instead of a "stupid doctor's advice and reading abstruse books, to drink real medicine." When Ivan begins to falter in his resistance to Pavel, the physician appears in the door and stops Pavel by asking him: "It is not enough to kill yourself – you would like to kill your sick brother too?!" To Pavel's silly remarks about the benefits of traditional medicine, the physician replies: "You can do what you want but remember you are the son of a father who had tuberculosis too, and you could thus suffer from the disease too." Pavel's reply is: "When you fall into the hands of a doctor, consider that you have passed away!" The second part of the film closes with optimistic dialogue between the physician and Jaga about the high probability that Ivan might be remedied by summer.

In the third part, Pavel becomes the center of the narration. Because of a lack of money, he decides to sell the only horse that he has, and despite his wife's protestations, rides away on the horse. Late at night, Pavel, now in torn clothes and totally confused, returns to the pub, where he orders a liter of *rakija* as usual, but he feels so poorly that even the *rakija* does not go down his throat; he cannot manage to take a sip. Completely destroyed, he returns home, where he bleeds out and dies quickly, without waiting for help from his brother, to whom Mara has rushed. While Jaga runs together with Mara back to Pavel, Ivan calls for the physician – only for establishing the fact of the death and for ascertaining the main reason behind it, namely, the drunkenness that had prevented timely examination, killing Pavel. Despite all the troubles he has brought to the family during his lifetime, Pavel is mourned by all his relatives – who unanimously call him an unfortunate victim of his own vices.

The film ends with a very emotive scene in which Ivan, healed and filled with strength, walks through a flowering forest in the early morning, waving a twig, stopping near the most beautiful trees. He is shown full of energy, mowing grass in the field while the unfortunate Mara mourns Pavel, one of the numerous victims of tuberculosis and drunkenness. The concluding moral of the film concerns the victimization of men who are unable to resist the temptations of alcohol: "How many victims of drinking and tuberculosis are there, and how easy would it be to avoid it"? This dual depiction of Pavel as both a victim and the main cause of his troubles aligns with the concept of toxic masculinity – a complex of prescriptions for men's behavior are connected with damage to society and to men themselves, a consequence of false ideas about what means to be "real men."

Exposure to toxic masculinity as a strategy of health propaganda

The concept of "toxic masculinity" is a product of the movement for delegitimizing traditional norms regarding men's behavior, developed in the 1980s within the struggle against misogyny and homophobia. Notwithstanding, historically, it stems from earlier attempts to differentiate regressive and progressive behavior among men with regard to the new, modern, norms introduced by demographic changes and expectations from the side of experts or authorities.[35] Critical reception of the division into "toxic" and "healthy" masculinity indirectly reflects the modern roots of this movement and its limits in addressing gender inequality, victimizing those men who remain aligned with traditional, conservative, or even toxic norms.[36] The opposition between toxic and healthy masculinity was easily recruited by medical experts, who started connecting the most disseminated issues of men's health with "toxic" masculinity.[37] Addressing the question of the historical continuity of using the motif of toxic masculinity in public health campaigns is beyond the scope of this book.[38] However, in Western Europe, the penetration of this concept into public discourses was directly connected to changes in attitudes toward drinking practices, especially in rural areas, one of the epicenters in producing discourses of modernity: "When the drunkard stopped to be described only as an affirmative figure, celebrating life, he became ever more disapprovingly depicted as a habitual drunkard, ... a negative figure soliciting pity as a dramatic fallen character."[39]

In Germany, Belgium and France, historians have traced a comparable dynamic, from an initial focus on drunkenness as an inseparable part of the festive atmosphere and rare moments for abandoning social conventions, through the differentiation of pride and laziness that should be punished because of a close link with drunkenness on the one hand and "sobriety accompanied by modesty and thrift would lead to life improvement," on the other, to constructing drunkenness as an unavoidable part of an individual's biological and hereditary make-up.[40] The latter trend reflected the increasing role of eugenics in constructing public intolerance to alcoholism as a social disease. The specific attitude of Štampar and other experts at the School of Public Health toward eugenics as limited due to the predominance of hereditary factors determined the centrality of the motif of moral choice in numerous campaigns against alcoholism. *Dva brata*, the culmination of this trend, opposes the behavior of siblings who should ostensibly have comparable complexes of hereditary factors.

Notably, in Czechoslovakia, where the impact of the eugenics movement on public health was stronger than in Yugoslavia, the motif of toxic masculinity as an issue of moral choice remained on the margins of health propaganda. One of the rare examples is the following task assigned within mathematics classes for fixing the attention of young men on their health:

Once upon a time, there were two brothers: one drunkard, who also smoked, and one abstinent. The drunkard drank 3 crowns a day, and smoked 2 crowns, for a total of 5 crowns. With this exception, both had the same income and spending. How much more could the abstinent man spend on vacation travel than his brother? How many vacation days could he afford if one vacation day costs 50 crowns?"[41]

Toxic masculinity, stemming from asocial or even criminal behavior, was seen by the ideologues from the School of Public Health as one of the main barriers to cooperation between rural population and public health representatives. In the film *Dva brata*, Pavel tries to contest the authority of public health representatives but Ivan is ready to accept the superiority of medical experts. In a notable scene depicting the confrontation between the physician and Pavel, Ivan asks his older brother to bow his head in front of the visiting physician, but his brother ignores this request. Moreover, Pavel balances on the boundary between delinquency and crime. Dependence on alcohol plays the central role in shaping this profile of undesirable behavior. From their very beginnings, public campaigns against alcohol addiction had introduced the interrelation between the unregulated consumption of alcohol and the primitive or, even more, violent, behavior of men as one of the main reasons behind the rural population's struggle against alcoholism.

The campaigns promoting abstinence often explained the growth in violent crimes against persons, especially on the periphery of the country, as a manifestation of the "savage" or "uncivilized" masculinity that included the unregulated consumption of alcohol: "The reason for the excessive use of alcohol is that our people do not know other ways to celebrate the holidays of our Lord than to get drunk, and, therefore, drunkenness destroys the lives, and the bodily and mental health and integrity of our people."[42] Among several artistic texts included in one of the first manuals against alcoholism,

Štampar chose a short poem by Serbian physician and writer Jovan Jovanović Zmaj titled *Nesretnik* (The unfortunate man), in which the decay of the personality of the drunkard is described:

> In his face, there was nothing left of the likeness of our Lord
> Now you see a picture that breaks your heart
> Man has sunk lower than any animal
> Lost pride, trampled shame[43]

The motif of alcoholism as a main cause of unhappiness and misfortune is evident in *Dva brata*: Ivan and Pavel mutually call each other *nesretnik,* and the film promulgates the popular idea that luck is one of the qualities attributed to a "real man": Not Pavel but Ivan is the bearer of healthy masculinity. This contest between "proper" and "improper" understandings of luckiness reverberates with the metaphors introduced by an earlier film targeted at the issue of alcohol, *Čarobnjaci* (Wizards, 1928). The film was produced using the technique of silhouette theater and tells the story of a struggle between bad wizards, Alcohol and Dirtiness, and good wizards, Fresh Air and Sun, for acceptance by the people in favor of their happiness.

Birtija (The pub, 1929 by Jozo Ivakić) connects masculinity, health and luckiness with the ability to resist the pressure from the side of those who translate toxic masculinity. The film tells the dramatic history of Anka and Franjo, whose happy marriage has been destroyed by the *birtija*, and those who seduce Franjo not to be "henpecked" but to be a "real man" and not to fear his wife. Other "real" men who live in the same village attack Franjo, who tries to avoid visiting the *birtija*, telling him that he is not a man but a *šeprtlja* (do-nothing, nobody).[44] While Franjo fails to resist the pressure, Ivan wins – along with the independence of his happiness from "backward" habits. *Dva Brata* introduces the motif of this manipulation through showing the communication between Pavel and a pub owner who indulges Pavel's addictions and is willing to search his pockets on occasion to embezzle money.

Dva brata embeds the multifaceted threats of tuberculosis into two mutually opposed profiles of men's behavior fixed in the characters of the brothers, explained not so much by their personality differences but by their acceptance or rejection of toxic masculinity. Ivan's ability to effectively cultivate the field and to care for livestock, along with a thoughtful approach to one's own health is contrasted to Pavel's irresponsibility regarding farming and health emerging from "wrong" ideas about masculinity, such as alcohol and tobacco dependence, overt verbal and physical aggression against women, and overly dominant behavior. While the film mentions the father of the two brothers only once, when the physician warns Pavel, it is easy to imagine that the father was a victim of toxic masculinity too. Remarkably, Ivan breaks the cycle and develops a healthy masculinity, moving away from his inability to communicate his disease to his wife and toward openness in sharing his troubles. Moreover, he stopped smoking and achieved impressive competency in the fields of health and disease. Indirectly, the film asks viewers, "What makes men inclined toward either healthy or toxic masculinity?"

The casting for the film reinforces the opposition of the two brothers as the embodiments of toxic and healthy masculinity: Kamilo Brössler, who had a public reputation for being a romantic hero, performs Ivan, and Mladen Širola, who had already played ambiguous characters, such as a wizard in children's films, embodies Pavel, who contrasts with the sensitive and thoughtful Ivan, and is squat and fat, with vulgar whiskers. Pavel is the embodiment of resistance to progress. His repulsive psychological and physical profile is supplemented by a very visible opposition between the poorly maintained house and yard and the well-organized space of Ivan's family life, suggesting that prosperity is maintained through sobriety.

At the beginning of the film both Ivan and Pavel are depicted for the viewer from the perspective of other characters, primarily their wives, the physician and the nurse, often shown as seeing the main characters with a very clear emotional expression, but by the end of the film, the audience can observe the beauty of a spring morning from Ivan's point of view, which only reinforces the idea of a man as a demiurge of the rural world.

The binary of toxic or healthy masculinity is the only driving force from the side of ordinary people who would like to prevent the spread of tuberculosis. *Dva brata*, a film about life choices and their consequences, presents the disease as "the consequence of ignorance and negligence," one of the first statements in the film, ascribing the right and duty to take responsibility for choices exceptionally to men. The destinies of woman and children depend on the rightness of men's decisions. While the lives of both wives are deprived of stability, only Jaga gets the chance to take meaningful steps toward triumphing over the disease, through her willingness to learn new skills and help her husband – because of the proper choice he has made to read a manual about people's health to his wife. Fertility is one of the main signifiers for opposing the brothers: The God-fearing Ivan is the father of two charming boys, but Pavel is a childless drunkard, and this difference once again stresses the prerogative role of men in achieving the ideal family. Indirectly, the film connects unhealthy marital relationships, as the reason for not having children, with men's domestic violence – in each of the five scenes featuring interaction between Mara and Pavel, he expresses either verbal or physical aggression toward his wife.

Besides the two spousal pairs, Ivan-Jaga and Pavel-Mara, *Dva brata* introduces one more pair meant to symbolize the unity of public health: The physician and the nurse. In the film, there are no scenes in which these public health representatives communicate with each other. The role of the physician is in fact modest in comparison to the impact of the nurse, who has consistently reorganized and transformed the life of Ivan's family. However, it would be hard to evaluate the central role of the nurse as a signifier of gender-based equality. On the one hand, the interwar projects targeted with developing public health in rural areas relied heavily on nurses. On the other hand, at the end of the 1920s, medicine had not developed a comprehensive strategy for treating tuberculosis, except for timely assessment and prevention. In the film, apart from a healthy daily routine, diet and rest, Ivan does not receive any visible treatment, a scenario that represented the reality at the time. The main aim is to provide new rules for stopping the dissemination of the disease, rather than to involve people in new assessment and treatment practices: How not to infect others is the central point of the film.

In much of the interwar world, including Yugoslavia, timely diagnosis and monitoring (from the second half of the 1930s through X-ray examination) remained the only medical strategy. The limitations of interwar Yugoslav medicine in solving the problem of tuberculosis were additionally determined by the insufficient number of physicians who would be able to organize timely assessment, especially in rural areas. These limits were reflected not only in the film but in numerous complex studies aimed at identifying the primary non-medical causes of the disease. Thus, it was found that the well-being of a peasant family, determined by the proportion of land in cultivation, did not affect the number of cases and deaths from tuberculosis, despite a significant difference in the organization of nutrition for more and less well-to-do villagers.[45] But along with this conclusion, sociological research conducted in a Serbian village in the Kragujevac district, where 80 percent of households had experienced tuberculosis, pointed to the indirect causes for preventing and treating tuberculosis as major factors, namely, the number of children and housing conditions. Notably, the comprehensive professional report about the research was complemented by a list of folk-medicine treatments against tuberculosis.

The ideologues of the fight against tuberculosis often claimed that solutions should be based on combining the interests of the sick individual and the village community,[46] but the question of what constituted the interests of the community remained unanswered in *Dva brata*. The shift from the opposition between the negative, "backward" influence of the environment and the progressive role of public health to the cooperation between public health and the rural community is reinforced in the film *Pošast: film o tifusu* (Pestilence: A film about typhus, 1931) in which the disease could be totally eradicated – with the efforts of all the villagers.

Manhood against infections in *Pošast: film o tifusu*

In the part "Društvena borba protiv zaraznih bolesti" ("The struggle of society against infectious diseases"), *Narodna čitanka o zdravljiu* (The people's health reader) asserts to its readers, "We can keep our house clean, but if the neighbors have dirt, then our cleanliness will not help prevent the spread of diseases."[47] Recruiting the rural population in collective actions aimed at preventing diseases was a kind of mission of the School of Public Health, and *Pošast: film o tifusu* can be regarded as one of the most outstanding achievements of the School of Public Health Film Laboratory in this field.

Aimed at introducing a complex approach to preventing endemic or flea-borne typhus, *Pošast* was shown not only in all parts of Yugoslavia, but also in several other countries, including Czechoslovakia, Turkey, Spain, Italy and Albania.

The film was made in the same year as the First International Conference on Rural Hygiene was organized by the League of Nations in Geneva, and the choice in favor of endemic typhus was aligned with the priorities of the Preparatory Committee, in which Štampar had obtained one of the leading positions.[48] Three other priorities, "treatment of garbage and manure to prevent fly-breeding; methods for testing and analysing water and sewage; and the hygiene of foodstuffs, in particular milk," were directly connected with the aim of eradicating endemic typhus. Over the following few years, in Eastern Europe, special retraining for physicians who worked in rural areas was organized to inform them about the proper organizational approaches to preventing endemic typhus.[49] The program was supplemented by showings of the film as a part of the planned campaign against endemic typhus. But it was not only the choice of disease and the prevention of its dissemination that ensured the film's success.

The film opens with a scene depicting the burial of young Kata, Mark's wife, who has died because of endemic typhus. Men and women in national costumes express their grief; some sit on the benches in front of the mayor's office. The mayor tells a recently arrived physician that there is now the first typhus death in their village. He condescendingly pats the physician on the shoulder when he expresses fear that the disease is about to spread throughout the village, saying that everything is God's will. In response, the physician replies that everything is in the hands of the villagers. He is concerned about the folk custom of holding a collective memorial in the local public house, and the mayor of the village proposes an order that would prohibit such events during the epidemic. The film then alternates between scenes of excessive grief among the relatives of the deceased Kata and the real fears of the physician, who, in his office, examines recommendations for preventing a typhoid epidemic. Further, the postal clerk, after a drum roll that attracts the villagers to him, reads out an order banning collective visits to the public house. But with a grin, he, along with the villagers, announces that no one can forbid them from visiting private houses.

The entire village gathers in the house of the deceased Kata's mother. Those who wish to commemorate Kata walk past the mayor's office, in front of which only the physician and the mayor are sitting on the bench, who immediately realize that all their efforts to prevent the epidemic have been in vain. The scene of the memorial not only shows the way the disease spreads but also the multiple forms of irresponsibility among the village inhabitants. Kata's mother, who has all the symptoms of the disease – clinging to her stomach and exhibiting a fever, sets the table without washing her hands after using the toilet. In the food and drink, visitors catch flies that emerge from a toilet too close to the house. The grief is drowned in alcohol, and after the memorial, two more deaths occur. Two weeks after that, during the incubation period of the disease, there are even more sick people in the village.

Tomo, the closest friend of the widower Marco, becomes so ill that the physician sends him to the hospital. Delirium and persistent diarrhea attract curious village inhabitants to Tomo's house, creating another opportunity to spread the disease. Flies transmit infection from Tomo's pot to food in the house, and one of the apples is eaten by the neighbor's young daughter. The mayor initiates the inspection of the village houses by the physician in order to stop the dissemination of disease. And the physician makes the decision to vaccinate the inhabitants. All of them are invited to the mayor's office, where the physician gives a lecture about endemic typhus, its symptoms and its dissemination. His narration is interrupted by the couple whose daughter has eaten the apple in Tomo's house and who is seriously ill. The physician promises to visit them after finishing his mission of enlightening and vaccinating. Unsurprisingly, the father of the infected girl makes the decision to be vaccinated first despite his obvious fear.

In the house of the sick girl, the scene very much resembles the scene in *Pomoć u pravi čas* (the character of the girl is even performed by the same actress, Ada Širola): The physician teaches the parents hygienic rules and helps to organize the care for their daughter. In addition to the more common rules, he shows them how to properly dispose of the urine and feces of a sick person. He overcomes the resistance of the mother, who would like to continue to sell milk in the nearby town, showing the father how to disinfect the toilet and the water spring. The film ends with the return of the recovered Tomo to the village and the recovery of the sick girl. All of the residents greet the physician in front of the mayor's office and congratulate him on the victory over the disease.

Those familiar with the various short stories by Guy de Maupassant, such as *Le Petit Fût* (The little cask) or *Le Baptême* (The christening), which denounce the tradition of collective drunkenness in the countryside will easily recognize similarities between the texts by the French writer and the scene of the memorial in *Pošast: film o tifusu*.[50] The film uses the same range of artistic devices to present excessive drinking as a source of the brutal neglect of the needs of the most vulnerable, such as children and women, and the main reason for the degradation of society. The genre of pathetic grotesque introduced into European literature by Maupassant and Victor Hugo connects characters to a repertoire of disturbing situations,[51] which creates the psychological plausibility of narration through the ease of recognizing the protagonists, "revealed in a few significant gestures"[52] without subtlety. Pathetic grotesque produces laughter as a springboard to comedy,[53] presenting viewers with familiar or even shared emotional patterns such as mockery of medicine, fear of vaccination and the horror of illness among beloved people in familiar cultural contexts. The most coherent application of this genre in the film is the character of the postal clerk, who is obliged to inform the villagers about the quarantine and other measures offered by the

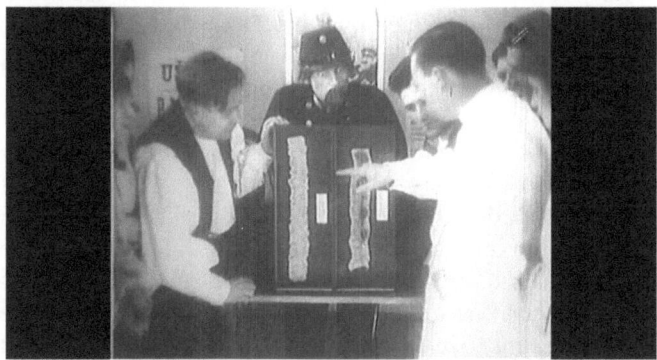

Figure 9.3 Pathetic grotesque in depicting retrogrades in *Pošast: film o tifusu* (Pestilence: A film about typhus, 1931).

Source: Kinoteka, HAD.

physician and the mayor and who obviously mocks his duties by adding his own interpretation of the warnings and restrictions he introduces in favor of collective drinking (see Figure 9.3). A ridiculous gait, a funny mustache and bulging eyes complement the image of someone who is accustomed to being a jester. Another easily recognizable character is the father of the infected girl, performed by Širola, which can be interpreted as an attempt to connect the character of Pavel from *Dva brata* with this luckier man who has a child in the name of whom he is ready to change (see Figure 9.4).

Like Maupassant's texts, *Pošast: film o tifusu* reproduces multiple cultural practices familiar to the audience as an integral part of everyday rural life, from drinking alcohol as a part of rituals to thinking about alcohol as

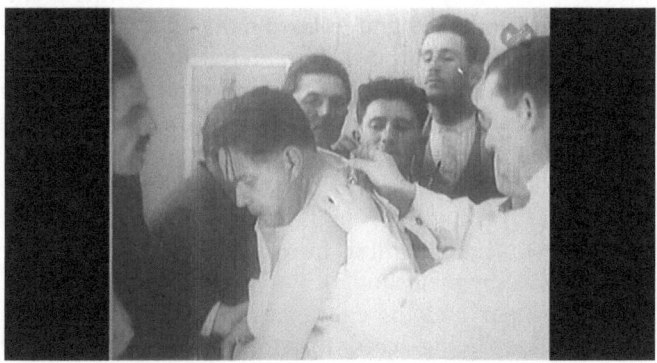

Figure 9.4 Readiness to change in *Pošast: film o tifusu* (Pestilence: A film about typhus, 1931).

Source: Kinoteka, HAD.

strengthening the ability to work. Undoubtedly, Yugoslav public health experts might have shared the view expressed by Mary Douglas: "Drunkenness expresses culture in so far as it always takes the form of a highly patterned, learned comportment."[54] Field research conducted in the 1930s indicated the involvement of all generations and genders in various collective practices of drinking or, even more, the collective production of distillates.[55] As for farmers in many other countries, for Yugoslav villagers "drinks act as markers of personal identity and of boundaries of inclusion and exclusion."[56] But the film tries to extend the native view on alcohol-related troubles. The remarkable scene in which Tomo and Marko are repairing the house, and Marko offers Tomo, who has fallen ill due to a developing infection, the advice to drink more *rakija* to regain his strength, aims to reinforce the analogy between alcohol and contagion.

The celebrations among farmers accompanied by the unlimited consumption of alcohol are posed as threatening to the authorities and to the social hierarchies that operate in favor of order and health. In contrast to Maupassant's texts, the film offers the hope to move away from mass irresponsibility and toward collective actions against disease. While the physicians in the texts by Maupassant are disenchanted cynical observers, in the film, the physician is a devoted citizen who not only possesses the competence to treat diseases but also knows how to heal the community.[57]

The narration in *Pošast* is organized around the changing position of the physician with regard to the village community. The scenes set in the space in front of the mayor's office are easily interpreted as signifiers of the dramatic development of the relationship between the community and the physician. The introductory scene provides an imaginable border between the unreliable majority of inhabitants on the one hand and the mayor, who tries to cooperate with the physician, on the other. The scene in which the physician and the mayor observe the crowd of inhabitants who are going to take part in the memorial only reinforces the feeling of this rupture. In the following scene, the villagers are invited to be vaccinated and to learn more about the disease. The distance between the inhabitants of the village and the physician narrows and, eventually, disappears, at the moment he presents the sanitation plan for the whole village, which receives everyone's approval. And the very last scene features a meeting of all the inhabitants, in particular, the men, who welcome the physician as the rescuer of the village. The film claims the victory of the village's "manhood" by constructing a new holistic rural community led by progressive medicine. The educational films produced for peasants were among the novelties introduced by the School of Public Health in rural areas. All the steps taken by Štampar and his colleagues aimed at achieving a balance between the task of providing access to public health for groups of poor people and maintaining the cultural, social and economic variety of rural life in the country. The institutionalization of public health was intended to ensure accessibility of health services for those limited by their economic condition and to edify them through films and other means of health propaganda.[58] Furthermore, the system of institutions and activities was expected to be aligned with the diversity of the Yugoslav nation.

This complex mission was implemented by establishing a network of regional Institutes of Hygiene, local health centers (*Dom zdravja*, and other types of ambulant assistance. Such an organizational approach aimed to bring together practical medicine and relevant scientific investigation, not only medical research but also sociological and ethnographic studies for better understanding the needs and behavioral patterns of peasants. Health films were part of this ambitious project, and by the end of 1930, both documentary and fiction health films started to be seen as "the most powerful and successful method of health education."[59] Meanwhile, the leaders that produced health films, such as Drago Chloupek, criticized other methods, for example, popular books, citing their lack of availability to the population.[60]

The mobilization of the rural population to take part in various practices targeted at improving hygienic conditions and establishing sustainable prevention of infectious diseases relied on an idealized image of the farmer, whose overall and family life would only be improved through the increasing role of public health. This regime of national authenticity put men at the forefront as the most responsible for accepting new public health rules. Involvement in public health activities ensured that men would achieve the position of political subjects, able to make decisions and to participate in their implementation. The films for women promoted the complementary role of women as those who accepted responsibility as servants of nation-building – the films' systematic institutionalization was determined by the multifaceted frustration regarding the risk of the extinction of the rural population, the soil of the nation.

Notes

1 We maintain the original orthography of Štampar's writing.
2 Andrija Štampar, The letter To Alice Masaryková 01.03.1933, HR-HDA-831, Andrija Štampar, HR-HDA-831 Andrija Štampar, Box 11.
3 Ibid.
4 Ibid.
5 Štampar was recruited by the League of Nations for several international projects targeted at improving public health in rural areas.
6 Andrija Štampar (1913) Izvešće o pošasti Kolere u Kotaru Novogradiškom [The report about Cholera epidemic in Nova Gradiška] Ditrict HR-HDA-831 Andrija Štampar, HR-HDA-831 Andrija Štampar, Box 1.
7 Ibid.
8 Ibid.
9 Andrija Štampar, The letter To Alice Masaryková 01.03.1933, HR-HDA-831, Andrija Štampar, HR-HDA-831 Andrija Štampar, Box 11.
10 Dom Narodnog Zdravja u Mostaru 1929 Ministarstvu socialne politike i narodnog zdravja. Sanitske odelenje u Beogradu Kredit od 50000 dinar iz Kralevog Fonda za izgradnu vodenich objekata u Hercegovini [The Letter to the Ministry of social policy and public health. The Department of Hygiene in Belgrade. Credit of

50000 dinars for building water supply system in Hercegovina] Andrija Štampar, HR-HDA-831 Andrija Štampar, Box 1.

11 More about the activities of the School targeted at the modernization of buildings, both rural houses and medical institutions, can be found in Dubravka Kisić (2014) Škola narodnog zdravlja "Andrija Štampar" 1926–1939. Arhitektura i sanitarna tehnika u službi napredka [The School of Public Health "Andrija Štampar" 1926–1939. Sanitary Engineering in the Mission of progress], Zagreb: Hrvatska Akademija Znatnosti i Umjetnosti Hrvatski Muzej Arhitekture and Tamara Bjažić Klarin (2015) Ernest Weissmann: društveno angažirana arhitektura, 1926–1939 [Socially Engaged Architecture, 1926–1939]. Zagreb: Hrvatska Akademija Znanosti i Umjetnosti, Hrvatski muzej arhitekture.

12 Fraser Brockington (1958) *World Health,* London: Penguin Book p. 182.

13 Doreen Warriner (1959) Urban Thinkers and Peasant Policy in Yugoslavia, 1918–59, *The Slavonic and East European Review* 38, 90, 59–81 p. 60.

14 Alex Toshkov (2019) *Agrarianism as Modernity in 20th-Century Europe: the golden age of the peasantry,* London: Bloomsbury, p. 10.

15 Doreen Warriner (1959) Urban Thinkers and Peasant Policy in Yugoslavia, 1918–59, *The Slavonic and East European Review,* 38, 90, 59–81 p. 60.

16 Alex Toshkov, ibid., p. 10.

17 Daniel Brett (2018) Indifferent but Mobilized: Rural Politics during the Interwar Period in Eastern and Western Europe, *Central Europe,* 16:2, 65–80, p.77.

18 Andrija Štampar Untitled and undated text 9.1.3.2 HR-HDA-831 Andrija Štampar, HR-HDA-831 Andrija Štampar, Box 7.

19 Ibid, p. 79.

20 Susanne Aschenbrenner (1996) Dr. med. Marta Fraenkel, Generalsekretärin der Gesolei: Organisatorin und Schriftstellerin in der Gesundheitaufklärung [Doctor of medicine Marta Fraenkel: General Secretary and the author of health education] *in* Christoph Meinel and Monika Renneberg *Geschlechterverhältnisse in Medizin, Naturwissenschaft und Technik [Gender patterns in Medicine, natural sciences and technique]* Bassum Stuttgart Verlag für Geschichte der Naturwissenschaften und der Technik, 83–88 p. 85.

21 Marta Fraenkel 07.12.1932 The Letter to An. Štampar HR-HDA-831 Andrija Štampar, box 9.

22 Ibid.

23 Ibid.

24 Ibid.

25 Andrija Štampar 10.12.1932 The letter to Marta Fraenkel HR-HDA-831 Andrija Štampar, box 9.

26 Paul Weindling (1995) Social medicine at the League of Nations Health Organization and the International Labour Office compared in Colin Jones, Paul Weindling, Charles Rosenberg (eds.) *International Health Organisations and Movements, 1918–1939,* Cambridge: Cambridge University Press,134–149, p. 135.

27 Grażyna Szelągowska (2019) Lutheran Revival and National Education in Denmark: The Religious Background of N. F. S. Grundtvig's Educational Ideas, *Scandinavica,* 58 1, pp. 6–30.

28 Thorstein Johannes Balle (2014) Myten om Grundtvigs indflydelse på den danske folkeskole [The myth of Grundtvig's influence on the Danish public school], *Grundtvig Studier,* 65 1, pp. 65–98.

29 Andrija Štampar (1926) *Pet godina socijalno-medicinskog rada u Kraljevini Srba, Hrvata i Slovenaca* [Five years of social-medical work in the Kingdom of Serbia, Croatia and Slovenia], Zagreb p. 3.

30 Jane Lewis and Barbara Brookes, A Reassessment of the Work of the Peckham Health Centre 1926–1951, *Health and Society* 61, 2, 1983, 307–350, p. 309.

Masculinity in health films for the rural population 161

31 Andrija Štampar (1931) Hygiene auf dem Lande: Aufteilung des Programms Štampar in einzelne Darstellungen [Hygiene in the rural areas: texts' supplement of the Štampar's program to special exhibition] HR-HDA-831 Andrija Štampar, HR-HDA-831 Andrija Štampar, Box 14.

32 Vladimir Ćepulić (1940) Smjernice za suzbijanje tuberkuloze u Banovino Hrvatskoj [Guidelines for tuberculosis control in Croatia] in *Organizacija zdravstvene službe na selu Zagreb: Zbirka separatu „Liječničkog vjesnika"* [Organization of the Health Service in the Rural area Zagreb: The collection of articles of the Medical Herald], p. 1.

33 This part was inspired by French documentary *Dispensaire Léon Bourgeois: La visiteuse D'Hygiène* [Léon Bourgeois Dispensary: Visiting for Hygiene, produced between 1916 and 1917] aimed at promoting new forms of public health, including the practical demonstration of the work of visiting nurse who comes into an apartment where a man is suffering from tuberculosis and shows the family how to put the place in proper order and teaches the use of various receptacles to avoid contagion. The film had been purchased by The Red Cross for disseminating around the world in the early 1920s: The League of Red Cross Societies Geneva Switzerland 1921 Conditions concernant le prêt des films par la Ligue des sociétés de la Croix-Rouge EMVZ box 106 SNA.

34 Ćepulić, ibid., p. 3.

35 Stephen M. Whitehead (2021) *Toxic Masculinity: Curing the Virus: making men smarter, healthier, safer,* AG Books.

36 Andrea Waling (2019) Problematising 'Toxic' and 'Healthy' Masculinity for Addressing Gender Inequalities, *Australian Feminist Studies,* 34:101, pp. 362–375.

37 One of the recent examples is the book *Masculine Norms and Men's Health: Making the Connections,* by Cody Ragonese, Tim Shand, and Gary Barker, published in 2019 by the Moveber Foundation, one of the global actors aimed at promoting new norms of men's health.

38 The main realms for producing and developing the contemporary concept of toxic masculinity include different public campaigns and even cultural wars, within which the historical echo of previous cohorts of propaganda is evident but rarely followed. The topic of the transnational and global circulation of toxic masculinity in the twentieth century remains one of the open calls for historicizing the inter-relation between public health, gender politics, and popular culture.

39 An Vleugels (2013) *Narratives of Drunkenness: Belgium, 1830–1914,* London and New York: Routledge, p. 14.

40 Vleugels *Narratives of Drunkenness,* 14–15, p. 22; Hasso Spode (1993) *Die Macht der Trunkenheit: Kultur- und Sozialgeschichte des Alkohols in Deutschland* [The power of drunkeness: Cultural and social history of alcohols in Germany], Opladen: Leske und Budrich.

41 Karel Driml (1927) Přednaška pro učitele škol přihlášených k dorostu Československého Červeného Kříže [Lecture for teachers of schools engaged with the Czechoslovak Red Cross]. *Příručky dorostu Československého Červeného Kříže No. 8* [Czechoslovak Red Cross youth manuals] Prague: Zdravotnická výchova na školách [Health Education at schools] p. 17.

42 Andrija Štampar (1919) Narodna čitanka o alkoholu [People's manual about alcohol] Knižnica protiv alkoholu [Library collection against alcohol] Zagreb: Društvo apstinenata u Hrvatskoj i Slavoniji [Union of the abstinents of Croatia and Slovenia], p. 31.

43 Andrija Štampar (1919) *Narodna čitanka o alkoholu* [People Guidance about alcohol], p. 42.

44 *Birtija* Subtitles to the film. Kinoteka of the State Archives of Croatia, Fond of Škola za narodnog zdravja, box 1.

45 Alexandar Petrović (1934) *Male Pčelice: tuberkuloza i narodna medicina* [Tuberculosis and folk medicine in Male Pčelice], Belgrade: Štamparija Centralnog Higijenskog Zavoda p. 36.
46 Ćepulić, ibid.
47 *Narodna čitanka o zdravljiu* (1930) p. 57.
48 Andrija Štampar (1932) Rural Hygiene: The Draft of the Report to the League of Nation. HR-HDA-831 Andrija Štampar, box 3.
49 Kurs o boji proti tyfu pro úřední lékaře na Slovensku porádaný v Košicích v únoru 1933 [Retraining for the district physicians about the struggle against endemic typhus organized in Kosice in February, 1933] HR-HDA-831 Andrija Štampar, folder Vaček box 14.
50 Some of the stories by de Maupassant were included in an attachment to the manual about the dangers of alcohol prepared by Štampar in 1919.
51 Alberto Godioli, (2015) *Laughter from Realism to Modernism: Misfits and Humorists in Pirandello, Svevo, Palazzeschi, and Gadda,* London and New York: Routledge.
52 Benjamin Mather Woodbridge (1922) Maupassant's realism, *Texas Review*, 8, 1, 7–20 p. 16.
53 Godioli, ibid.
54 Mary Douglas (ed.) (1987) *Constructive drinking: Perspectives on Drink from Anthropology,* London and New York: Routledge p. 4.
55 Petrović *Male Pčelice* p. 83.
56 Douglas, ibid., p. 8.
57 Algirdas Julien Greimas (1988) *Maupassant: the Semiotics of Text. Practical Exercises*, Amsterdam: John Benjamins Publishing Company.
58 Dom Narodnog Zdravja u Plevlu (1929) Ministarstvu socialne politike i narodnog zdravja. Higienicke odelenje [The letter to the Ministry of Social Policy and Public Health. The Department of Hygiene] Andrija Štampar, HR-HDA-831 Andrija Štampar, Box 1.
59 Andrija Štampar (1925) *Socijalna medicina. Uz saradnju jugoslovenskih socijalnih lekara* [Social medicine: From the experinece of Yugoslav physicians] First volume Zagreb: Institut za socijalnu medicinu p. 281.
60 Željko Dugac (2010) *Kako biti čist i zdrav. Zdravstveno prosvjećivanje u međuratnoj Hrvatskoj* [How to be clean and healthy. Health education in interwar Croatia], Zagreb: Srednja Europa p. 70. In 1929 Milan Marjanović filmed the exhibition about hygienic rules for making it more accessible for rural population: *Higijenska izložba* [Hygienic exhibition] ŠNZ 1929 Subtitles to the film. Kinoteka of the State Archives of Croatia, Fond of Škola za narodnog zdravja, box 1.

10   Health films in the service of eugenic surveillance over women

Eugenic patriarchalism in child welfare propaganda

-No girl will refuse us, choose any!
-I want the best, father!
-Who is the best?
-Well, who has the prettiest face?!
-Well, no, son, this is not enough, a girl should be the best in everything.
-I want Yoka, she has a pretty face
-Yes, but she has scrofula marks.
-But in clothes it is not visible.
-Even a latent disease remains a disease.
-What about Yela?
-She is pretty, but she has no breasts, she is all of twenty, and she is flat as a board.
-Well, Marie, beautiful and sweet as a green flower
-Just about green, bent, as if not a drop of blood is present – this one will give birth to two children for you and become an old woman![1]

This dialogue, between the rich farmer Ilja Gotovac and Nikolica, his first-born, written by Dinko Šimunović,[2] continues further – in the very first pages of *Narodna čitanka o zdravlju* (*National book of health*), the book aims at educating the rural population of Yugoslavia regarding how to be healthy. One of the possible interpretations of this text is "making women directly placed on the edges of the symbolic order"[3] in interwar Yugoslavia. But the eugenic pathos of this text, as well as the many other products of health propaganda addressed to women, stress their physical condition; features of their figure and their habits are assessed in terms of readiness to give birth to healthy children.

Women were not on the margins of health propaganda – they embodied the position of the primary "others," whose submission would ensure the salvation of an entire people. In 1933, Štampar was welcomed by Czechoslovak authorities and experts to present lectures for the public as well as for those in

DOI: 10.4324/9781003272267-14

the medical professions. Personally, Štampar prioritized women as his key audience and highlighted women's issues, not only within Yugoslavia but also abroad. In his letter to Bohumil Vacek, the head of the Institute of Hygiene in Prague, he wrote: "In Zlín, as well as in Turčiansky Martin, I will exclusively speak about the topic 'Woman and the people's health,' for female audiences. I have prepared new films that shed light on the everyday issues of people's health that are important."[4]

The films that addressed women stemmed from the mission to educate them, as well as the practical task of making them more obedient to new hygienic rules. In Yugoslavia, women, especially those in rural areas, represented the most uneducated part of the population: In 1926, in rural areas, more than 80 percent of women were illiterate, and in some areas, there were no educated women at all.[5] Despite the complex causes underlying the high rates of infant mortality and decreasing natality, health propaganda brought forward the illiteracy of women and their lack of health competencies as the central obstacles to ensuring child welfare. Štampar situated the level of education of mothers among such factors as income, legal status and place of birth for explaining the mortality of infants,[6] which was comparable among poor mothers and illiterate mothers, 30 percent and 25.6 percent, respectively. According to his data, only 10 percent of children among educated workers died before one year, but the proportion rose to 20 percent among workers who were not educated. Health films aimed at teaching women to care for children played a central role in the overall strategy for auxiliary medical education targeted at rural women.

It is difficult to judge whether propaganda outstripped institutionalization or the films intended to delegate some competencies to mothers because of the systematic lack of institutionalized childcare in the first half of the 1930s.[7] The films *Terenska sestra* (Visiting nurse, 1929), *Seljačko sveučilište Škole narodnog zdravija: ženski tečaj (*Peasant's university of the School of Public Health: Women's course 1929*), Blago kući gdje se žena uči* (Wellbeing of home where women are learning, 1936) directly taught rural women to utilize certain elements of medical knowledge.

Endowing a woman with the competence of a doctor was not a novelty of the interwar period. *Die Ärztin im Hause* (The house doctor, 1910) by Jenny Springer was translated into Czech, Serbo-Croatian and Polish, and enjoyed great success in Eastern Europe. Along with guidance prepared by physicians, since the last quarter of the nineteenth century, magazines for women published short instructive articles of conduct fiction aimed at educating their readers (mainly middle-class women) on how to apply the most progressive practices of proper care for children.

The institutionalization of childcare, which began in Western Europe and North America in the late nineteenth century, and reached its peak during the interwar period, was accompanied by various strategies of health education targeted at reaching women from the most vulnerable social groups. The institutionalization of caring for young children went hand-in-hand with films on relevant topics, which not only disseminated new information, but also motivated both women and the public to become part of the institutionalization process.

Bringing it home (1919), one of the first films aimed at propagating the *infant welfare station,* a new organizational approach to caring for not only poor children but for all children in the periphery,[8] tells the story of retrogradely thinking Mr. Clarkson, a wealthy business owner. Clarkson is opposed to the establishment of an infant welfare station. When he visits a local fair, he bypasses the exhibition on care for children because all his attention is devoted to livestock, as long as his granddaughter is healthy, that is. But when she becomes sick, and the physician says that the issue could have been prevented if the mother of the child would have been taught to properly care for the child, Mr. Clarkson offers financial support for childcare in his homeland. The documentary part of the film presents the activities of the infant welfare station, juxtaposing examples of unsanitary methods of care with proper care such as dressing, bottle-feeding and protecting children from flies.[9]

Our children (1921), commissioned by the Child Welfare Bureau in Gadsden, Alabama, "shows various types of community work for child welfare and a children's health conference by representatives of the children's bureau."[10] The film introduces to mothers the work of visiting nurses, teaching them to measure the height and weight of their children and familiarizing them with the operation of Babies' Days, a regular action by the Red Cross, during which babies could be measured at the Red Cross nursing office.

Parentage (1919) tells the story of two boys and their destinies, as determined by their early education and care. It presents two families, the Smiths, whose love for their son manifests in providing proper care for little Robert, and the Browns, whose son, Horace, is stunted in mind and body, a pale shrinking boy because he is not welcomed or cared for by his parents. The film follows the difference in the development and growth of both boys up until the moment they should take responsibility for their families and become successors to their fathers. The film emphasizes the role of cooperation with public health institutions as the signifier of a responsible attitude toward their own health and the health of future generations: When Robert and Horace decide to marry, their future fathers-in-law asks both to pass a premarital examination, and Horace refuses. The incredible success of *Parentage* can be explained by its realistic approach in depicting "purity, love, unselfishness. It is a portrayal of everyday life in the home - a chance to see ourselves as others see us."[11]

Being included on the list of films recommended by the Red Cross for international dissemination, *Parentage* and other two films[12] inspired the authors of *Dvije seke: film o njezi dojenčadi,* (Two sisters: A film about caring for infants, 1932), to adapt emotive realism in depicting the differences between proper and improper care. *Dvije seke* was one of the most popular films produced by the Film Laboratory of the School of Public Health. By the end of the 1930s, this film was shown in the majority of Balkan countries, as well as in Czechoslovakia, the United States, Germany and France. The film consists of three parts and continues for more than 35 minutes.

Sentimental health education in *Dvije seke: film o njezi dojenčadi*

The first part of *Dvije seke* introduces the farmer Joža, who has twins. Mara and Bara have grown up in the shadow of the premature death of their mother. They move with scythes on their shoulders through the field belonging to their father – toward their maturity: The camera shows young girls, then teenagers, and, finally, two young women who smile at each other and at their father. They happily fall in love, and the schoolteacher approvingly asks Joža: "Will they soon expect an addition to the family in your house?" Not occasionally, this dialogue occurs with a church in the background, and the teacher's proposal to send the girls to a family preparation school should be seen as a continuation of his approving attitude toward developing relationships in a "proper" way. The hesitation of the father, who takes off his hat, scratches the back of his head, and replies thoughtfully, "This is something to consider," creates the opportunity for the teacher to showcase for the father and for the audience the main goals of the school.[13] The father practically orders his daughters to go to the school, to which Mara reacts: "How great that we will spend time there!" Meanwhile, Bara grows gloomy and refuses to attend – she fears for her relationship with her prospective bridegroom. In response to Bara's fears, that Ivan will leave her while she prepares to become an ideal wife, Mara replies: "And for me, if Pero leaves me, let him be carried away! It is better now than later that the man deceives!" This exchange, likely the first mutual contest, is accompanied by a sarcastic comment in the film's subtitles: "Bara stays to guard the guy." Mara, in turn, travels to the big city to be trained as a perfect mother and housekeeper.

In the second part of the film, Mara arrives at the school. The camera work takes on a significant symbolic load - Mara is shown from top to bottom and, gradually, the camera moves in on a close-up – as she progresses in mastering the intricacies of housekeeping and caring for a child. The audience is invited to live with Mara during a lecture on the main causes of death of young children, along with classes in gardening, sewing, weaving, cooking and caring for sick members of the family. The most dramatic facts are accompanied by a close-up of Mara's bewildered, frightened or worried face. The lecture attacks the most disseminated (according to the experts) unhealthy practices, such as coughing on a child, kissing a child even if ill or suspicious of being ill, wrapping the child up and restricting movement and treating with a distillate to calm a child. The motto, "mothers who do not know and do not apply hygienic rules sow death over their children," is central. Mara sends a letter to her family, which Joža shares with Bara in the hope that she will change her mind about the school, but to no avail. This part of the film ends with a wedding scene that mixes fiction and documentary content about the traditions of collective celebration, featuring dances and music. Then, the viewers witness the pride of Joža in being the fresh grandfather of two young boys.

In the third part of *Dvije seke*, the contest between the two sisters reaches its zenith because of their mutually opposed approaches to caring for their sons. One of the encounters, which begins with Bara's question concerning whether Mara bathes her son everyday, develops into a conflict. Bara reproaches her sister for striving to rise above all the women in the village, saying that no one needs her sermons and everyone is tired of her. Mara only states the fact that her nephew would benefit from the best care and that he is currently weakened. The offended Bara claims that her child is no worse off than others and quarrels with her sister. Mara is upset by the confrontation with her sister, but her worries about her child and her husband consume all of her attention. The viewers then observe the outputs of proper and improper care for children. Remarkably, the film devotes more than twice the screen time, nine minutes, to positive examples than for a negative example, taking up only about four minutes. For instance, for more than two minutes, the camera follows how Mara bathes and wipes the baby. The audience can observe the unbridled enthusiasm with which Mara puts into practice her acquired knowledge – the expression on her face mixes pride and joy. The feeling of self-confidence is reinforced by the constant close-ups of the baby being bathed, walked and fed, presenting a persuasive scenario of a realistic picture of happiness.

Bara makes only "improper" decisions – she breastfeeds her son without giving him complementary foods and then gives him cow's milk. But her key mistake is not to seek help from a doctor or her sister but instead to ask for advice from rural healers. The old women healers convince Bara that Mara has jinxed her son and put a curse on him. In despair, Bara chews a piece of bread, wraps it in a napkin, soaks it in brandy and gives it to her son, who continues to cry hysterically but sucks the "medicine." Then, he dies. Mara consoles her sister: "When the apples are ripe, you will have a new son, and you will take care of him properly." The sisters reconcile – and together they harvest wheat. At the very end of the film, a happy Mara feeds her son with cherries against the background of a wheat field.

Dvije seke should be seen as not only a part of the propaganda about new competencies needed for responsible mothers but also as embedded in the massive public campaign aimed at promoting motherhood. Despite all her mistakes, Bara is a devoted mother who just needs to be more educated and emancipated from the "backwardness" of previous generations of rural women, in favor of "natural" progress. Healthy maternal instincts among women started to be seen as a main precondition for the proper care of biological and fostered children, especially young children.[14] This message is reinforced by multiple analogies between children and plants. For instance, in exploring the importance of the sun for the prevention of rickets, the nurse at school shows two plants, one growing with sunlight and one without. The cycle of giving birth is harmonized with the change of seasons: When the cherry trees blossom, when the wheat is ripe, when the apples are ready.

The naturalness of "proper" care reverberates with another message of the film, namely, the call for women to achieve and maintain peace of mind through the acquisition of competencies. The main difference between the two sisters is the measure of their psychological stability. While Mara is self-confident and ready to take risks, Bara has a long way to go in the task of becoming a balanced woman. Notably, Mara is performed by Krunoslava Ebrić-Frlić, the actor often recruited to represent such confident characters in other films: The teacher in *Spas male Zorice* (Save little Zorica), Anka in *Birtija* or Maca in *Griješnice: Macina i Ankina sudbina* (Sinners: Maca and Anka's destiny, 1930). Bara is more often portrayed as crying or trying to deal with difficult situations from the position of a dependent child, rather than a responsible woman. Connecting new competencies with the psycho-logical comfort of women, a main motivational component of the film, cre-ates a dichotomy of healthy and toxic femininity, reinforced in another film that addressed women and their mission to reproduce the nation – *Griješnice: Macina i Ankina sudbina*.

Criminalizing abortion in *Griješnice: Macina i Ankina sudbina*

The motto, "Not the owner who has a bull, but one who has a son," with which *Griješnice: Macina i Ankina sudbina* opens defines the main idea of abortion as a betrayal of men's vital interests by irresponsible women. The reason behind the dramatic decrease in natality around the world was, according to the interwar experts, a consequence of the Great war and the economic crisis.[15] But in *Griješnice*, as in many other products of pronatalist propaganda, the selfish behavior of women, who are afraid to lose their beauty after giving birth, was the main explanation for "depopulation," a risk that had started to be ex-pressed by many European experts since the late 1920s.[16]

The film is set in Slavonia, a Croatian region considered one of the main centers for migration, which was not welcomed by the experts in the School of Public Health: "These immigrants for the most part settled in primitive dwellings and had no knowledge of modern methods of agriculture. As a consequence, they suffered many setbacks."[17] This totally alarmist sentiment is presented to viewers as a part of the *Narodna čitanka o zdravlju*: "As soon as a woman stops giving birth, this leads people to the abyss and [the nation] is filled with foreigners." But the main protagonists of the film *Griješnice*, the young widow Maca and her friend Anka, who is in a *pokusni brak*[18] with the handsome Stipa, only scoff at the *Čitanka's* declaration (see Figure 10.1) as opposed to proper, serious, reading of this manual by future mothers of the nation (Figure 10.2). In response to the call to have at least three children, or four, or even a maximum of six, Maca exclaims: "God forbid me six [chil-dren]; that would definitely be God's punishment." In the end, she, along with Anka, is punished for not wanting even one child.

The film tells the story of the moral fall of both women – Maca because of her irresistible desire to please and Anka because she has been corrupted by

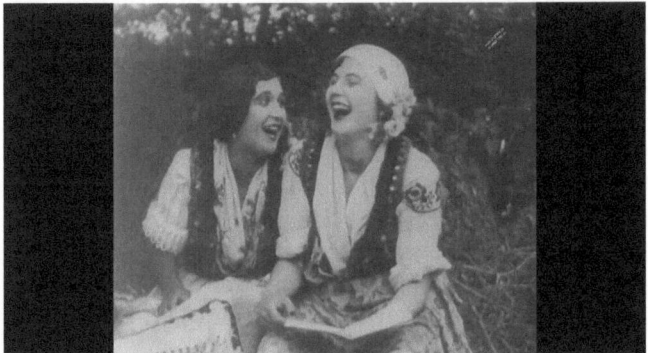

Figure 10.1 Ignorance of knowledge as a sin in *Griješnice: Macina i Ankina sudbina* (Sinners: Maca and Anka's destiny, 1930).

Source: Kinoteka HAD.

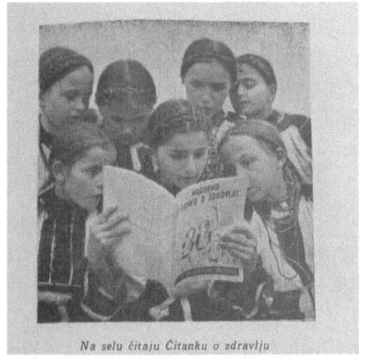

Figure 10.2 Commitment to health knowledge: rural girls read *Narodna čitanka o zdravlju*.

Source: Andrija Štampar Zdravlje i društvo (Health and society, 1929) p. 129.

Maca and convinced to have an abortion. In the film, Maca rushes between two partners. One is Boža, a reveler and womanizer who is not married. The name of her probationary husband remains unknown, which only stresses the disorder in Maca's life, persistently noted by Manda, Maca's mother, who characterizes her daughter as "unrestrained." Boža seduces Maca when she is washing clothes in the river – frankly erotic flirting, depicted in detail, aims to persuade viewers that lust is the only motive for their relationship. At some point, the camera focuses on the reflection of both in the river – which is carried away by the current, reinforcing Manda's dramatic prediction that Maca will be carried away and nothing will be left of her.

While Maca is nearing her imminent moral decline, Anka is enjoying her new life as Stipa's probationary wife –she takes care of the livestock, cleans the house and loves Stipa. Anka becomes pregnant and Stipa is happy with the prospect of being a father, but when she shares her fears that "children steal a mother's beauty," Maca convinces her to have an abortion. The dialogue takes place in the same location in which Maca first met Boža and where their relationship began, which only emphasizes one of the moral precepts of the film: Women are corrupted by men in order to corrupt other women. In her time, Maca was corrupted by Malča, a woman who trades in clandestine abortions and who is described as a sinner and a procuress. Self-interest and profit are Malča's main motives, and when Maca explains to Anka that she must pay to "get rid of the burden," the audience sees a satisfied Malča, who surreptitiously watches the young women, and, in anticipation of the money she will earn, strokes herself on the chest.

Another man in the village, Jole, becomes a witness to how Maca practically drags Anka into Malča's yard, and he easily understands what is about to happen. The following Sunday, when Anka goes to church, Jole starts extorting money in exchange for his silence about the abortion. Because she does not have any money, Jole asks Anka for her necklace made of ducats (silver or gold coins), one of the elements in traditional women's costumes. The documentary part of the film shows how prestigious it is to wear a well-decorated necklace of ducats, and viewers observe the flow of young women wearing such necklaces, with obvious pride in possessing one. Anka surrenders her necklace as a pledge of Jole's silence, but the next day, when she comes to buy back the jewelry, the blackmailer takes the money and refuses to return the necklace, saying that he is not a fool. Anka belittles him but without result. Moreover, Stipa catches them together and creates a scene of jealousy.

Anka is waiting for punishment, leaning against an unfinished fence – which only reinforces the perception of her as a victim crucified by her own mistakes. To shed the suspicion of betrayal, she confesses that she has had an abortion. Stipa is disappointed, and Anka wants to become pregnant again. In despair, she rushes to Malča and asks for her help to become pregnant again; Malča advises "folk remedies," in which even a desperate woman dares not believe. Then Anka turns to a doctor, who confirms the terrible diagnosis – she will never become a mother. Even Anka's prayers do not help – and the previously spontaneous happiness with Stipa disappears. In his every gesture, look and word, both Anka and the audience recognize condemnation and anger at Anka, who has betrayed him. Anka is totally deprived when Stipa abandons her with the words that there is no meaning in marriage without children. In the following scene, Anka discloses that Stipa has relationship with another girl, who would like to bear him a son. The last word from Stipa to Anka is *nerotkinja,* "infertile," and Anka rushes into the river – at the very same place that Boža flirted with Maca, and Maca persuaded Anka to have an abortion. Maca dies of blood poisoning after another abortion; in her dying scene, the viewers discover that she is Manda's only child, which only reinforces the message that one must have more children.

The film exploits a wide range of analogies for demonstrating to the viewers how fine the line is between vice and innocent entertainment, which becomes dangerous "if only the heads of young people are busy with this," an exhortation by the old men of the village when they observe Maca and Boža. *Griješnice* includes two scenes of collective dancing; one is a round dance initiated by Boža in front of the local pub, to celebrate the seduction of Maca, and the other occurs in front of the church on Sunday. The dance near the pub, emphatically polished, with a solo performed by professional dancers, is clearly perceived as overkill, which symbolizes a false sense of femininity. In contrast, the round dance at the church – in which Maca does not participate, unlike the pub dance, is rather a collective practice of togetherness, clearly evocative of true femininity.

The exaggerated drama of *Griješnice*, aimed at convincing viewers that abortion is a crime against the nation, is compatible with the expressiveness of another film about abortion, *Frauennot – Frauenglück* (The misery and fortune of women, 1930), produced by Soviet filmmakers Sergej Eisenstein and Grigori Alexandrov for the Swiss film company Praesens-Film AG. *Frauennot – Frauenglück* attacked the practice of illegal abortion, defined by the unhappiness of women, as compared to the perfectly organized and safe procedure for interrupting a pregnancy in a clinic. Verging on a Malthusian approach, *Frauennot – Frauenglück* presents safe abortion as the only option for women of the working class who already have more than enough children or who lose their family's breadwinner.[19]

The scandalous popularity of *Frauennot – Frauenglück*, which attracted the attention of female activists in many European countries,[20] inclines us to interpret *Griješnice* as a response to the Swiss film, in which the message was diametrically opposed to the pronatalist stance of the Croatian film. Moreover, the intention to subject women to new medical practices depicted in *Frauennot – Frauenglück* was compatible with the aims of health propaganda produced by the School of Public Health. In contrast to the totally misogynistic *Griješnice, Frauennot – Frauenglück* does not construct the dichotomy of "proper" and "improper" femininity. Abortion was constructed not in terms of a crime against nations but against humanity: The statistical data presented at the beginning of *Frauennot – Frauenglück* describe the consequences of clandestine abortions for the health and life of women in all of Europe.

The coexistence of these films in the interwar European cinematic space cannot be separated from the struggle between two approaches to birth control, which had engulfed both the national and global levels of the health security regime since the late 1920s. While female activists and some physicians, especially those affiliated with leftist movements, promoted access for women to regulate their desire to have children,[21] pro-natalists worked at criminalizing abortion.[22] Notwithstanding the strong position of pro-natalists, including Štampar[23] himself, interwar Yugoslavia introduced at the end of the 1920s, quite liberal legal regulations regarding abortion that seriously limited the options for punishing women and those who helped them.[24] The echo of this defeat is evident in *Griješnice*, in which the village community remains totally powerless in their attempt to call Malča to account: Old men try to stop her by threatening to go to the police, but she responds with a threat to the threat and nothing happens.

Remarkably, some restrictions on abortion, such as tougher punishment for unmarried mothers engaging in abortion or infanticide, were introduced within the regulations on children without legal representatives in 1934. This regulation fostered the conservative backlash in the politics of birth control provided by *Ustaaše*,[25] accompanied by a flourishing discourse on the naturalness of motherhood and true femininity. Czech health films that addressed women adapted this discourse for approaching not rural but urban working-class women.

Eugenic pronatalism in *Manželství pod drobnohledem*

"The first of our children will replace the father, the second perhaps me, and the third - this will strengthen our nation. We won't die out."[26] These final words of a nameless Czech mother, the main character in *Manželství pod drobnohledem* (Marriage under the microscope, 1940), facing the rising sun after a sleepless night at the bedside of her ill first-born, sum up the main message of the population policy typical (not only) of the Second Republic.[27] *Manželství pod drobnohledem*, "a film calling for population growth,"[28] tells the story not of people – but of informal institutions such as the family or childhood, and formal institutions such as maternity hospitals, centers for maternal and children's health, or vocational counseling centers, which should be aligned with each other for implementing the mission of reproducing the population.

One of the most remarkable features of this film is the anonymity of the protagonists, who remain "she," "he" and "son," as opposed to the public care institutions, which have names and addresses. One of the movie posters depicts a doctor who is watching "him" and "her" under a microscope. The film's protagonists are described by three interrelated social roles: Gender, family membership and professionality. Even the little boy has a professional dream, to become a pilot; he is sent by his father for vocational consultation. Only one personal detail matters: The number of siblings the protagonists have, representing an argument in the contest for having more or less children.

The opening of the film features shots of human legs walking in the park from different angles; the story starts from the moment when two pairs, "his" and "hers," meet. The courtship phase is the shortest section of the film, but during these five minutes, the audience learns that "she" is a seamstress and "he" is a worker, and that the main gift for their future children would be better knowledge about health and reproductive functions. The recommendation to undergo a premarital medical consultation is depicted through the rotation of the two bodies against the background of the physician's eyes.

On the morning after the wedding, the newlyweds, who have settled in the suburbs, are walking and observing the triumph of fertility in nature: A duck with chicks and a pig with a brood of piglets suckling their mother's milk. The viewers then witness the passionate kiss of a young couple, and the camera delicately pans toward the tall trees and the sky. As in stories with a dual focus narrative, in *Manželství pod drobnohledem*, "Human rhythms are no longer subservient to those of nature; nature instead reflects the decisions of each individual. The world becomes a speculum, a mirror in which men and women see the values of their own consciences reflected."[29] With a modest smile, "she" informs "him" that they will become parents, and during one of the first visits to the gynecologist, the future mother asks the physician: "How will the life of my begin?" The answer takes more than 32 minutes. This one-third of the film is devoted to a detailed description of the development of the fetus, including various comments on potential deformities and the role of the mother in preventing such deformities during the intrauterine development of the child. This part of the film features many visual and discursive matches with the famous U.S. film, *Birth*, produced by a eugenic film company in 1917[30] and well-known among Czech public health experts.[31]

The detailed reproduction of the procedure for preparing a doctor to deliver a child cultivates trust in public care and its power. Critics enthusiastically described the realism achieved by the film in depicting the birth, including the fact that Eva Listová, the performer of the role of the mother, as well as the film's production crew, were constantly in the maternity hospital in order to depict the moment of birth.[32] Mentioning the fact that Listová's mother was congratulated on the addition to the family[33] only reinforced the link among the film, reality and the behavior of women desirable for the nation.

In contrast, the detailed depiction in *Dvije seke* of the hygiene procedures conducted with a newborn as the basis of his health shifts the focus from the decisive role of the mother to the role of medical staff and institutions. Even the introductory words stress the important role of public health: "The main threats to the child are the mother's ignorance of basic hygiene rules and the limited prerequisites for the healthy development of poor families." There are no instructive scenes featuring a mother caring for a child, except for a demonstration of breastfeeding, accompanied by information about devices for feeding weak children. This scene almost immediately turns into a story about helping sick and premature babies who must be placed in an institution. The detailed description of care ends with a depiction of the training for nursing the child, including its aims and duration, "decisive for efficient operation of maternity and child care."

Instead of scenes depicting caring, the mother sings a lullaby that attracts the attention of a passerby, an elderly person who quietly sings while standing at the window and gazing with tenderness at the stroller with the baby. This peaceful family scene contrasts with the one just prior, in which an older couple is seen spending time in a restaurant - without joy, but instead with boredom and mutual irritation. Like *Pramen lásky*, another health film by Kokeisl (see Chapter 8), *Manželství pod drobnohledem* contrasts the older generation, poisoned by unhealthy habits and unable to save the nation, with the younger generation, which shows hope. The film was intentionally opposed to the previous so-called "sexual films," defined as an "an aphrodisiac for older gentlemen, films that were made for commerce rather than science, from which fragments had to be cut in order to preserve morality."[34]

The film then approaches its central issue, the number of children in a family. While the mother, following her healthy instinct, seeks to give birth to a second child, the father, fearing economic difficulties, sharply objects: "I don't even want to talk about it." And only the unexpected illness of the son, who nearly dies, may make him reconsider and become an ally of his wife. The fading of hope, and then its return due to the successful outcome of the disease, is portrayed through the analogy of life with a candle burning more or less intensely and then blurring with the daylight. This analogy, in combination with the lack of information on what kind of disease the boy has experienced, only reinforces the approach to the family as an informal institution that passes through particular situations determined by formal institutions.

The scene depicting the celebration of Mother's Day is a remarkable example of constructing family life as an informal institution aimed at translating "proper" regulations. The main character calls her mother to ask that she visit them, and upon her arrival, gives her a bouquet of flowers; the son, seeing a gesture of affection, gives his mother a flower in a pot. While the filmmakers weigh in on the side of the mother's instinct, they demonstrate perfectly the operating system for institutional support of children and mothers, even those who are poor.

The film takes six minutes to introduce the counseling center for mothers and children, designed to convince the audience of the need to rely on the hands and heads of specialists. A daycare center, a sanatorium and a special care unit for premature infants are shown as machinery that should persuade "a modern woman to find her mission in the family and children and to win despite all the hardships and uncertainties of society."[35] The participation of the father in raising his son is also embedded in the institutional design of care: He is interested in the professional choice of his child and in the proper evaluation of the child's abilities. The scene portrayed in a psychotechnics laboratory, which alternates between showing several children and several types of psychological tests to determine different abilities, becomes another element of "the institutional empire caring for children and their future."

The institutional power of childcare is aligned in the film with the long-term consequences of images of collective childhood aimed at establishing a strong analogy between children and the people on the one hand, and childcare and the state on the other. The mode of collective identity dominates in depicting the children: More than seven minutes are devoted to showing the various group activities of children in the park. Like the protagonists, the groups of children are shown through the lenses of gender and age difference: The film presents the most suitable group activities for older and younger boys and girls. Even the tempo of the musical accompaniment changes: Slow for girls and fast for boys.

Manželství pod drobnohledem continues to implement the mission of routinizing the institutions that aim to provide surveillance over reproduction and childrearing introduced by another film for women, *Procitnutí ženy* (Recognizing the woman, 1925). This film mostly focuses on womanhood as an informal institution that would require systematic institutionalization from the birth of the woman until her death, through the strong affiliation of women with different services and entities. *Procitnutí ženy* does not introduce any particular person – but women of different age groups united within particular institutionalized practices (see Figures 10.3–10.5). According to the

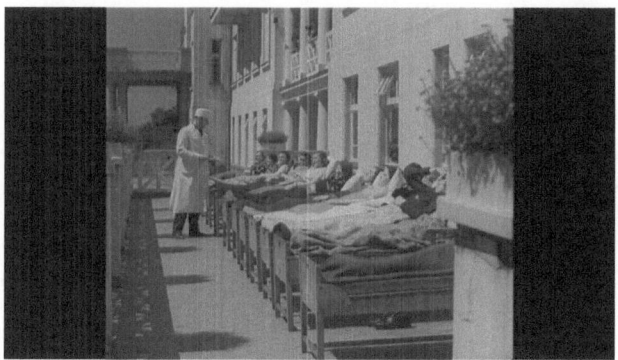

Figure 10.3 Physician supervises women in sanatorium *Procitnutí ženy* (Recognizing the woman, 1925).

Source: NFA.

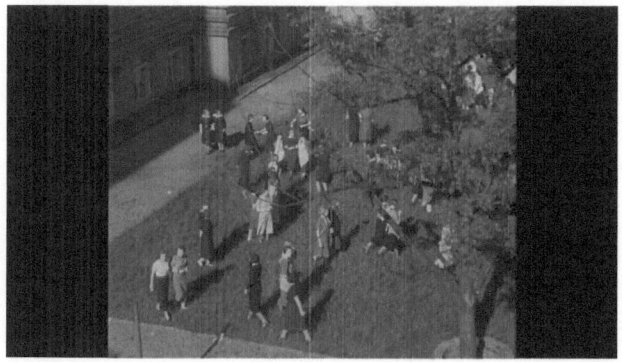

Figure 10.4 Městská odborná škola pro ženská povolaní (City school for female occupations) *Procitnutí ženy* (Recognizing the woman, 1925).

Source: NFA.

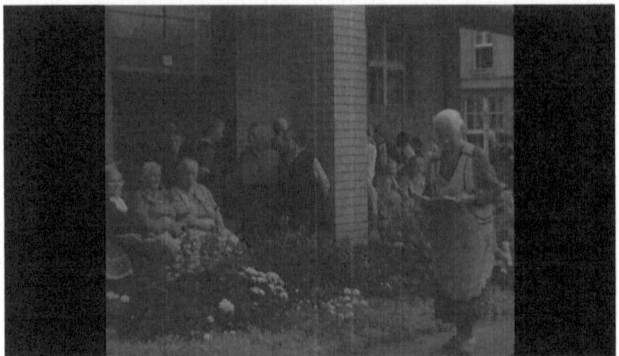

Figure 10.5 Residential care institution for elderly women in *Procitnutí ženy* (Recognizing the woman, 1925).

Source: NFA.

film's authors, it was inspired by the idea of producing a film that would act as a journal for women: "Unlike heavy German films, our directing tries to present the scenes vividly and diversely; for example, after the scientific part, examples are immediately given. To connect science and life – not to address only a cold fact to the brain, but also a warm word to the heart – that was the idea of our authors."[36]

In late 1933, Procitnutí ženy was purchased by Bayern authorities with the goal of educating the public, and women in particular. The film was censored to exclude any overly explicit display of internal organs,[37] but the main content remained, which only reaffirms the suitability of this approach for audiences in different countries. Subjecting informal practices and institutions such as childhood, family life, or womanhood to public health was reflected in the depersonalization of the main characters and their transformation into ant personalities that differed only slightly from each other. This way of constructing the other had achieved its peak in the films produced for the periphery.

Notes

1 *Narodna čitanka o zdravljiu* (1930) p. 10.
2 Dinko Šimunović (1873–1933) was a Croatian teacher and writer famous for his overtly patriarchal views and their promotion in fiction and public activities.
3 Dejan Durić (2012) Patrijarhat, rod i pripovijetke Dinka Šimunovića [Patriarchat, gender, short stories by Dinko Šimunović] *Croatica et Slavica Iadertina* 8 1, 259–276.
4 Andrja Štampar Letter to Vacek 11.01.1933 HR-HDA-831 Andria Štampar, box 14.
5 Andrija Štampar Maternal and child welfare in Yugoslavia. The updated draft of the presentation HR-HDA-831 Andrija Štampar, box 3.

6 More about the complex causes of infant mortality in rural areas can be found in Kristina Popova (2011) Combating infant mortality in Bulgaria Welfare activities, national propaganda and the establishment of pediatrics 1900–1940 in Christian Promitzer, Sevasti Trubeta and Marius Turda (eds.) *Health, Hygiene and Eugenics in Southeastern Europe to 1945,* Budapest: CEU Press, pp.143–164.

7 The rural population was not protected by social insurance. Only in Zagreb and Ljubljana were consultation clinic for mothers established before 1918. In fact, until the middle of the 1930s only four institutions, in Skopje, Zagreb, Belgrade, and Ljubljana, were able to provide sustainable assistance to mothers and children. See more in Alojzia Štebi (1935) Les devoire et la collaboration des *banovinas,* des districts, et des autres institutions administratives et autonomes pour la protection des enfants de la campagne [Collaboration of banates, districts, and other administrative and autonomous institutions for the protection of rural children] Archiv of Yugoslavia Fond 39 Ministarstvo Socijalne Politike a narodnog zdravlja 1919–1945, box 7, folder 2.

8 Frederic J. Haskin Better care for babies. Altoona Tribune (Altoona, Pennsylvania), 13.05.1916, p. 8.

9 Programmer for Child welfare week. Buffalo Morning Express and Illustrated Buffalo Express (Buffalo, New York), 21.09.1919.

10 Many fail to clean alleys. Inspection shows germ breeding places yet untouched warning issued. The Republican News Journal (Newkirk, Oklahoma), 28.04.1922, p. 1.

11 Lawrence Daily Journal-World (Lawrence, Kansas), 25.12.1920, p. 5.

12 The League of Red Cross Societies Geneva Switzerland (1921) Conditions concernant le prêt des films par la Ligue des sociétés de la Croix-Rouge EMVZ, box 106 SNA.

13 *Megu idniti domakinki* (Among future housewives), produced by the Institute of Hygiene in Skopje, was another example of men's benevolent paternalism regarding the health education of their daughters. The documentary was accompanied by subtitles written not for school-aged girls but for those who had sent their daughters, granddaughters or sisters, namely, men: "Our grandmothers studied with their grandmothers and our youth can study in the school." The film ends with a scene in which the students bring the pies they have prepared at school to their grandmothers, who taste the pastries with approval and thanks. Megu budućim domaćicama [Among future housewives] Subtitles to the film. Kinoteka of the State Archives of Croatia, Fond of Škola za narodnog zdravja, box 2.

14 Mica Trbojević (1935) Le rôle de la paysanne dans le placement familial rural des infants [The role of rural women in the substitute family palcement of infants] Congrès *balkanique* de *protection* de l'Enfance, Archiv of Yugoslavia Fond 39 Ministarstvo Socijalne Politike a narodnog zdravlja 1919–1945, box 7 folder 2.

15 The causes of infant mortality and depopulation varied from region to region, but lack of education remained one of the central concerns that connected "proper" care for children and "proper" pronatalist behavior: "There is, of course, a general tendency towards a falling birthrate, but data covering the period 1930–34 tend to show that the worsening of social-economic conditions affected the birthrate; an abrupt decline occurred during this period. The birthrate was 35,50 in 1930 and only 31,45 in 1934". Andrija Štampar (1936) Maternal and child welfare in Yugoslavia the draft of the presentation HR-HDA-831 Andrija Štampar, box 3.

16 Friedrich Burgdörfer, an influential German demographer, attracted the attention to decreasing natality and his monumental monograph, *Volk ohne Jugend. Geburtenschwund und Überalterung des deutschen Volkskörpers. Ein Problem der Volkswirtschaft - der Sozialpolitik der nationalen Zukunft* [People without youth. Declining birth rates and aging of the Germans. A problem of the national

economy - the social policy of the future of nation] (Berlin, Vowinckel. 1932), was adopted by several Eastern European experts, including Slovak pediatrician Alojz Chura, who published a two-volume study with practically an identical title *"Slovensko bez dorastu?: sociálne-paediatrické štúdium"* [Slovakia without youth: socially-pediatric study] in 1936 or by Andrija Štampar, who not only enthusiastically accepted the appoach to collect data regarding demographic changes but also expressed general alarmism typical of the publications by Burgdörfer. The visible influence of this German expert on increasing pronatalist stances in the international agenda remains an open field for exploration.

17 Andrija Štampar (1936) *Maternal and child welfare in Yugoslavia*. The draft of the presentation HR-HDA-831 Andrija Štampar, box 3.

18 Trial marriage, cohabitation without official registration of relations until the birth of a child, was common practice for rural Croatia and Slovenia; see more in Vera Ehrlich (1964) *Obitelj u transformaciji: studija u tri stotine jugoslavenskih sela* [Family in Transformation: Study in Three Hundred Yugoslav Villages], Zagreb: Naprijed, pp. 140–144.

19 This motif was not exclusive to the film. In the second half of the 1920s, the fiction genre began to address birth control and to draw public attention to the unresolved issue of how to preserve the dignity, health, and life of a woman who did not want to have children. It is noteworthy that one of the first popular writers to touch on this topic was an American of Slovenian origin, Louis Adamić: Beth Widmaier Capo (2004) Can This Woman Be Saved? Birth Control and Marriage in Modern American Literature, *Modern Language Studies*, 34, 1/2, pp. 28–41.

20 Kai Nowak (2012) Mütterlichkeit und Mutterschaft. Der Filmskandal um "Frauennot-Frauenglück" (1929/30) [Motherliness and Motherhood. The scandal around The Misery and Fortune of Women (1929/30)], *Ariadne. Forum für Frauen- und Geschlechtergeschichte* 27 62, pp. 32–40.

21 Dorothy McBride Stetson (2001) *Abortion Politics, Women's Movements, and the Democratic State: A comparative study of state feminism,* Oxford: Oxford University Press.

22 Interwar France, Soviet Russia, Great Britain, and Germany (after 1933) were the leaders in pronatalist policy and the struggle to criminalize abortions: David Hoffmann (2000) Mothers in the Motherland: Stalinist Pronatalism in its Pan-European Context, *Journal of Social History* 34:1, pp. 35–54; Siân Reynolds (1996) *France between the wars: Gender and politics* London: Routledge. In the second half of the 1930s, pronatalist policy acquired all the features of a global movement. In 1937, one of the French ideologues of pronatalism, Robert Henri Hazemann, became an expert for the League of Nations and, in cooperation with the experts of British Inter-Departmental Committee on Abortion, initiated an inter-country, comparative overview of the regulations concerning birth control. More in the correspondence between Hazemann and Štampar: Robert Henri Hazemann The letter to A.Štampar 22.12.1937, box 10.

23 In his report for the comparative research on maternal and child welfare politics conducted for the League of Nations in the late 1930s, Štampar explained the changes in the regulation of abortion made in Soviet Russia through the "real equality between men and women, and abolition of capital exploitation and the raising of the cultural level." Andrija Štampar (1937) Visit to the State Institute for Maternal and Child Protection, Moscow HR-HDA-831 Andrija Štampar, box3.

24 Gordana Drakić (2011) Prekid trudnoche prema krivichnom zakonu kraljevine Jugoslavije i proektima koji su ga prethodni [Abortion Under the Criminal Code of the Kingdom of Yugoslavia and the Projects that Preceded it] *Zbornik radova*

Pravnog fakulteta Novi Sad [The collection of works of the Faculty of Law of the University Novi Sad], 45(3), pp. 533–542.

25 Rory Yeomans (2008) Fighting the White Plague: Demography and Abortion in the Independent State of Croatia, 1941–1945 in Christian Promitzer, Sevasti Trubeta, Marius Turda (ed.) *Health, Hygiene and Eugenics in Southeastern Europe to 1945* Budapest: CEU Press pp. 385–426.

26 *Světozor:* časopis pro zábavu i poučení [*Světozor:* a magazine for entertainment and instruction] 1940 40.

27 The production of the film started to be planned in 1937, which was relevant to the changes in the official aims of demographic policy: Manželství pod drobnohledem (1937) *Film Orgán Svazu kinematogr. industrie ČSR v Praze* [Film Organization of the Union of cinematography in Czechoslovak Republic, Prague] 17 20 p. 3. Along with a few other short films, *Manželství pod drobnohledem* was part of a demographic campaign aimed at recruiting women to give birth more: Lucie Česálková (2014) *Atomy věčnosti. Český krátký film 30. až 50. let* [Atoms of Eternity Czech short film of the 1930s and 1950s], Prague: NFA.

28 Filmová kartotéka: týdeník pro kulturní využití filmu [Film archive: a weekly magazine for the cultural use of film], 1940 3, p. 2.

29 Rick Altman (1999) *Film/genre* London: British film institute p. 116.

30 The film, also shown under the slogan "better babies," presented the duties and privileges of motherhood as embedded in various services, based upon the idea of improving the quality of children: "Birth to be shown whole week again" The Washington Herald (Washington, District of Columbia), 5.05.1918, p. 14.

31 Karel Driml, who cooperated with Kokeisl, was able to watch this and other films commissioned by various eugenic associations during his stay in the United States as a fellow of the Rockefeler Foundation in 1921.

32 O filmové naději bez drobnohledu [About film hope without microscope] (1940) *Expres* 102, p. 3.

33 Pressa Filmová tisková služba [Pressa: Film Press Service], 1939 11, 218, p. 1.

34 Otakar Hanuš (1940) Manželství pod drobnohledem *Filmový kurýr* 14 3, p. 5.

35 Co nového ve filmu [What is new in film production] 1940 *Český deník* 29 142, p. 8.

36 Nový český film z oboru hygieny [New Czech film in the field of hygiene] (1925) *Zdraví lidu: Zdravotnický měsíčník Čsl. Červeného kříže* 9 3, p. 71.

37 Das Staatsministerium des Innern 1933 Der Brief an die Filmoberprüfstelle [The letter to Film supervision office] Berlin. Betreff: Widerruf des Bildstreifens "Geschlecht und Leben; die Gesund der Frau" [Subject: Revocation of the cutting the images in the film "Sex and Life: the health of the woman"] BayHStA.

Part 4

Health films for the interwar periphery

11 *Stín ve světle* as the first health film for the periphery

The birth of the canon

Crossing the border of the periphery as a deadly and dangerous trap of individuality

Juro and Jano, rivals in love, are both trying to win the favors of Maryša. Juro leaves to do seasonal work and when he returns, he decides to marry Maryša. Jano also leaves, along with other villagers. They all live together in a stable and a number of them catch an eye infection – trachoma. Jano wants to be cured but Juro refuses medication and decides to go off to America. There he is held for a medical inspection and is sent back, and must pay his own way. Meanwhile Jano, now recovered, has married Maryša. Juro becomes blind and lives as a beggar in his native village.[1]

This description comes from a film that had four different titles *Stín ve světle/Tvrdošijný Juro/Slepý Juro/Tvrdohlavý Jura* (The Shadow in the Light/ Stubborn Juro/Blind Juro/Hardheaded Juro, 1928). As one of the most successful health films[2] produced in interwar Eastern Europe, it reflects considerable similarity with the plot of a typical Western health film, embedding desirable patterns of healthy behavior in a love story and the competition between "good" or educable and "bad" or uneducable heroes. Notwithstanding this first impression, an attentive viewing persuades one to accept this film as a great step away from the double-focus narrative as a canon of health propaganda, a detailed description of the social, cultural and psychological prerequisites for becoming healthier through opposing the lifestyle, childhood and personal choices of those who are "good" and "bad." Viewers know virtually nothing about Jano, the positive character who has won his health and the love of beautiful Maryša. But they are taught a great deal about the tragic destiny of Juro, a bright and gifted individual who has lost his health, love and human dignity because of being too self-centered, too stubborn to accept hygienic rules and the necessity to be treated by a physician. In terms of structural-linguistic logic, traditional health films focus on primary motifs as the grounds for individual patterns of conflict and resolution; instead, *Stín ve světle* has introduced "systems of differences" and "bundles of relations," which should be interpreted in terms of larger cultural

DOI: 10.4324/9781003272267-16

paradigms, rather than the psychological explanations introduced by traditional health films.[3]

Stín ve světle aligns with the canon of the crossing-borders story, typical of many cultures, the myth that ascribes to borders the power to destroy human lives and kill those who cross them. The central line of the plot is Juro's crossing of all possible types of moral, cultural and geographical borders. At the beginning, he tries to take possession of Maryša, who loves him and tries to stop him by encouraging him to follow the word of God. He is nearly ready to cross borders in the conflict with Jano and brutally attacks him. He then crosses physical borders, traveling to Bohemia to earn money for his marriage and moving to the United States in search of a better life when Maryša refuses to marry him. When he returns, being rejected by the U.S. authorities because of visible symptoms of trachoma, he visits a Jewish hostelry and spends the night with a prostitute, contracting a venereal disease. But the point of no return in this long history of crossing-borders between "proper" and "improper" behavior occurs when Juro has rejected the treatment for trachoma. Remarkably, the scene of the trachoma diagnosis is presented as a division between people who are separated from the employer who asks workers to be medically treated and the physician on one side of the belt of the hay harvester, and the reluctant workers on the other side of this belt. Those who are diagnosed positively and accept treatment move to the side of the employer and the physician. Obviously, Juro is not happy to cross the "line" and move to the side of those who have agreed to be treated against trachoma (see Figure 11.1).

In contrast to those who have obeyed civilization in the face of medical treatment, Juro remains "the human being, over whom some animal sense receives full control, in the end becomes the victim of his lost higher human nature; he is a creature humiliated below the levels of true human nature."[4] He not only remains in the shadow of the light of progress but also represents

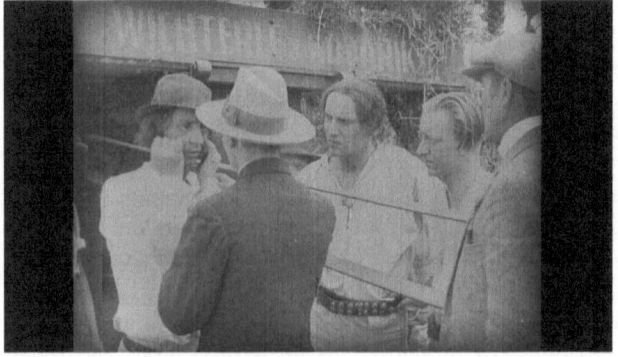

Figure 11.1 Rejecting to be civilized in *Stín ve světle* (The Shadow in the Light, 1928).
Source: NFA.

the "primitive men who piss on [the] fire" of advanced culture introduced by Prometheus.[5] *Stín ve světle* is an especially apt title for a film about trachoma, which can gradually deprive a person of sight – including the ability to differentiate light and darkness. In a figurative sense, Juro loses this ability much earlier than he loses his sight. Along with underscoring this risk, the title establishes a strong association between the risk of losing sight and the risk of being so bright that one inevitably drifts toward the shadow of their own personality. An entire range of analogies between individuality and disease is provided by the cascade of four different titles, including *Slepý Juro* (Blind Juro) – who is at the beginning "blind" to the risks of his behavior and then actually loses his sight. *Tvrdošíjný Juro* (literally Hard-neck Juro) accentuates other characteristics, a lack of readiness to accept the new rules of civilization, leading Juro to the fact that becoming blind can really "break his neck" and his life.

The multilayered analogies between disease and behavior in the titles of the film reverberate with the ambiguous intertextuality of *Stín ve světle* with other health films aimed at captivating the "center," namely, Czechs and, mostly, men (more in Part 3). Juro is performed by Roman Roda-Růžička, an actor who had played all the main roles in each of the Czech health films[6] and some popular fairy-tales. For instance, in the first filmed version of the most popular Czech fairy tale, *O Popelce* (About Cinderella, 1929) made the same year as *Stín ve světle*, he plays the Prince while the same actress performs Maryša and Cinderella, and the actor who performs Jano also performs in *O Popelce* as Cinderella's father. Roda-Růžička firmly embodies the position of one of the "princes" of Czech interwar cinema. This status makes the character of Juro more plausible as too bright and too individualistic, due to several depictions of the re-education of his characters, who at the beginning have lost their way (including being physically infected) but then accept the call to become responsible for their health, listen to wise physicians and identify their own "proper" way. Moreover, it adds one more border to the ones crossed by Juro, the border between center and periphery – not in geographical but in cultural and socio-political terms – despite his organic belonging to the periphery, Juro, as performed by Roda-Růžička, behaves as a person from center, and he has been punished for this.

Embedding diseases into undesirable patterns of behavior is at the foundation of all health films, but the novelty of *Stín ve světle* lies in linking these undesirable patterns of behavior with the analogy of crossing the border, not only the border between responsible and irresponsible behavior but also the border of belonging and not-belonging to the periphery and being a part of its regime of authenticity. Juro is opposed not to Jano but to the "proper" regime of authenticity for his periphery, Slovakia. He is a Slovak who rejects the task of being an obedient son of his people. The aim of presenting his dramatic destiny is to demonstrate the consequences of non-belonging to the periphery – by crossing borders that denote the boundaries of the periphery and its regime of authenticity. In this motif, it is easy to recognize one of the central themes of interwar literature in continental Europe – the unfunny futility of embracing individuality[7] and rejecting the call for people without characteristics or ant personalities – one of the central messages in the literature of the former Austro-Hungarian Empire disseminated among various social groups and nations.

The ant personality as an agent of progress for the periphery

Through recounting the history of alienation from belonging to the periphery, *Stín ve světle* introduces and fixes a particular régime of authenticity based upon the inseparable interconnection between the periphery and the ant personality, a non-personalized agent of civilization and the new practices targeted at preventing diseases. The film presents Jano as the only type of personality suitable and reasonable for efficient operation of the periphery, including the mission to combat trachoma. In contrast to the bright, handsome and sexually attractive Juro, Jano does not have a memorable appearance. Viewers do not have the same opportunity to examine his appearance and understand his emotions as they do with Juro's feelings and affect.

As the ant personality of Jano merges with the crowd, he is indistinguishable from the majority, and only a close-up or a pointed camera shot indicates that he is also a main character. Juro is the only one who remains different from the beginning to the end, and the film confirms the impossibility of remaining different but healthy and wealthy simultaneously or being a part of the periphery. But the invisible ant, Jano, who appears at the end of the film together with Maryša working in their garden and pausing their labor for a moment to cross themselves and thank God, represents this desirable personality profile.

In this turn, *Stín ve světle* has reversed the pessimistic or, even more, the dystopian image of ant people shaped by "highbrow" literature about the mass urban population. Joravsky synthesizes all these negative cliches by exploring this pattern as one of the keys to interpreting interwar literature, noting the "vehicles or pedestrians in city traffic, molecules of air in cyclonic swirls … sanitary engineering: Pedestrians [who] have no more understanding of the system that directs them than drops of sewage have of the pipes that channel their flow."[8] The ironic and negative view on mass participation had been well known among Czech intellectuals, reflected in one of the most consistent theatrical performances, in a play by the Brothers Čapek, *Ze života hmyzu*, (Pictures from insect life, 1921). The protagonist, a bystander without specific features or even a name, but obviously a Czech, has gained the unique possibility to interactively observe the routine of different insects: Upper-class butterflies, who obviously represent the anti-hero of the Czech national movement in the nineteenth century, the pseudo-noble Czechs, for whom exquisite pleasures and refined experiences are the most important in life;[9] middle-class dung beetles, who with their priority of family interests, represent the majority of Czech society as limited by an overly selfish and narrow understanding of welfare; and ants, who are pictured as loyal followers of the ideology of progress. The sarcastic and negativist tone regarding each of these three groups allows us to interpret the play as a cautionary tale, whether against the internal enemies of the new nation or against any attempts to map the world in terms of enemies and aliens. But how humanist was the view on humanity translated by the Čapeks in their play?

Since the earliest attempt by Roman Jakobson[10] (1963) to identify the play by the Čapeks as a case of the multilayered adaptation of their pessimism and dystopian view on progress and humanity, the play has remained a kind of complex enigma that needed to be solved. Following Jakobson, B. R. Bradbrook[11] (1986) interprets these motifs as a novelty introduced by the Čapeks to the plot of the more neutral short story *Ceho tu nebylo* (What did not happen, translation into Czech in 1898) by Vsevold Garshin and stresses the shift from the ideas in the Russian text to the morality in the play by the Čapeks. Milada Blekastad[12] (1976) embeds the play in the common European trend to look upon the issues of humanity through the lenses of absurd black comedy, in which there is no clear boundary between reality and dreams. She generally describes the play as one more adaptation of *Az ember tragédiája* (The Tragedy of Man), a play about the never-ending reproduction of the myth about the expulsion of humans from paradise, written by the Hungarian author Imre Madách in 1861, who puzzled viewers with the impossibility to decipher whether it had happened with Adam and Eve or was only Adam's nightmare.

The intertextuality of the play seems inexhaustible if analyzed as a part of the movement for emancipation from the German view on culture and human progress. Heavy irony in establishing multiple analogies between humans and insects directly opposes the play by the Brothers Čapek to the novels *Die Biene Maja und ihre Abenteuer* (The adventures of Maya the bee, *1912*) and *Himmelvolk, ein Märchen von Blumen, Tieren und Gott* (People of the sky, 1915) by Jakob Ernst Waldemar Bonsels, who romanticizes German nationalism through the story of the young bee Maja, the future queen of the bee nation, and her coming-of-age journey, accompanied by meeting various insects and other animals. In the Čapeks' play, the ants could be easily associated with the German middle class, mainly represented by professionals: Engineers, physicians and lawyers. Remarkably, those ants who answer the protagonist's question about why they engage in a never-ending war with other "races" of ants are named "engineers." The ants are labeled black, red, or yellow, which adds one more argument in favor of connecting ants and Germans, seen as overt racists since the early 1920s.

But along with the possibility to recognize in the Čapeks' ants the satirical image of somebody preoccupied with nationalist and racist ideology (as many Czech intellectuals depicted Germans), it is reasonable to recognize not only satire against particular ethnic groups but also a more general negation of ideologies as a part of the Čapeks' predominant idea about the necessity to reinforce the responsibility of science.[13] The ants mention a myriad of possible reasons for sacrificing their own lives and others' lives, from progress to the intention to obey the time. But the protagonisteasily moves from the ideological veil to the distribution of power between individuals and society:

> Common unit! I have caught you now,
> human thought! We are just grains
> a great harvest that belongs to all.
> Little "I," there's something above you,
> name it either nation or humanity or state,
> whatever you want to name it, but just serve:
> you are nothing. The biggest price of living
> is sacrificing life.[14]

Among many other, if not all, possible ideological platforms of the interwar period, the ants with their obsession of social unity (*spolecný celek*), in the name of which they act uncritically, accept the idea by Johann Heinrich Pestalozzi, which had received a second wind during the interwar period, namely, that the participation of the mass creates civilizations. "All civilization is nothing but that which acts on the great majority, on the masses of people and which leads to the widespread mood that we are actually united in economic, technical, etc. unity";[15] the influential German social pedagogue Artur Buchenau (1924) underscores these words by Pestalozzi for introducing the difference between culture and civilization, and the necessity to face the possible confrontation between them.

According to Joravsky, the interwar contest between culture and civilization stemmed from viewing culture as evading active civic virtue, instead relying on progress or advanced nations and civilization, "which included democracy as a distinguishing mark of developed nations."[16] This difference was aggravated by the contest between the German tradition of exploring the development of humanity in terms of culture and the focus on civilization in French literature and philosophy, echoed later in British and U.S. American traditions of social thinking. The skepticism of the Brothers Čapek, expressed by their protagonist who remains tobe a bystander, perfectly fits with this explanatory model:

Bystander:	We have, for example deputies, members of parliament; this is democracy. Do you have MPs too?
First engineer:	No. We have the unity.
Bystander:	And who speaks for the whole?
First engineer:	The one who orders. The unity speaks only orders.
Second engineer:	He lives in the laws. It's nowhere else.[17]

These dynamic tensions between literature and social formation gained traction within the public reflections on the periphery in terms of culture and civilization. The long-term representative of Subcarpathian Ruthenia (another part of the Czechoslovak Eastern periphery), lawyer and sociologist Stanislav

Severynovič Dnistrjanskyj, published in 1927 the article "Kultur, Zivilisation und Recht" (Culture, civilization and right)[18] targeted with differentiating culture and civilization for different nations and ethnic groups. For solving the task of explaining the multiple ways in which culture and civilization interrogate each other, Dnistrjanskyj introduced the concept of rights as "inseparable from the mission to bring together culture and civilization."[19] The main methodological approach of Dnistrjanskyj is boundary work, different approaches aimed at explaining the interconnection between culture and civilization. He underscores various criteria introduced by other thinkers, such as mental and material culture, "natural people" (*Naturvölker*) who connect culture with nature, and "cultural people" (*Kulturvölker*), who differentiate humanity and nature in order to ultimately unite them for dividing the task of reproducing culture and civilization between people and the politics of the state, respectively.

This central argument regarding the division of the functions between the people and the state is nuanced by Dnistrjanskyj in three interrelated pillars of civilizing the people: Action (*Handlung*), originally agrarian and religious practices that emancipated humans from total dependence on nature; the sustainability (*Stabilität*) of these activities, which could not be short-term and accustomed people to constant practicing civilizing activities; and order (*Ordnung*), which introduces the rules for regulating civilizing activities in favor of connecting people through the collective practice of the coherence between a more global civilization and local culture, namely, agriculture and religion for the people of the periphery.[20] These three points introduced by Dnistrjanskyj nuance the idea of human bondage reinforced in interwar Europe after the triumph of the similarly titled novel, *Of Human Bondage*, by William Somerset Maugham (1915). The novel tells the story of young Phillip's coming of age, a story that can be interpreted (among many other possible interpretations) as a move from the position of patient (Phillip has a congenital defect of the foot) to the position of physician. After several attempts to find his professional way as an artist, Phillip becomes a rural doctor.

Human bondage in the periphery: A way of civilizing "nature people"

The *bildungsroman* by Maugham reintroduces a strong ethical division between emotions operating either in the name of good or evil, but remains a manifestation of "human infirmity in moderating and checking the emotions" or "human bondage" in Baruch Spinoza's terms.[21] Maugham, who was informed not only by the psychoanalytic approach but also by his own ambiguous sexual desires, consistently reconstructs the primary idea of Spinoza toward understanding the role of society and referent people in constructing human bondage and becoming emancipated from it.[22] In the very same way, *Stín ve světle* not only fixes Juro as a man who, "prey to his emotions, he is not his own master, but lies at the mercy of fortune: So much so, that he is often compelled, while seeing that which is better for him, to follow that which is worse"[23] but also provides an explanation for the destructivity of human bondage through the inevitable isolation of Juro from the social opportunities of civilizing under-scored by Dnistrjanskyj.

Joravsky links the renaissance of the idea of human bondage in European literature between the 1910s and 1940s with the politically desirable and mas-sive popularization of a psychoanalytical understanding of human bondage as connected "to sex and family down here, to Kultur as the realm of universal progress far above, with disdain for political in-between,"[24] which ought to fix a particular type of servility to Western civilization sanctified by many interwar intellectuals. Barbara Hannan, who focuses on different strategies to leading a person out of love-induced bondage as culturally and socially determined, underscores that the choice of a more complex route, namely, the replacement of bondage by a contrary passion, is possible for those who, like Philip, have gained the option for becoming subjects of their own lives,[25] or in Enlightenment terms, have accepted authenticity as an axiological principle.[26] This solution does not imply the subordination of authenticity to instrumental rationality. But a second, a less complex route, conquering human bondage by means of a reasoned emotion, is possible only within interconnecting authen-ticity and local or community culture, including the acceptance of collective interests as predominant.

In the film *Die Biene Maja und ihre Abenteuer* (The adventures of Maya the bee, 1926), based on the novel by Bonsels, the threat of becoming a victim of such bondage and the unique role of community is presented through the story of young bee who has been rescued from a web prepared by a villain spider, a symbol of human bondage in European culture, by those with whom she is connected, and who has taken her back to her kingdom and community. Human bondage is seen as a selfish betrayal of community – or, even more, the nation. Spinoza's relativism in differentiating "good" and "bad" feelings has been replaced by the strong opposition between individuality and the collective. This antinomy between the very personal, or even asocial, nature of human bondage and the monopoly of community in the cure for the feeling of hope-lessness frames the relations among ant personalities in *Stín ve světle*, produced two years later.

Stín ve světle opens with a cascade of the landscapes typical of Slovakia: Mountains covered by forests and flocks of sheep, fast mountain flows traversing into the slow rivers of the foothills. In terms of Jakobson's communications paradigm, these very first moments of the virtual meeting between the sender, the authors of the film and the receivers, the viewers who are the people of periphery, are obviously decisive for establishing good communication and achieving recognition of the film's message. Using landscapes as a part of the *phatic function*, "specifically geared to establishing an initial connection and ensuring a continuous and attentive reception,"[27] points to an ethnic-genealogical conception for defining the identity of Slovaks. applied within a "nation-formation approach which combines the formal recognition of polyethnicity with efforts to forge a common national identity along civic lines."[28]

Stín ve světle only underscores this commonality by referencing one of the most Slovak places, indeed a symbol of Slovak nationalism, *Turčiansky Svätý Martin,* which was also presented as one of the most vulnerable due to the spread of infectious diseases, including trachoma. Not only the documentary part of the film but also the landscapes are filmed in this district. The landscapes aim not to impose a bucolic picture but to underscore the risks and difficulties that Slovaks face because of the beautiful but almost uncontrollable forces of nature. Remarkably, the report of the local physician, Šulc, obliged to prepare the plan for developing public health in *Turčiansky Svätý Martin,* starts with describing these climate and geographical conditions:

The Tur district is located almost in the middle of Slovakia. It covers an area of 946 km. It is bounded on all sides by mountains, on the ridges of which its border runs. The mountain wall is broken by the river Váh, which flows through the northern part of the district from east to west. The altitude range varies between 360–1700 m above sea level. Thus, the district forms a basin from the neighboring districts separated by natural boundaries, so that all its parts have a natural gradient to its center and nowhere to the neighboring district. From south to north, it is crossed by the river Turiec, which flows into the Váh. Its basin measures 927 km, length 50 km. The river is unregulated, it runs in numerous and steep bends, the riverbed is shallow, not fixed anywhere, the bottom has numerous and sudden changes in the slope - the depth fluctuates between 70 cm–3 m. As a result, even in less heavy rains, the water immediately rises and floods the surrounding landscape. The groundwater stands high and with its considerable mobility in the local gravelly soil; this is often due to the frequent appearance and rapid transmission of some infectious diseases.[29]

In contrast to the nationalization of nature and the civic-territorial conception of the Czechs, which viewers could observe in the films that addressed the Czech, or dominant, audience, men, the naturalization of Slovakia immediately starts with the first seconds of *Stín ve světle* through depicting the landscape as an expression of the national cultural character and the seat of the country's national virtues.[30] The spectators observe the first depictions of Juro and Maryša, dressed in national costumes as they meet each other on the bank of the river. This visualization fixes the timelessness of national character – viewers may not know which historical period the characters represent but they know from the very beginning that the characters are Slovaks. According to Eric Kaufmann and Oliver Zimmer, lacking a distinct ethno-historical past is one of the main reasons for practicing the ideal of ethnic homogeneity and taking pride in their polyethnic composition and civic values. Natural analogies and a preference for the "primitive" nature that opens the film are continued by visualizing the patriarchal culture and the predominant role of men ascribed to the periphery as its organic feature. The men of the periphery are those seen as the key figures in both the dissemination and prevention of disease.

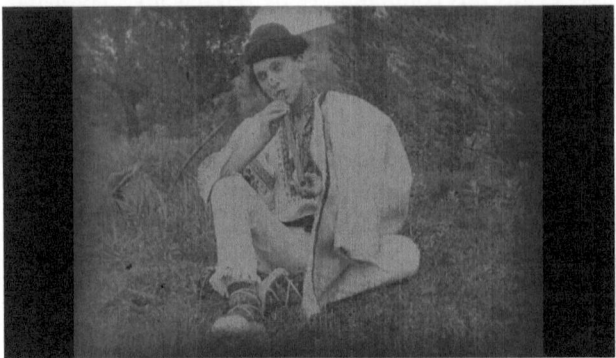

Figure 11.2 Male geobody in *Stín ve světle* (The Shadow in the Light, 1928).
Source: NFA.

Accepting the patriarchal order with the predominant role of the father figure as its central characteristic shapes a particular type of embodiment, the geobody of the ant personality: "a living embodiment of authenticity appears to be able to move."[31] Visualization of a purported authenticity is coined in the folk costumes that all the characters wear – but not during their seasonal work far from their home, when they have abandoned their periphery. The motifs of rootedness and the timelessness of peasants are exercised through the systematic analogy between the flow of time and the flow of the river. The film begins with a scene in which Juro sits on the bank of the river and plays the flute – young, healthy, full of strength – and ends with the same scene, this time depicting the prematurely aged and blind Juro (see Figure 11.2).

While men are those who act either "properly" or not, women are aimed at embodying the nation but not as active agents in shaping it.[32] In contrast to the other characters, Maryša is the only one who has not crossed the borders of her community. Her passivity is only underscored during the scene in which Juro is reading her letter, which describes how she spends her time without her lover. The viewers can see how Juro's imagination works: He sees Maryša sitting with a fawn on her knees, a typical cliché for presenting the pacifying power of female beauty (see Figure 11.3). Maryša's devotion to her people culminates in the moment when she rejects marrying Juro, despite her love for him. This act becomes a performance of "civilizational truth," a choice in favor of health of the people. She continues to care about Juro and to be sorry about losing her love but not at the expense of the health of her people. In this way, Maryša remains a soul of tradition-within-modernity and the evolutionary way of civilizing the periphery seen by Pestalozzi and his interwar successors as the most desirable: "Not revolution, but evolution, that is, the development of internal social forces, Pestalozzi insists incessantly, is necessary for the fatherland."[33]

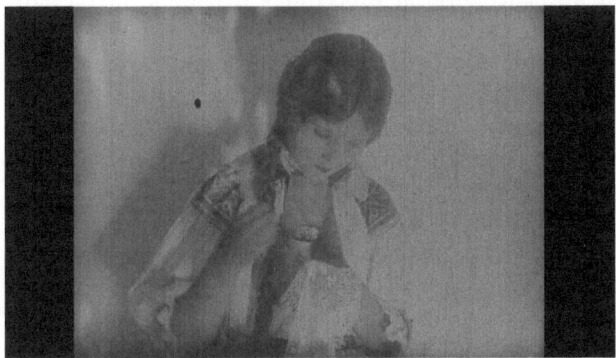

Figure 11.3 Female geobody in *Stín ve světle* (The Shadow in the Light, 1928).
Source: NFA.

The success in solving the task to captivate the peripheral audience depends on the possibility to produce a visual "text" with a code that would be shared and accepted by viewers. After establishing contact through demonstrating the belongingness of the main characters to the typical landscapes and patriarchal order as a "natural" and timeless social construction, the film introduces other performances of human bondage, the growing contradiction between the obvious sensuality in the relationship between Juro and Maryša and Christian morality. The mutual sexual attraction of the main characters is a predominant motif in the first part of the film, before Juro's departure; moreover, with the increasing contradictions between Juro and Maryša, the role of Christianity and Church is strengthened. The performance of these contradictions shapes the ensemble of communication functions.

The daily presence of Christianity in the life of the characters implements the conative function aimed at legitimizing commands or interdictions – in the fictional part of the film. The religious rules require Juro to ask Maryša to be married, not to seduce her. From the very beginning, Juro is presented as not aligned with Christian morality, and only the purity and innocence of Maryša temporally save Juro from a moral fall. Maryša tries to persuade Juro to be treated against trachoma in the name of God. Perhaps the most emotional scene with Jano is the moment he tries to win the interest of Maryša by giving her a present, a plate with an image of the holy Virgin Mary, later pitilessly shattered by the jealous Juro. Christian charity is the only option available to the blinded Juro at the end of the film. While the film opens with a cascade of landscapes, it ends with a scene of all the villagers attending a Sunday church service – except for Juro, who remains outside, waiting for alms.

In the documentary part of the film, the conative function is ascribed to visualizing the different stages of trachoma and its medical treatment, from early and timely examination to surgical procedures inevitable in the late stages of the disease. The pedagogical "weight" of the message is reinforced by showing not only adults but also children in the different stages of suffering from trachoma. New medical practices are presented as non-disruptive to the microcommunity or family, as long as the disease does not become a source of severe restraint for infected people. In this way, disease is constructed as a direct threat to human bondage, and the visits of nurses, along with regular medical examinations at the medical station, represent new forms of protecting the community and the relations inside it.

Along with cautionary narration about the risks of late intervention, the documentary part of the film shapes the idea of the risky situation of contamination and those "aliens" who are dangerous carriers of trachoma. If, in the fictional part, only the insufficient hygienic conditions of migrants are seen as a risk for being infected, in the documentary part, entertainment, of not only questionable quality but also hazardous to health (such as "Gypsy" circuses or "Gypsy" music bands) could lead to infection (see Figure 11.4). "Gypsy" musicians are depicted in the film as careless and oblivious to their illness – which not only reverberates with the irresponsible and alien behavior of Juro but also with one of the primary discursive practices brought forward by the authorities in order to introduce tough surveillance over the Eastern periphery and its population. Instead of "unhealthy" entertainment, the film offers puppet theater and a play about combating trachoma as an alternative, healthy type of entertainment. The happy and smiling faces of children and adults who observe the performance of one of the many plays written by Karel Driml for the simultaneous dissemination of new hygienic competencies and national

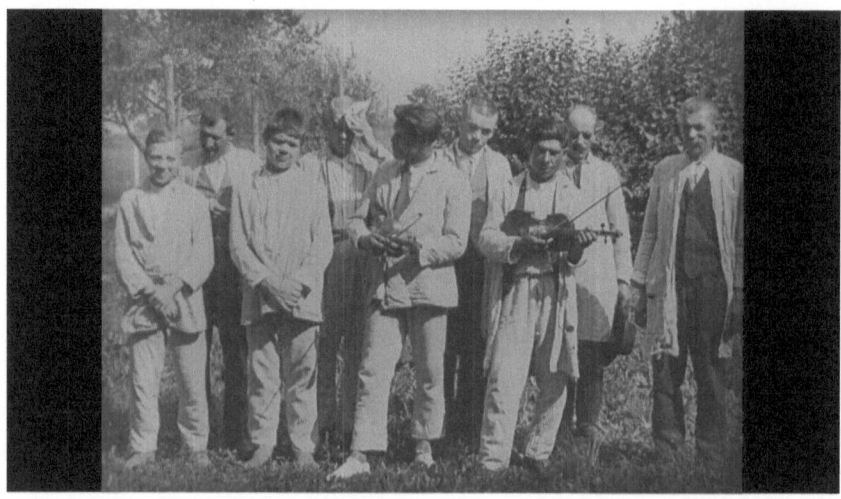

Figure 11.4 "Gypsy" orchestra infected by trachoma in *Stín ve světle* (The Shadow in the Light, 1928).

Source: NFA.

ideals contribute an emotive function targeted at expressing and describing the emotions of the authors of the film to the peripheral audience. But not only health propaganda was presented in the film as a part of human bondage for the people of the periphery. The film, in both the fictional and the documentary parts, aims to introduce public health as an inseparable part of the regime of authenticity for Slovakia.

Public health as a part of the new régime of authenticity: Uniting people in the fight against trachoma

The history of Juro's ordeals reflects the contradictory history of regulations regarding infectious diseases as a part of Czechoslovak politics concerning labor migration. In the early 1920s, the authorities called for better quality of medical examinations from the side of local physicians, who were responsible for granting permission to the locals for working abroad, mainly in France. The multiple cases of those examined by French authorities as infected or unable to work because of disability led to tensions between Czechoslovakia and France. Consequently, the Czechoslovak government increased control over Slovak physicians in order not to lose the option to provide the opportunity to work for the people from the periphery. Later, these tensions were reproduced in the relations with the authorities of South Morava, which had become the main destination for seasonal agricultural workers from Slovakia.[34] The requirement of a three-week quarantine for those who arrived from places already indicated as heavily contaminated by infectious diseases was accepted as impossible and thoughtless by the Slovaks. Multiple cases of transmitting infectious diseases by Slovaks occupied Czech mass media. The authorities in Bratislava reported to the Ministry of Social Affairs in Prague: "The next issue of *Péče o mládež*[35] will publish the article by Dr. Krystýn concerning trachoma in Slovakia, which, for the first time, will describe how awfully this dangerous disease has been disseminated, and how large insecurity threatens the population of other part of our republic."[36]

Indeed, Josef Krystýn, a physician from Brno, conducted medical examinations among the children placed in three institutions, one for deaf and mute children in Kremnica, an orphanage in Slovenská Lupka, and a Catholic orphanage in the monastery at Znimov. The documentary film made during these examinations was later used in the documentary part of *Stín ve světle* in order to demonstrate the misery of the local population. In the middle of the 1920s, trachoma started to be seen as a signifier of the Eastern periphery due to the enormous number of cases in Slovakia and Subcarpathian Ruthenia (more than 12,000) in contrast to just a few in Bohemia (less than 30).[37] Labor migration was posed as the main and virtually only carrier for spreading trachoma. Obtaining the status of a social disease, trachoma engendered the label "socially blind people" (*sociálně slepí*) and Czech experts took on the task of how to persuade the population to visit a physician despite the long-term and painful treatment. By the end of the 1920s, the authorities started recruiting teachers for the campaigns against trachoma. The multiple gaps in public health started to be seen as "natural consequences of economic and cultural backwardness as well as poverty common for Slovakia,"[38] leading to the expansion of internal colonialism as a main frame for the policy regarding the Eastern periphery since the mid-1920s.

Presenting Juro as sentenced to lose everything because of their reckless attempts to find a better life beyond his "natural" borders can be read as a cautionary message to the Slovak audience, well known for its mobility. By the end of the 1920s, the negative public view on labor migration started resonating with the restrictions introduced by the United States for migrants from Eastern Europe. Labor migration began to be viewed as a part of irresponsible behavior for the citizens of the new state, and improving hygienic conditions represented a step toward the desirable civilization of the region to make it as good as "America." Intensive migration operated as one of the central arguments of authorities to pay special attention to public health in the *Turčiansky Svätý Martin* district, where, according to the authorities, "*drotárs*,[39] well known around the world, had a house, and in America many compatriots live, who transferred there. The majority of our domestic population moves away for seasonal work because of the misery of life and in order to save money which they need during winters."[40] The documentary part of *Stín ve světle* heavily relied on the data collected by Slovak authorities in this district. Trachoma was posited as the most widespread infectious disease in *Turčiansky* Svätý *Martin*, along with tuberculosis and smallpox. A graph from the documentary part aimed at presenting the uncontrolled growth of the cases of trachoma reproduced the data collected by local physicians.

Clearly, one of the motives to make the film aimed at addressing the Eastern periphery of trachoma was the dissatisfaction of the authorities with the involvement of the local population in medical examination and treatment:

From time to time, the district is visited by an ophthalmologist, who examines as much as possible the entire population of the infected communities and compiles a register of patients, who are then to be treated free of charge by district doctors. It takes place very haphazardly, because patients do not receive treatment, especially where it is quite far to the doctor. The population is very indolent about the disease - the disease is spread mainly in the western, culturally backward part of the district, and therefore all previous attempts to at least prevent the disease have failed.[41]

While the destiny of Juro challenges the neglect of the population concerning the task to prevent trachoma or treat it in a timely manner, the documentary part of the film aims to present various options for avoiding the risk of repeating Juro's mistake, including the special centers for treating those infected by trachoma (*Trachomová ambulance*), visiting nurses who not only monitored hygienic conditions but also provided initial treatment, and surgery for those who had an advanced case of trachoma. The physician at the center and the nurse who visits her patients reproduce the advice and information provided in a leaflet containing the basic hygienic rules aimed at preventing the dissemination of trachoma, prepared in the three languages: Slovak, Czech and Hungarian, for dissemination in Slovakia. This intertextuality between various media is only reinforced by the pictures on the walls of the center, which are obviously copies of the images used for hygienic exhibitions.

The film indirectly mentions other predispositions for improving the approach to eliminating trachoma. The railway station from which Juro and Jano move to the Czech part of the country is presented in the film as a stronghold of civilization and this depiction is not accidental. *Vrútky*, the biggest railway station in *Turčiansky Svätý Martin,* was posed as the epicenter of trachoma. At the same time, the expectations regarding health propaganda and the involvement of the local population in medical examination, prevention and treatment were optimistic, according to the opinion of local experts, "because 90 percent of the population are employed by or directly dependent on the railway station. And with great understanding of the railway station's headship regarding the actions [health examination] it would be easy to lead many inhabitants not only to testing but also to correction of their behavior [toward better hygienic conditions]."[42] The shared responsibility of authorities and employers for the health of the local population was consistently promoted in the film, e.g., the Czech who organized seasonal work immediately calls for the doctor when he recognizes the first symptoms of trachoma among Slovak workers.

But, according to authorities, notwithstanding all efforts to combat trachoma, this disease remained "a stubborn enemy of the poor Slovak people" (*urputný nepriateľ chudobného slovenského ľudu*) who lived in *Turčiansky Svätý Martin.*[43] The stigma of "stubborn" Slovaks who would be unable to combat a "stubborn" disease started to be a part of the regime of authenticity, which should captivate not only the local population, including physicians, but also international organizations such as the Rockefeller Foundation and the Red Cross who were asked to financially help to transform this district into an exemplary one (*vzorný okres*) in terms of local public health.[44] The reports, along with the film, presented Slovakia and *Turčiansky Svätý Martin* in particular as the border between the civilized West and the dangerous barbarian East (Subcarpathian Ruthenia), highlighting the desirable profile of the ant personality on the front line of the mission to promote civilization and humanity.

Stín ve světle coherently manifested the "otherness" of Slovakia in terms of its culture, situated between West and East, and called for civilizing Slovaks through cultivating the ant personality – ready to accept and implement new, Western rules. This canon not only aligned with the intentions of the Czechoslovak government aimed at establishing efficient political surveillance over the Eastern periphery but also with the expectations translated by the new, global order of health security. Moreover, *Stín ve světle* was aligned with the expectation of "[t]he best films for hygiene propaganda [which] have no need to ostentate their purpose; they are more likely to carry conviction when the onlooker spontaneously realizes their purpose."[45] The challenge to produce health films suitable for the periphery started to be articulated in the late 1920s by international experts:

> It is a thankless task to show the peasants of Latin European Countries the measures taken in America to combat tuberculosis and malaria. The conditions of life and work of the North American farmer are not akin to those of the Italian, Roumanian, or Spanish peasant. For this reason, we hold it necessary to depict the general conditions of the Italian, Roumanian, or Spanish peasants themselves, and to show how these conditions might be improved by the adoption of simple rules of hygiene, easily applicable in the countries in question.[46]

The key frames of *Stín ve světle,* namely, the ant personality, its specific human bondage, and public health as an indispensable part of community life, reverberated with the renaissance in social medicine and its view on society as an organism that formed the concepts of social disease, social pathologies and social therapy. Not individuals but society and its singularities, antpersonalities, should be treated. This approach was adopted and modified by Croatian educator Kamilo Brössler, often called the "Yugoslavian Pestalozzi,"[47] who had written the plot for the film *Ikina sudbina* (Ika's destiny, 1933) and Drago Chloupek, a physician, who had created another film, *Dobro za zlo* (*Good for evil*, 1936), which addressed the population of Bosnia and Hercegovina, the Eastern periphery of Yugoslavia, and aimed to involve them in the prevention and timely treatment of infectious diseases.

Notes

1 This is a period description, used for the film's advertisement (https://www. filmovyprehled.cz/cs/film/395450/stin-ve-svetle).
2 The film was distributed in Slovakia for more than five years and presented the achievements of Czechoslovakia in the progress of public health at many international events, including the *first International Hospital Congress* held in Atlantic City in 1929, the Hygienic exhibition in Dresden, 1930, and *The European Conference* on *Rural Hygiene* in Geneva, 1931.
3 Robert Stam, Robert Bugoyne and Sandy Flitterman-Lewis (1992) *New vocabularies in film semiotics Structuralism post-structuralism and beyond,* London and New York Routledge, p. 20.
4 Artur Buchenau (1924) *Kultur und Zivilisation. Eine Studie zur Geschichte der Sozialpädagogik* [Culture and civilisation. One study of the History of social pedagogy], *Natorp-Festschrift* p. 13.
5 David Joravsky (2019) *Great nations of the West: Conflicting mind-sets* Unpublished manuscript, p. 128.

6 *V blouzeni* (In delirium / When Frost Creeps into the Nest … 1928); *Osudná chvile,* (Fortuitous Moment, 1935); *Pramen lásky* (The Seed of Love, 1928) and *Bataljon* (1927).
7 Joravsky Ibid., p. 224.
8 Ibid p. 220.
9 This pattern was a central target of the disciplinary humor introduced by Czech female writers in their *Bildungsromans* for Czech girls; more in Victoria Shmidt (2020) Female bildungsroman in Czech conduct periodicals: The inception of the genre *History of Education & Children's Literature* XV, 2, pp. 407–428.
10 Roman Jakobson (1963) Russkiy istochnik cheshskoy komedii [Russian source of the Czech comedy], *Ricerche slavistiche,* I, 331–335.
11 Bohuslava. R. Bradbrook (1983) A Russian Model for the Čapeks' "The Insect Play"? *The Slavonic and East European Review,* 61, 3, 411–415.
12 Milada Blekastad (1976) Probleme der Originalität in *Ze života hmyzu* der Brüder Čapek, [The issue of originality of *Ze života hmyzu* by Čapeks], *Scando-Slavica,* 22:1, 79–91.
13 Ibid p. 89.
14 In both English translations of the play, produced by Paul Selver (1922) and Owen Gould Davis (1933), this strophe is omitted, and the translation into English is ours. The Czech original is as follows:

Spolecný celek! Nyní te už mám,
myšlenko lidská! My jsme jenom zrna
veliké sklizne, která patrí všem.
Malické já, je neco nad tebou,
jmenuj to národ, lidstvo nebo stát,
jak chceš to jmenuj, ale jenom služ:
ty nejsi nic. Nejvetší cena žití
je život obetovat.
Bratří Čapové (1921) *Ze života hmyzu* Praha: Aventinum p. 54.

15 Buchenau Kultur und Zivilisation. p. 15.
16 Joravsky Ibid. pp. 134–135.
17 Bratří Čapkové Ibid. p. 57.
18 Stanislav Severynovič Dnistrjanskyj (1927) Kultur, Zivilisation und Recht," [Culture, civilization, and right] *Archiv für Rechts- und Wirtschaftsphilosophie,* 21, 1 pp. 1–17.
19 Ibid p. 1.
20 Ibid pp. 13–14.
21 Benedict de Spinoza (1883) *The Ethics,* Part IV Of Human Bondage, or the Strength of the Emotions available online: https://www.sacred-texts.com/phi/spinoza/ethics/eth04.htm.
22 Barbara Hannan (1997) Love and Human Bondage in *Maugham,* Roger E. Lamb (Ed.) Spinoza and Freud *Love analyzed* New York: Routledge.
23 Spinoza Ibid.
24 Joravsky Ibid. pp. 134–135.
25 Hannan *Love and Human Bondage,* p. 102.
26 Ori Schwarz (2016) The Symbolic Economy of Authenticity as a Form of Symbolic Violence: The Case of Middle-class Ethnic Minorities *Distinktion* 17 (1), pp. 2–19.
27 Robert Stam, Robert Bugoyne and Sandy Flitterman-Lewis (1992) *New vocabularies in film semiotics Structuralism post-structuralism and beyond,* London and New York Routledge p. 16.

28 Eric Kaufmann and Oliver Zimmer (1998) In Search of the Authentic Nation: Landscape and National Identity in Canada and Switzerland *Nations and nationalism,* 4 4, 483–510, p. 496.

29 Vzorná zdravotní demonstrace v okresu Turč. Sv. Martin [Exemplary public health demonstration in the district Turč. Sv. Martin] M.U.Dr. M. Šulc 1927 p. 9 Box 107 Expositura Ministerstva veřejného zdravotnictví Slovenský narodný archiv [Slovak National Archive SNA].

30 Kaufmann and Zimmer Ibid. pp. 489–490.

31 Prasenjit Duara (1998) The Regime of Authenticity: Timelessness, Gender, and National History in Modern China *History and Theory,* Vol. 37, 3, pp. 287–308.

32 Ibid. p. 298.

33 Buchenau *Kultur und Zivilisation* p.15.

34 Zavlékání nakazlivých němoci ze Slovenska v Brně [Dissemination of infectious diseases in Brno] 10.04.1926 Protitrachomová akcia školské děti, skolníci [Anti-trachom action, school children] 1010–27. Box 107 Expositura Ministerstva veřejného zdravotnictví SNA.

35 *Care for youth* was one of the most influential interwar periodicals.

36 Dopis Ministerstvu sociální péče v Praze [Letter to the Ministry of Social affairs in Prague] Opatření proti trachomu v státních a statem subvenovaných sociálních ústavech pro mládež na Slovensku [Measures against trachoma in the state and by state supported social institutions for the youth in Slovakia] 24.01.1924 Protitrachomová akcia školské děti, skolníci [Anti-trachom action, school children] 1010–27. Box 107 Expositura Ministerstva veřejného zdravotnictví SNA.

37 Záboj Bruckner (1927) Příčiny a prevence slepoty v dětském věku [The causes and prevention of blindness in child ages] in Cyril Stejskal (ed.) *Třetí sjezd pro výzkum dítěte. V Praze 30., 31. října 1. a 2. listopadu 1926* [The third congress for the studies of child. In Prague 30.10.1926-02.11.1926] Praha: Pedologický ústav 351–390.

38 Župný úrad v Turč. Sv. Martine [District authorities in *Turčiansky Svätý Martin*] Organizovanie vzorného okresu na Slovensku [The organization of an exemplary district of public health in Slovakia] Číslo 51.555/125 7. novembra 1925 Box 107 Expositura Mnisterstva veřejného zdravotnictví SNA.

39 *Drotar* was a home repairer of kitchen utensils, or a manufacturer and seller of wire and sheet metal products; it is possible to say that the *drotar* is a symbol of Slovakia.

40 Župný úrad v Turč. Sv. Martine [District authorities in *Turčiansky* Svätý *Martin*] Organizovanie vzorného okresu na Slovensku [The organization of an exemplary district of public health in Slovakia] Číslo 51.555/125 07. 11. 1925 Box 107 Expositura Mnisterstva veřejného zdravotnictví SNA.

41 Vzorná zdravotní demonstrace v okresu Turč. Sv. Martin [Exemplary public health organization in the district of Turčianský sv. Martin] M.U.Dr. M. Šulc 1927 p. 7 Box 107 Expositura Mnisterstva veřejného zdravotnictví SNA.

42 Šulc Ibid.

43 Dopis Referátu ministerstva školství a národnej osvety v Bratislave Obezník č.135 [The Letter to the Board of the Ministry of Education and People's enlightenment in Bratislav].

Protitrachomová akcia na Slovensku učiteľov v smyslue preventivnaj pečlivosti [The action agains trachoma in Slovakia: the role of teachers in prevention].

Bratislava 22.IX.1927 Box 107 Expositura Mnisterstva veřejného zdravotnictví SNA.

44 More about the long-term attempts to include this Slovak district among the locations chosen by the Rockefeller Foundation for introducing the model of "public health demonstration," in Victoria Shmidt (2018) Public health as an agent

of internal colonialism in interwar Czechoslovakia: shaping the discourse about the nation's children, *Patterns of Prejudice,* 52:4, 355–387.
45 Bernardo J. Gastelum (1930) The cinema and hygiene propaganda *International review of educational cinematography* 3 155 2.
46 Stationary and moving pictures for hygiene propaganda (1930) *International review of educational cinematography* 1, 53–54, p. 54.
47 Ćiril Petešić (1991) Kamilo Brössler - naš Pestalozzi: pedagoško-socijalni rad i bibliografija objavljenih i neobjavljenih članaka, knjiga i filmova K. Brösslera [Kamilo Brössler is our Pestalozzi: pedagogical-social work and bibliography of known and unknown articles, books and films by K. Brössler] *Zbornik za povijest školstva i prosvjete,* 24, 145–165.

12 *Ikina sudbina* and *Dobro za zlo*

Extending the canon of health films to the Muslim periphery

Endemic syphilis as a long-term enemy of the Yugoslav periphery: The socialist upgrade of colonial motives

Ika, a young Herzegovinian, is a main character in *Ikina sudbina*, aimed at educating the population of Bosnia and Herzegovina about how to prevent the dissemination of endemic syphilis – often labeled as "rural" or "primitive,"[1] and one of the oldest and the most stubborn "enemies" of the region. Endemic syphilis and the history of attempts to combat it had become a part of the regime of authenticity attributed to Bosnia and Herzegovina before filming *Ikina sudbina*. "Bosnia as a region where syphilis known to be endemic for many centuries"[2] was a part of the discursive practices introduced by Austro-Hungarian authorities during the occupation of Bosnia in the last third of the nineteenth century. Explaining the dissemination of syphilis as introduced by the Ottomans started to resonate with the many complaints by occupational authorities regarding the resistance of the population to compulsory examination and mercury treatment.[3] The post-war call for reinforcing the health standards of the entire Yugoslav population only reinforced the stigma of the "medical Orientalism" associated with endemic syphilis; its dissemination continued to be explained by the cultural and hygienic "backwardness" inherited from the Ottoman Turks.[4]

Interwar Yugoslavia perpetuated this view on disease as a negative part of "human culture" (*ljudska kultura*) and the inevitable shadow of technical progress.[5] Along with the widely disseminated view on the transmission of endemic syphilis through sharing commodities and between family members,[6] *Ikina sudbina* connects the issue of syphilis with labor migration, a new risk for efficient surveillance over the Eastern periphery. Like the male characters of *Stín ve světle*, Ika travels far from his home for seasonal work to earn enough money for a wedding with his girlfriend, Janja.

Like Juro and Jano, Ika has been infected due to unsuitable hygienic conditions – by drinking from a common water jug. But instead of the psychological opposition of unique individuality to the ant personality, the main hermeneutical code of *Stín ve světle*, *Ikina sudbina* opposes the ordinary person to the selfish and not-humanist order of the economy, only aggravated by labor

DOI: 10.4324/9781003272267-17

migration. In *Ikina sudbina*, despite the spread of endemic syphilis among seasonal workers and its visible symptoms, nobody is interested in treating the people until Ika has returned home. Only the local physician, a role performed by Kamilo Brössler himself, has finally rescued Ika's entire family from the disease – in cooperation with older generations. In this way, not male selfishness but the absence of public interest in health is highlighted for the viewers.

The extraction and processing of stone "for the construction of large cities," as spectators are informed by the titles, the main activity of Ika, is presented as hard work – opposing the people of the periphery to the pressure of urbanization. The visualization of labor at the quarry as exhausting and dangerous fits with one of the main messages from the side of the key experts on public health in Yugoslavia, Andrija Štampar:

> [I]n a capitalist economy man possesses some economic value, but he himself it is of no economic value, if it does not use its labor power, or loses it. We are appalled today by the games in the Roman arenas, and do not see, that today the place itself has changed, for the masses of the working people are perishing in the factories, which are many times worse from the arenas themselves.[7]

Štampar, who was under the influence of the ideas espoused by Rudolf Goldscheid, an Austrian sociologist with moderate leftist views,[8] had introduced into the ideology of Yugoslav public health the main ideas of socializing public health through spending a larger part of the state budget on the needs of workers, as presented by Goldscheid in his program texts *Staatssozialismus oder Staatskapitalismus: Ein finanzsoziologischer Beitrag zur Lösung des Staatsschulden-Problems* ("State socialism or state capitalism: A sociological contribution to solving the national debt problem," 1917) and *Sozialisierung der Wirtschaft oder Staatsbankrott: Ein Sanierungsprogramm* ("Socialization of the economy or national bankruptcy: A program of renovation," 1919). Goldscheid had brought forward the idea that public health should operate not as protection for the weak but rather as protection *against* weakness.[9] He blamed the current politics for undermining the task of preventing disease, calling "glossing of over the degeneracy work of politics," one of the "greatest sins in the politics regarding the health of people." Goldscheid criticized Austro-Hungarian politics regarding public health and, thus, his arguments were easily accepted by the Yugoslav experts after 1918.

Štampar was armed with an argument designed by Goldscheid to attack the neglect of public health because of the rule of natural selection: "It is said that our health efforts are affected by the decline, the decadence of peoples and races. With that objection, we must remember that this is a matter of social, not natural, selection. Social selection or rather social misery destroys for the most part just healthy people."[10] Aligned with Goldscheid's approach, Štampar conceptualized infectious diseases as a problem of "health deficit" (*zdravstveni deficit*), which directly influenced the "capitalization" of the nation through rationalizing politics regarding people's health. The argument by Goldscheid was reinforced by the idea developed by Heinrich Potthoff in his *Krieg und Sozialpolitik: Handelspolitik und Wehrkraft* ("War and social policy: Trade policy and military forces"), on the economic importance of workers and the necessity to exert more effort toward improving human capital. Štampar argued against an improper, capitalist, view of health as a privilege through attributing to health the role of one of the main sources: "Undoubtedly, man also represents capital, and in every member of our people capitalized is a great economic value."[11]

This socialist view significantly transformed the benevolent paternalism emblematic of the Austro-Hungarian Empire regarding its Eastern periphery, including Bosnia and Herzegovina. Štampar brought forward the concept of "social medicine," developed and disseminated by Rudolf Virchow in his periodical "Medical Reform," issued between 1848 and 1849: "Physicians are the natural advocates of the poor and the social issue falls largely within their jurisdiction. Public concern for public health has the main say in most social difficulties as still relevant today, but it has not been implemented."[12] Notably, Virchow developed the concept of social medicine after making his field observations of the typhus epidemic in Upper Silesia in 1848, one of the German peripheries, and preparing a report for the government.[13] In his report, Virchow embedded social medicine in the revolutionary trend that he declared "a spring for the nations."[14] Along with freedom and independence, Virchow promoted economic equality as a main prerequisite for combating infectious diseases. In line with Virchow's concept, not the innocence of the naive indigenous population but the impossibility of winning the battle between individuals and the capitalist order started to be seen as one of the main signifiers for building the régime of authenticity within the periphery.

Despite the many obstacles to implementing this approach in practice, in the health films developed by the School of Public Health, social medicine, with its focus on hygiene and enlightenment, in combination with sustainable protection from the side of medical professionals, reached its apex – in promoting the cooperation between physicians and the community as the foundation for the sustainable prevention of disease. The lack of such cooperation is at the center of the critical view on Ika, who reproduces the behavior of the man who has infected him, and who simply ignores the symptoms of syphilis, such as ulceration on his lips, which are shown close-up several times. Ika continues ignoring his disease even after meeting the physician who has immediately recognized that Ika has been infected and could infect other people. As an educational aim, the film reproduces the same dialogue between an already infected person and those still not infected three times: "What is it?" – Ika asks his colleague about the ulceration. Ika's brother then asks Ika and Ika's betrothed, Janja, asks Ika. "Nothing serious, I must have caught a cold" – the already infected characters reply.

The vicious circle of carelessness has been stopped by Ika's father, old Marić, who goes to the physician immediately after recognizing the first symptoms of his youngest son, a six-year-old boy. The physician immediately shares with Ika's father his worries regarding Janja. Acting as a united front, these men have combated the disease. The physician decides to visit Ika, who is now married. The physician indicates that Janja has been already infected and observes the threatening progress of the disease in Ika. The physician persuades Ika, in the presence of Janja, to begin treatment. The speech of the physician is accompanied by documentary shots aimed at illustrating the various risks of untreated syphilis: Giving birth to a child with a severe mental disability, losing mental health, being unable to have children. The next day, Ika and Janja visit the medical center and receive their first treatment. The film closes with a visit by the physician to Ika's house and meeting his newborn son, who is healthy and happy in the embrace of his cured mother.

Ikina sudbina reproduces all the main features of the canon introduced by *Stín ve světle,* and even the differences between the films point to their common core, namely, establishing a régime of authenticity for those who are seen as "other" by the authors of the film. The major differences between *Stín ve světle* and *Ikina sudbina* can be explained by the obvious difference in the visions of the periphery among the Czech and Croatian ideologies of public health, as well as their different positions regarding national governments and supranational organizations. Constructing the messages aligned with the cultural and historical specifics of periphery represented a shared strategy for making the film able an efficient and persuasive tool of health propaganda.

All the characters of *Ikina sudbina*, except the physician, fit with the profile of the ant personality: They are shown as an inseparable part of their community. As in *Stín ve světle*, the spectators observe the collectives of Herzegovinians within the borders of their land and beyond, when they work at the quarry. During the crowd scenes, when they are working or having fun, the main characters are indistinguishable from the extras. Remarkably, all characters except the physician are performed by local inhabitants. In comparison with *Stín ve světle*, the boundary between fiction and documentary is blurred; the film tries to persuade the viewer that the history of Ika is one of many compatible histories, and Ika is just one of many inhabitants of Herzegovina.

In *Ikina sudbina*, the unity of the periphery and its identities is presented through a range of cultural practices compatible with *Stín ve světle*; *Ikina sudbina* stresses a positive, or even admiring, view on Herzegovina. The cascade of wonderful but dangerous landscapes at the beginning is supplemented by the title: "How beautiful is our Herzegovina!" Seconds later, the viewers see an older, mature man in folk costume and read the following title: "And how handsome is our Herzegovinian!" Ika's looks very much resemble this man – only younger. *Ikina sudbina* provides an ethnographic "portrait" of the region and the people living there. The men and women wear different folk costumes, depending on the situation and their social status. *Kolo*, the national round dance, in which a happy and reunited Ika and Janja participate (see Figure 12.1), continues for more than 25 seconds, and the viewers have a chance to observe all the aspects of this dance from different vantage points.

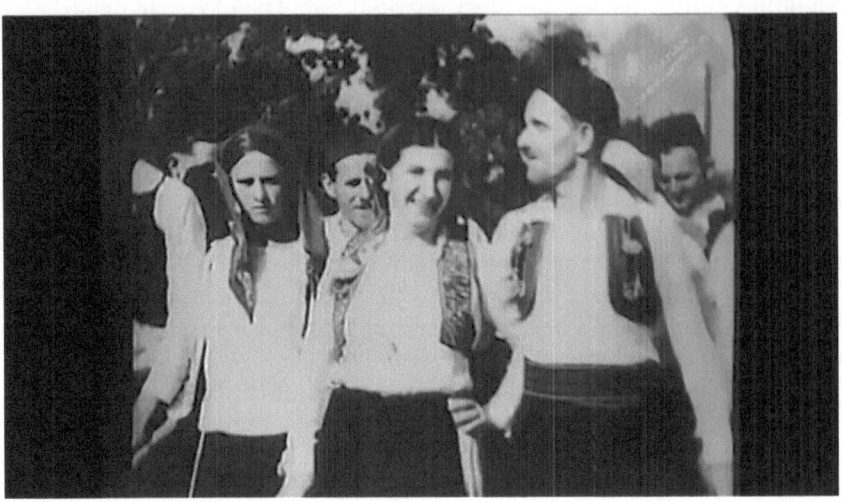

Figure 12.1 Ika and Janja dance in *Ikina sudbina* (Ika's destiny, 933).
Source: Kinoteka HAD.

Ikina sudbina presents the Herzegovinian community as patriarchal: While men are active members of the community, women achieve the most consistent performance of the national spirit. The traditionally female crafts, such as embroidery and weaving, connect Janja and Ika's mother, who discuss the return of Ika and the future wedding while engaging in their handwork. Janja remains a passive victim of Ika's irresponsible behavior, whose remedy totally depends on the involvement of Ika. The scene in which they visit the medical center underscores the different social status of women and men: Janja stays for the treatment but maintains her distance in communication with the physician (see Figure 12.3).

The patriarchal order is stressed by the presence of the Catholic Church in the life of community: The viewers do not necessarily know which religion Ika practices, but the Church plays an important role in the daily life of all inhabitants. The main characters meet each other near the Church after the Sunday service; the Church people are in the habit of spending their free time in the yard. *Ikina sudbina* was filmed in Široki Breg, the Franciscan Province of Herzegovina (see Figure 12.2). The long-term fight of the Franciscans against the pressure of the Catholic Church for keeping their independence and decisive role in the life of the local community in Herzegovina[15] can be seen as a possible precondition for including the church in the film. *Ikina sudbina* was produced during a period of obvious antagonism between the Orthodox Church and Catholic Church, as a part of the increasing influence of centrifugal forces from both sides, Serbian and Croatian nationalists, since the end of the 1920s.[16] The main message of the film, or in terms of Jakobson's communication paradigm, the emotive function, is the unity of Yugoslavs.

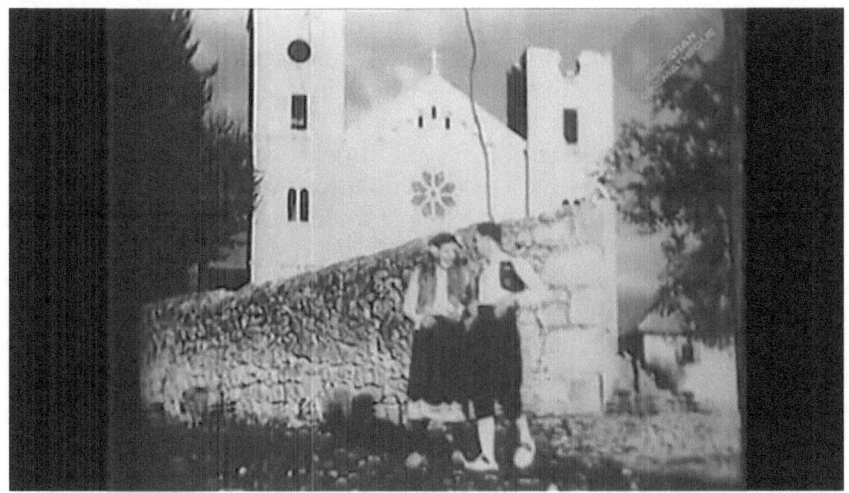

Figure 12.2 Ika and Janja make a decision about wedding in *Ikina sudbina* (Ika's destiny, 1933).

Source: Kinoteka HAD.

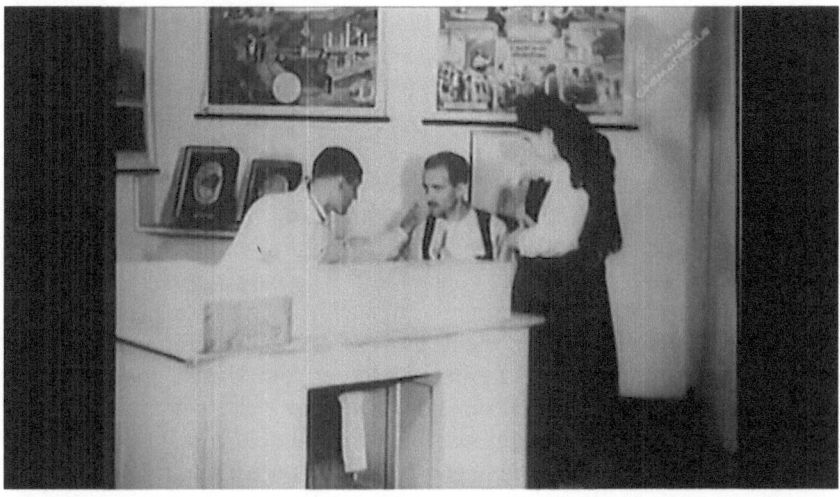

Figure 12.3 Ika and Janja visit the physician in *Ikina sudbina* (Ika's destiny, 1933).

Source: Kinoteka HAD.

Kamilo Brössler has infiltrated the film with one of the main messages for Yugoslavs, the pseudo-opposition between individuality and the universality of humans in the dimension of nation-building. Like Rudolf Goldscheid, who defined culture as a tool representing whether harmony between unity and individuality can be achieved or aggravated by this conflict,[17] Brössler put forward the idea by Miljenko Vidović, one of the Yugoslav ideologists of nation-building and educators for illiterate adults. Vidović introduced the concept of the immensity of human individuality (*neizmjernost čovjeka*) as "an achievable force for the human pursuit of joy, the main and common intention for all human beings."[18] In 1930, Brössler collected and published some of the short articles by Vidović written earlier for various regional newspapers. The main criterion for selecting the texts was the presence of the idea of a new, integrated Yugoslav nation. In the early 1930s, this collection challenged the political reaction started in Yugoslavia, positing the School of Public Health as a part of the opposition to the political regime. The first part of this collection is made up of articles targeted with the concept of "sun people" (*sunčani ljudi*), adopted by Vidović from the play by Maxim Gorky *Deti solntsa* (Children of the sun, 1905).

In contrast to the doubts of the Russian writer concerning the possibility to overcome the rupture between intellectuals, children of the sun and ordinary people, Vidović remained full of optimism and presented the desirable image of Yugoslav nation as "an army of progress, for it fights the light of reason and the light of culture and enlightenment."[19] The metaphor of the "new previously unknown army of peace which brings people together" fits with the role of the physician who is obliged to lead this army. In a text entitled *Tražite čovjeka* (Look for a man), Vidović directly appeals to teachers, physicians, engineers and priests as those who must accept the role of supervisors over the new people.[20] Vidović reproduces the call of Andrija Štampar, who had stressed in his report to the Ministry of Health the necessity to involve a wide range of professionals in solving the task to develop social medicine.[21]

Vidović reinforces the metaphor of sun people by adding the characteristic "fiery people" (*ognjeni ljudi*) and directly connecting this particular personality profile with the myth of Prometheus: The light of enlightenment should warm those frozen by the lack of education.[22] The entire professional biography of Brössler represents an exemplar of such a fiery person. The fact that in the film he, a representative of the Red Cross, an educator, and, even more, a future hero who had rescued Serbian children from Ustaše concentration camps, performs the role of a devoted physician, whose image is easily associated with the noble knight on the horse, should eliminate skeptical doubts in the appearance of a new generation of sun people.

The ant personality as a "sun" person: An unattainable ideal of the peripheral individual in *Dobro za zlo*

The next film aimed at addressing Eastern periphery, entitled *Dobro za zlo*, develops the motif of a medic who has rescued people from epidemic typhus, while being one of them. The choice of epidemic typhus was not coincidental. In terms of the number of typhus cases, Bosnia continued to dominate by an enormous margin over other Yugoslav territories. Out of 16,124 cases of the disease in Yugoslavia in the first half of 1920, more than 10,000 occurred in Bosnia. There were also considerably more deaths in Bosnia: Out of 1,970 deaths throughout the country, 1,203 died in Bosnia.[23] But the most alarming was the slow decrease in cases of the disease compared to other territories. While in Serbia, which was second only to Bosnia in the number of infected people at the beginning of the 1920s, the number of cases of typhus by the end of the 1920s had become isolated, significant foci of infection remained in Bosnia.

The propaganda aimed at equipping the rural population with the necessary competencies and preparing it for cooperation with epidemiologists included exhibitions and leaflets but it was not enough. Previous documentary films about epidemic typhus had reproduced many elements found in exhibitions and direct education, and *Dobro za zlo* aimed to introduce more persuasive, emotionally laden arguments.

The beginning of the film stresses a behavioral issue shared by two brothers: They live under the power of affect and lack rationality. As in *Stín ve světlě*, a love triangle triggers the events of the film. Meho and Ahmed fight for the same girl, pretty Zuleika, and Meho tries to kill his brother, who survives. Because of the argument with his brother, Meho "leaves his family, village, and ancestral coffins."[24] Twelve years have passed, and the audience recognizes that Meho has not changed and continues to behave presumptuously. Meho, who tries to look brave and handsome, is extremely vulnerable in front of the doubts in his masculinity. Coming back to their village, Meho and his friend, sober Ibro, decide to spend the night with their old neighbor, Suljo. Suljo, an elderly man, whose whole family seeks answers to the worries of young men, especially Ibro, exhibits the symptoms of *pjegavac* – epidemic typhus – and he believes that it is all the will of Allah. Ibro instead asserts that it is not God's will but "ours." Suljo accuses Ibro of being a coward and asks Meho if he is a coward too. Ibro tries to remind his friends that previous epidemics have killed more people than "cannons kill in a battle" but this appeal works neither for Suljo nor Meho. While the prudent Ibro goes to spend the night in the hayloft, away from the house, Meho, stung by the remark of Suljo about his cowardice, remains in the house.

On the following day, when they arrive at their village, Ibro suggests that Meho change his clothes to avoid the risk of transmitting the disease. But Meho refuses and jokes that some infectious sore has stuck to Ibro in the hayloft during the night, and condescendingly hits Ibro on the forehead. In response, Ibro, who is not inclined toward jokes, speaks grimly: "Take care of yourself and your own." In a play on words, Meho jokes one more time that it is Ibro's brain that has been "spotted" (in Bosnian, the word for epidemic typhus also means spotted). At this moment, the boyish enthusiasm with which Meho walks through the tobacco field to his house, knocking down the leaves with his hat, is highlighted.

Ibro takes all the safety precautions: He does not allow his wife to approach and asks her to bring clean clothes and a boiler to boil the ones he was wearing while in the infected house of Suljo. And after two weeks of quarantine, he is healthy. He learns that Meho, his family and their neighbors are all sick with typhus. He then goes for medical help and accompanies the doctor and his assistant (responsible for disinfection) to the village where the epidemic is raging. The film's viewers witness a remarkable scene aimed at stressing that real "heroes" who have the power and knowledge to rescue people are not an example of typical masculine dexterity. The doctor cannot climb onto the mule the first time. His assistant wears glasses, and his image does not have any features attributed to the standard of masculinity. During the conversation, the medical assistant learns that Meho is patient zero and asks Ibro if Meho has a brother, Ahmed. From Ibro's reply, he understands that people have forgotten all about Ahmed. The assistant confesses to the physician that he is actually Meho's brother, Ahmed, and asks if they can help his family and village.

The doctor shows Ibro, Suljo and other men all the symptoms of epidemic typhus, and in response, they ask how the disease spreads. Ahmed, grinning replies: "He is already on your lap," and removes some typhoid lice. The village men sarcastically say that "this stuff is in bulk here." The physician explains the transmission of disease through a lice nit, and remarkably, all the subtitles are accompanied in the film by relevant images in order to improve the audience's understanding. For instance, the dialogue about typhoid lice is illustrated with a large louse on the back of the subtitles.

In his short and energic speech, the doctor proclaims: "If you have ears, then you will rid yourself of epidemic typhus!" The audience of his speech is comprised of young men and boys, but in the next shot, the viewer sees all the village women disinfecting clothing. Ahmed organizes proper washing of the clothing; then, he shows the women how the typhoid lice settle in the seams of outerwear, and how to get rid of them with an iron. But the culmination of the disinfection ritual is the moment a disinfectant centrifuge appears in the village to clean mattresses and other bedding. These centrifuges had been purchased for different Yugoslav regions in the first half of the 1920s, becoming a part of epidemiological mobile services established at about that same time.[25] After disinfecting their houses, the inhabitants start to liquidate the lice in their hair (*depedikulacija*). Ahmed helps the men to shave their heads and gives soap and petrol to the women.

In fact, this work was often carried out by nurses and female assistants, who started working in Bosnian bacteriological stations from the early 1920s. The elimination of lice required teamwork among specially educated assistants, not one "hero" as is presented in the film. The exhibitions aimed at promoting hygienic procedures, and the institutions responsible for proper disinfection, often included images of these female assistants, but their faces were blurred and unrecognizeable, in line with cultural norms. But the film does not transgress beyond the boundaries of the genre of health films directed at make audiences and featuring men as the main characters.

The film does not reproduce the entire procedure for disease intervention, which was applied in interwar Yugoslavia in the event of a typhus epidemic.

For example, the film does not mention the bacteriological tests or the direct treatment of patients because it would attract attention to the figure of the physician, rather than to Ahmed. Moreover, the film presents the services of the epidemiologist and his assistant as permanent services, seen as the most desirable organizational approach for Eastern periphery but in reality, such a set-up was not widespread. But the detailed portrayal of the disinfection process depicted in the film echoes the visual approach of multiple exhibitions prepared in the 1920s. This approach was utilized in other documentary films disseminated in Balkan countries with a predominance of Muslim populations, such as Turkey and Albania.

After the end of the disinfection process, Ahmed devotes himself fully to caring for his brother. Meho, only having recovered, is shown as a weakened person with nothing remaining of his boyish enthusiasm. The moment of recovery coincides with the moment of Ahmed's confession and Meho's repentance, to whom Ahmed was reminded of a stab in the stomach and an attempt to kill him, but most importantly – depriving Ahmed of all ties with his family and his native village. The film ends with a reconciling hug and a call to be human – to respond to evil with good.

The inevitability of close-ups, the need for an entertaining and emotionally rich plot and the belief in the need to follow the pattern of popular films not only distanced the film from reality but significantly distorted the distribution of gender roles, both among the rescuers and those being rescued. But along with the limits produced by juxtaposing the expectations from Muslim audiences and popular movies, the motif of the ant personality should be taken into account. The transformation of Ahmed into a European-looking medic bridges the ascription of the ant personality as a part of collective identity and the typical European idea of coming of age through building an individual identity. Ahmed is able to combine both sides in the extreme example of the sun and ant personalities – one among many who are called to rescue their periphery. In the figure of Ahmed, who has returned to his village, it is possible to recognize another opposition consistently discussed by Štampar, who systematically opposed the physician who, because of an interest in personal enrichment, remains a servant of capitalism[26] and the physician as the head of the process of rooting hygienic culture.[27]

A major part of the film presents new hygienic skills for preventing infectious disease, translated by Ahmed to his community.[28] Chloupek utilizes the frames of traditional health films, a contest between two closely connected characters who have mutually opposed views on health and medicine. It was typical of the films produced by the Film Laboratory of the School of Public Health to situate siblings on the extremes of pro-healthy and anti-healthy behavior. Underscoring the kinship of opposing characters reflects in the film titles, which often included "Two brothers" or "Two sisters." (see Chapters 9 and 10) Clearly, this artistic device aims to stress that nothing like origin, childhood, or early education could influence the choice in favor of either health or sickness.

Furthermore, in contrast to a major portion of the health films by Chloupek, built on the opposition of siblings, which ends with the total demise of the character who has made the "wrong" choice (normally, the death of those who remain on the wrong side or the death of their relatives because of the irresponsibility of the main character), the contest between "good" and "bad" brothers in *Dobro za zlo* results in a happy ending for both sides. Even more, Chloupek doubles the opposition through introducing a contest between Meho and Ahmed, as well as between Meho and his friend, Ibro, too. This opposition in *Dobro za zlo* connects healthy and unhealthy patterns with true and false male maturity, stemming from collective, or even civil, responsibility. This transformation of one of the key frames of Croatian health films for men can be explained by the specific prescription for desirable human bondage in the films produced by the School of People Health for the Muslim periphery.

In 1952, Chloupek wrote a draft script for a film aimed at preventing trachoma, which exploited this idea in the new post-war and socialist contexts.[29] The characters in the film are not young people: The middle-aged Croatians, Janko and Anka, are survivors of the war who lost their partners but saved their children, and they are in search of a better life. They meet each other in Međimurje, destroyed by Nazi troops. While some of the inhabitants would like to stay and renovate their houses and make an effort to return to their previously peaceful lives, Janko and some of his friends would like to abandon this densely populated region and search for a better life in Istria. Together with his friend Mirko, Janko, after selling his house in Međimurje, moves away to start a new life with Anka. But before moving, they must be tested against trachoma. Janko thinks that it only wastes their time and thus he fraudulently, without proper medical examination, confirms that he is not sick.

After arriving in the new village, in a few days, the schoolteacher informs the village inhabitants that some children have trachoma, including Janko's children. This fact inclines Janko to go to the anti-trachoma medical office, where he learns about the disease and its different stages. He and his children obtain some drops, and after a few months, they are healthy again. Anka, who abandons Janko after recognizing his deception, comes back and shares how many people were infected very probably by Janko. Janko goes back to his village in Međimurje and offers a public apology, distributing health propaganda among his former neighbors. The two-page film draft is reminiscent of *Stín ve světle* but with a focus on the peripheral community as a social organism, one of the central points of health propaganda for the Muslim territories in Yugoslavia.

The peripheral community as a social organism: The power of intergenerational responsibility in Yugoslav films

Like *Stín ve světle*, *Ikina sudbina* and *Dobro za zlo* construct the idea of human bondage around the love story but not in the ambiguous attitude toward intensive eroticization as in the relationship between Juro and Maryša. The different approach to visualizing romantic relationships can be explained by other cultural norms ascribed to the periphery. Perhaps, only a happy ending comprised of marriage, cured disease and giving birth to a healthy baby makes it possible to present in *Ikina sudbina* the development of the romantic relationship between Ika and Janja – from a restrained hand-shake when Ika bids Janja farewell before migrating for seasonal work to the close embrace after Ika's return and the presentation of a wedding ring – when they embark together into the fields. Ika's strength of sexual attraction partly explains his disobedience to the doctor's advice to postpone the wedding until cured of syphilis. In this turn, Ika's behavior plays the same role as the entire story of Juro and his negative human bondage. In contrast to Juro, Ika is able to accept the alternative, positive, human bondage, including his attachment to the parental family. In *Dobro za zlo*, Meho gets a chance for reconciliation with his brother, and Ahmed in his turn is happy to be useful to his parental community which he had abandoned.

In contrast to *Stín ve světle*, *Ikina sudbina* extends the role of inter-generational relationships. While the love story as a frame for the plot of health films was not typical of the School of Public Health, the relationship between parents and children underpinned most of the collisions and the most dramatic situations in the films that addressed either the rural center, Slovenia or Croatia, or the periphery – Bosnia and Herzegovina. In the many films produced in Zagreb, the rescue of children was the dominant motif for the emotive message from the authors to the audience. The vicissitudes of children's lives were a main source for producing dramatic plots, but in the films for Bosnia and Herzegovina, such discourse was only supplemental.

Ika's parents are presented in the film as totally positive and responsible members of the community. The father, old Marić, is sensitive to the threats of disease and cooperates with the physician, and the mother supports Janja during the period of awaiting Ika's return. In contrast, the irresponsible behavior of Ika threatens not only his beloved Janja but also his parental family, including the younger siblings. After returning, Ika asks his mother about Janja and hopes for a chance to meet her and propose to her, and his mother totally supports Ika in his marital plans. The film underscores the responsibility of Ika in front of the next generation – as a father too, and the majority of examples of non-treated syphilis address irresponsible parenting. However, the child–parent connection does not exhaust the specific, familial, human bondage of *Ikina sudbina*. Suljo in *Dobro za zlo* is reeducated and participates in activities aimed at preventing the dissemination of typhoid fewer.

Emphasizing multi-generational relations reverberates with one of the pillars of public health ideology introduced by Štampar, who called for focusing on society as an organism, not the organism of individuals, in matters of public health.[30] Štampar defines the mission of medicine as "social therapy" or treating "constitutionally sick societies" (*konstitucionalne bolovanje društva*). Aligned with the model of the economics of development (*Enwicklungsökonomie*) introduced by Goldscheid, at the very beginning of his career as a public politician, Štampar stresses the impossibility of curing a disease among the wealthy without preventing it among the poor – because of social origin and mutual interconnection among social groups. In 1928, Štampar replaced the economic focus with a more political vision of class conflict and a directly opposed past, aristocratic medicine made "within the walls of laboratories," and the obsession over the idea of diseases, promoting instead a new, democratic medicine aimed at improving the health of people.[31] Along with this long-term call for a socialist approach, Štampar stresses some expectations from the periphery – regarding more consistent rationalization of behavior.

The social etiology of diseases includes not only the unsanitary milieu in which the periphery lives but also the vacuum of a rational approach to health at each of the levels of community life. This rational view stems from the optimistic persuasion in the naturalness of focusing on progress and the public good among the people. Social hygiene, eugenics and social therapy are seen by Štampar as three pillars for rationalizing the behavior of people. Social hygiene shapes new habits. Eugenics should ensure a rational approach to reproductive behavior. Social therapy aims to equip people with the "proper" strategies of nutrition, care for children, and the organization of labor. The lack of a rationalized approach to the health of society started to be seen as a social pathology, and "proper" human bondage should eliminate it. This view stems from another definition of culture given by Goldscheid, namely, the proper conversion of external work (*äußere Arbeit*) to the internal labor of rationalization. The main mechanism of such a conversion, according to Goldscheid, is adding value, whether economic or spiritual, through the deliberate redeployment of the outputs of human progress.[32] And the irrational behavior of Ika, who rejects being treated against disease, blocks this process in his community. The very same motive of irrational behavior constructs the plot of *Dobro za zlo*, in which Meh at the beginning rejects treatment because of his belief in disease as a part of fate. In both films, physicians have cured the communities – first of irrationality, as the core of social pathology, and then – of disease.

The films produced for Bosnia and Herzegovina reproduced the main semantic structure of health films for the periphery but in other cultural and political contexts or in Altman's terms, in other pragmatics. Far broader political and social enterprises, including the vicissitudes of public health and other extra-filmic events, led to generic changes that saturated the genre of health films for the periphery with new discursive practices. In 1934, the School of Public Health presented, among other films aimed at educating people, *Ikina sudbina* at the Congrès international du Cinéma d'Education et d'Enseignement in Rome. It is notable that for international audiences, the film was presented as targeted at sexually transmitted diseases, not endemic syphilis. Štampar arranged showings of both films during his international trips to the United States and Canada.

The films created for the periphery gained considerable attention from the side of the National Tuberculosis Association, which had started to point to suitable strategies for disseminating their preventive politics among minorities. Together with *Stín ve světle*, *Ikina sudbina* and *Dobro za zlo* shaped the semantics and syntax of three films developed by Edgar Ulmer for three different minority groups of the United States, African Americans, Latin Americans and Native Americans. In each of the films Ulmer produced, the effort to reconstruct a relevant regime of authenticity for each of the minorities was evident. Moreover, the set of these three films reproduced the racial hierarchy of the interwar United States. In this way, the logic of developing the genre of health films for the periphery, extended to the films targeted at reproducing racial hierarchy, rearranges our historical imagination about producing a racialized gaze on the periphery and minorities and the agents of this process regarding the role of Central Eastern Europe.

Notes

1 Brigitta Fuchs (2016) Škerljevo, Frenjak, Syphilis: Constructing the Ottoman Origin of Not Sexually Transmitted Venereal Disease in Austria and Hungary, 1815–1918 in Jörg Vögele, Stephanie Knöll and Thorsten Noack (eds.) *Epidemien und Pandemien in historischer Perspektive/Epidemics and Pandemics in Historical Perspective,* Geneve: Springer, VS p. 60.
2 Stefano Petrungaro (2019) The Medical Debate about Prostitution and Venereal Diseases in Yugoslavia (1918–1941) *Social History of Medicine*, Volume 32, Issue 1, February, 121–142, p. 128.
3 Brigitta Fuchs Ibid.
4 Petrungaro, Ibid, p. 129.
5 Andrija Štampar (1911) Socijalna medicina [Social medicine] *Zora,* 3, pp. 126–131.
6 Fuchs Ibid., p. 7.
7 Andrija Štampar (1919) O zdravstvenoj politici Jugoslavenska [About public health in Yugoslavia] *Njiva,* 29–31 pp. 1–29.
8 More about Rudolf Goldscheid and his role in developing "productive" eugenics in Cheryl Logan (2013) *Hormones, Heredity and Race* New Brunswick, N.J.: Rutgers University Press, pp.113–116; Veronika Hofer (2002) Rudolf Goldscheid, Paul Kammerer und die Biologen des Prater-Vivariums in der liberalen Volksbildung der Wiener Moderne [Rudolf Goldscheid, Paul Kammerer and the biologists of Prater-Vivariums in liberal education for all in modern Vienna] in Mitchell G. Ash and Christian H. Stifter (eds.) *Wissenschaft, Politik und Öffentlichkeit* [Science, Politics and Openless], Vienna: WUV, 149–184.
9 David Goldscheid (1909) *Darwin als Lebenselement unserer modernen Kultur* [Darwin as a decisive part of our contemporary culture] Wien und Leipzig, Hugo Heller, p. 99.
10 Ibid.
11 Štampar O zdravstvenoj politici Jugoslavenska.
12 Andrija Štampar (1925) *Socijalna medicina. Uz saradnju jugoslovenskih socijalnih lekara* [Social medicine: From the experinece of yugoslav physicians] First volume Zagreb: Institut za socijalnu medicinu.
13 Rex Taylor and Annelie Rieger (1984) Rudolf Virchow on the typhus epidemic in Upper Silesia: an introduction and translation *Sociology of Health and Illness,* 6 2, 201–217..
14 Ibid p. 202.

15 Ahmet Alibašić (2020) History of Inter-Religious Dialogue in Bosnia and Herzegovina From Force-Feeding to Sustainability? *Interdisciplinary Journal for Religion and Transformation in Contemporary Society* 6, 343–364.
16 Vjekoslav Perica (2002) *Balkan Idols: Religion and Nationalism in Yugoslav states,* Oxford: Oxford University Press, pp. 19–20.
17 Goldscheid Kulturperspektiven.
18 Miljenko Vidović (1927) *Ideje i problemi: članci i rasprave* [Ideas and issues: articles and discussions] Sarajevo: Obod.
19 Miljenko Vidović (1926) Dolaze sunčani ljudi [Sun people are coming] *Novi čovjek,* 2, p.1.
20 Miljenko Vidović *(1927)* Tražite čovjeka [Look for a man] *Uzgajatelj* 2 p.1.
21 Andrija Štampar (1920) O socijalnoj terapiji [About social therapy] Glasnik Ministarstva narodnog zdravlja [Newslatter of the Ministzr of Public health], 7, pp. 261–271.
22 Miljenko Vidović (1927) Ognjeni ljudi [Fiery people] *Novi Čovjek, 62,* p. *1.*
23 Štampar 1925 *Socijalna medicina.* p. 105.
24 Drago Chloupek 1936 Subtitles to the film "Dobro za zlo". Kinoteka of the State Archives of Croatia, Fond of Skola za narodnog zdravja, box 1. Notably, some versions of the film included the details of the love triangle but for some regions this part of story was excluded from the narration.
25 Štampar (1925) *Socijalna medicina.*, p. 81.
26 Štampar (1911) Socijalna medicina p. 126.
27 Ibid. p. 131.
28 Zoran Tadić (2004) Zaboravljeni Chloupek [Forgotten Chloupek] Dokumentarni film – uvod: Škola Narodnog Zdravlija available online: https://www.matica.hr/vijenac/279/Zaboravljeni%20Chloupek/.
29 Drago Chloupek (1952) Nacrt zdravstveno-prosvjetnog filma o trachomu [Draft script of the health-enlightening film about trachoma]. Kinoteka of the State Archives of Croatia, Fond of Skola za narodnog zdravja, box 2..
30 Štampar O socijalnoj terapiji 271.
31 Andrija Štampar (1928) Naša ideologija [Our ideology] *Nova Evropa* [Our Europe] 229–231.
32 Goldscheid Darwin 96–98.

13 Films of the National Tuberculosis Association

Rooting health films for the periphery in the racial hierarchies of the interwar United States

Films against tuberculosis for ethnic minorities: A case of multiple pragmatics

> No attempt is made to cover the whole complex domain of present-day sickness prevention. Instead, work is concentrated on certain diseases where there is a reasonable expectation that they can be transferred from the non-preventable to the preventable class.[1]

This approach, with its great potential to reinforce inequality among those with preventable and less preventable diseases, framed the global politics concerning health security in the second half of the 1930s. Timely medical examination started to be seen as bridging the most advanced outputs of scientific progress in understanding infectious diseases and the field work of health workers. Educating people through health propaganda represented a mission to shape collective responsibility for preventing preventable diseases, including tuberculosis.[2] The project of the Rockefeller Foundation targeted at the spread and frequency of disseminating tuberculosis was implemented in two southern US states, as well as in Austria and Jamaica.

The main concern of the project, "to determine the success of segregation, nursing care, and other measures that may influence the spread of the disease,"[3] tended to profile risk groups that needed more attention from the side of public health. In the United States, the predominance of "whites" or "blacks" was brought into analytical lenses as the most decisive factor. One of the two states included in the sample was Alabama, where the National Tuberculosis Association (NTA) and The Tuskegee Institute, led by Booker T. Washington, an industrial training school for African Americans, but also an institution for "character formation," stressing hygiene, or as Washington put it, "the gospel of the toothbrush,"[4] implemented certain steps toward preventing tuberculosis. Within the project, new types of medical examinations, such as roentgenography and the TB skin test, were explored. This experience of international participation drove the next steps by national bodies, including the idea to make the films as a part of the campaign aimed at involving communities in new practices of medical assessment.

DOI: 10.4324/9781003272267-18

By the 1930s, the NTA had already obtained the position of one of the most influential national organizations that contributed to the institutionalization of public health across the country and involved the majority, "white" population in the programs aimed at preventing tuberculosis.[5] The New Deal pursued, among other goals, improving access to public health, which reinforced the politics of the NTA aimed at the prevention and timely treatment of tuberculosis among the youngest generations. Edgar Sydenstricker, one of the New Deal ideologues, emphasized the threat of tuberculosis for people between the ages of 20 and 30 as the predominant cause of death.[6] The NTA had responded to this call with the idea to produce a cluster of films that would address young people from different ages, social and ethnic groups, generally those "too young for the vital spark to be dim."[7]

The films, intended to "reach the specific communities where the disease still lingered,"[8] namely, the ethnic minorities who were seen at risk for "spreading misinformation" and whose susceptibility adopt the content and esthetics to the mentality of minority" was discussed in terms of racial differences:[9] African Americans, Native Americans and Latin Americans. For many interwar experts, "tremendous disparities in death rates from tuberculosis remained to be a matter of not only socioeconomic status, but also race."[10] This intersectionality between age, social class and ethnicity reverberated with the interests of other actors who had a pragmatic interest in producing and disseminating such health films, first among them the activists of ethnic minority groups, "who, like their white counterparts, also hailed from middle-class origins, founded organizations through their churches, local women's clubs, or fraternal organizations."[11]

For instance, African Americans brought forward the idea of "Negro self-help" to the programs aimed at preventing tuberculosis, instead of the benevolent paternalism of the "whites," who were interested in preventing the spread of tuberculosis among those Blacks who cared for their children, served their dinner and worked at their factories.[12] The Tuskegee Institute was involved in the production of a film for young African Americans: the students performed all the roles, the film was made in the interiors of the Institute, and the choir, under the supervision of William L. Dawson, performed the gospel music which reinforced the messages of the film. One of the main concerns of Black activists was to protect and disseminate "a firmly fixed policy that blacks would be treated within segregation, and encouraged to teach and care for their own people."[13] This policy echoed in the production of films too; for example, Orson Welles made his *Voodoo Macbeth* using only African American casting.[14] The choice of this strategy was dictated by the long-term uncertainty of whether health care was a "privilege" or a "right,"[15] which solidified class-based disparities in health care and brought about the necessity to accept the compromise for those whose "political activity and 'the agitation of questions of social equality' were definitely discouraged."[16]

Governmental bodies, international medical experts and minority elites were interested in increasing surveillance over populations through disseminating new and healthier standards for coming of age and presenting the risks of being infected and treated in a timely manner as "a consequence of an outmoded, dangerously traditional way of thinking."[17] Georgina Feldberg has interpreted the efforts to control tuberculosis between the 1860s and 1960s as a part of "the varied social and scientific challenges that gave rise to the US American middle class."[18] Disseminating missionary medicine through health films about tuberculosis was the case "[w]hen the diverse groups using the genre are considered together, genres appear as regulatory schemes facilitating the integration of diverse factions into a single social fabric."[19] Being one of "the sites around which the middle classes formed,"[20] tuberculosis reinforced the hierarchical nature of this process and the necessity to reflect this difference in the films.

The choice in favor of films for the periphery as a suitable genre launched the process of attaching new adjectives to an already established canon and other existing genres as indispensable for creating a new cycle of six films for the youngest "others": *Diagnostic Procedures in Tuberculosis (1940)*, an educational documentary about the medical tests necessary for the timely diagnosis of tuberculosis; three films for various minorities, *Let My People Live* (1938), *Cloud in the Sky* (1939), *Another to Conquer* (1941); *Goodbye, Mr. Germ* (1940), a film with the elements of animation for children; and *They do come back* (1940), for young "white" people from the lower-middle class who could achieve a better life as part of the upper-middle class through efficient and timely treatment of disease.

Devin Orgeron underscores the difference, or, even more, the "otherness" of these films in comparison with the mainstream health films produced in the United States generally and for the NTA in particular. He explains this through the personality of Edgar Ulmer, a filmmaker especially capable of reaching niche or ethnic audiences.[21] Ulmer's sophistication in reconstructing the ordinary life of minorities[22] and his "transcendental homelessness ... a vital strain in Ulmer's aesthetic and cultural sensibility"[23] represent the main historical explanations for his cooperation with the NTA, along with his reputation of producing attractive films on a low budget[24] and with a sense of social responsibility.[25] It is reasonable to add one more historically relevant explanation to this typical focus of the films, a faith in the auteur's "addiction to directorial identification,"[26] namely, the affiliation of Ulmer, born in the Czech lands and making his filmmaking debut in Austria, with Central Eastern Europe as a global periphery in establishing the global regime of health security.

More health films for "others": Ulmer's "poaching" of films produced for the periphery

The analogy between minorities, especially between Latin Americans and Central Eastern Europeans, as racially inferior and threatening to the "American" nation, achieved its extreme among medical experts in the 1920s when the intensity of labor migration from Central and Eastern Europe to the United States reached a new peak.[27] At the same time, medical experts from Central Eastern Europe started to translate their experience with developing public health in rural and peripheral areas to the international level. Andrija Štampar not only visited the United States in 1931, within the international program of the Rockefeller Foundation, but also became an influential member of the League of Nations and conducted a trip to China for exchanging experiences in disseminating new models of health care. Health films produced for the periphery started to become a part of the international representation of the success of health propaganda in the region. This ambivalent position of the Central Eastern European experience fully reverberated with Ulmer's biography and his life situation at the moment of being recruited by the NTA. For the NTA, Ulmer was a person with a particular affiliation to the Eastern periphery, in several different meanings.

Ulmer, the oldest son of secular bourgeois Jewish parents, was born in Olomouc, the second center of the Moravian province of the Austro-Hungarian empire, and grew up in Vienna. After his emigration to the United States, he cooperated with migrant groups, most of all with Jews and Ukrainians, and his debut in Hollywood was a health film based upon on a French play produced for Canada.[28] At the time that he began his cooperation with the NTA, Ulmer's cultural in-betweenness resonated with his own prag-matic interests. Ulmer accepted the offer by the NTA in the midst of a most urgent need for funds and orders. He had lost the option to make Hollywood films, due to his love affair with Shirley Castle, the wife of Max Alexander, the nephew of Carl Laemmle, head of Universal Studios. It made Ulmer *persona non grata* in Hollywood.[29] Being consigned to the fringes of the US motion picture industry, Ulmer specialized first in "ethnic films," both in Ukrainian – *Natalka Poltavka* (1937), *Cossacks in Exile* (1939) – and in Yiddish – *Green fields* (1937), *The Light Ahead* (1939), *Americaner Shadchen* (1940), developing the reputation of an expert in ethnic minorities. Ulmer described this period as "a time of torture due to the necessity to sell himself to producers."[30] This vulnerable position made the candidature of Ulmer more attractive, not least because of reasonable expectations from the side of the NTA that would oblige the film director to make the best efforts to produce what the NTA needed – missionary stories for the periphery that would impose a particular behavioral pattern without the risk of systematic resistance from the side of minorities. Although Ulmer did not directly confirm it, the health films for the periphery produced in Czechoslovakia and Yugoslavia would seem to have been an ideal source of inspiration for this purpose. Understanding history, especially its cultural aspects, not only in terms of known events but also probabilities,[31] leads us to consider this option.

The probability of adapting Central Eastern European health films pro-duced for the periphery is determined by a multilevel composition of pre-dispositions. The level of interpersonal and inter-departmental relations, such as very probable connections between Ulmer and his Czech colleagues,[32] the attention to international trends from the side of the NTA, which had already produced health films, could play an important role in transferring the Central Eastern European experience to the NTA films made for US minorities. But there was more to the story. Like Czechoslovakia and Yugoslavia, two nations that relied on synthetic, "super-national" ideology (Czechoslovakism and Yugoslavism), the United States faced the dilemma of culture vs. civilization, which was entirely connected to the debates regarding the relation between human individuality and civilization in terms of the role of "man" in constructing a new social order on a worldwide scale aimed at fostering a sustainable civilizing process.[33] The semantics of health films produced in Czechoslovakia and Yugoslavia reconstructed the subordinated position of peripheral culture to global civilization, and the syntax of these films presented a wide range of options for solving the opposition between culture and civilization in favor of a global order of health security.

A linear model of human progress, well disseminated in the United States, stemmed from the stance that "civilization is culture, but not all culture is civilization."[34] Viewing the relation between civilization and culture in terms of instincts and intelligence shaped a kind of hierarchy of minorities, based upon the degree of conflict between instinct and intelligence. A more or less "organic" or "natural" connection between minority culture and global civilization reverberated with the inter- and intra-racial hierarchies that framed political and social life in the interwar United States.[35] The intensive formation of the foundations of racial assimilationism that besieged the interwar period involved not only inter-racial hierarchies, but also intra-racial hierarchies - ranking within one group.[36] This optic nuances the already established interpretation of Ulmer's films as producing an ambivalent discourse, one that brings together the recognition of minority cultures and a consistent call to integrate them into the "American" nation through the submission of such minorities to the know-how of practitioners, the key to their final assimilation.[37]

In each of Ulmer's films, regimes of authenticity are forged as multilayered constructions that encompassed the official rhetoric of inclusion, benevolent paternalism, which varied from film to film, and the presentation of collective cultural practices. The periphery presents in each of three films not as a particular region but as a social milieu or even a reservation to which the particular ethnic group belongs. In *Let My People Live* and *Another to Conquer*, this milieu presents as a rural area full of shtetl life, especially in opposition to the larger, "white," urban world from which the reeducated and surviving "ants" come back in order to help their relatives, communities and ethnic groups survive through educating them. In each of the films, collective identity and its progress due to the acquisition of new preventive health practices prevails over individuality and private life. In particular, combating tuberculosis is presented as a new historical challenge to each of the minorities. But along with this shared semantics, the films vary in the perspective on minority communities and the role they might play in their own fate.[38]

Cloud in the Sky presents the traditional collective cultural practices of Latin Americans as totally positive and deserving of admiration from the side of the "white" majority. However, the cultural practices of the indigenous population in *Another to Conquer*, such as nomadism after the death of family members or certain funeral rituals, are presented as a relic of the past incompatible with new progressive practices of public health. The films vary in the degree of the expectations placed on minorities to be aligned with new, healthier practices of preventing tuberculosis. In *Let My People Live* and *Cloud in the Sky*, the main protagonists have not abandoned their communities to being cured but in *Another to Conquer*, the main character is isolated in boarding school for the task of achieving a level of hygienic skills sufficient for educating other members of his community. Each of the films practice specific visual and audial tools for establishing clear boundaries between the "white" majority and the "non-white" minority as the grounds for crossing such boundaries, traversing the "bigger world" in order to get a carefully measured dose of progress. This theme is one of the main shifts in the generic changes to the films made by Ulmer for the NTA – in contrast to the health film produced for the periphery that aimed at legitimizing "white" penetration into the world of the periphery.

Altman's analogy between the development of a genre as "poaching" on established genre territory[39] aligns with the way in which Ulmer filmed missionary medicine for the NTA. The semantics of the health films produced for the periphery were adapted in line with racially based differentiation among minorities. Ulmer introduced a wide range of visual tools and intertextualities to reproduce the hierarchy of minorities that operated in the interwar United States.[40] This hierarchy not only generated new syntactic structures within already established semantics, but also significantly transformed and supplemented the original canon of health films for the periphery. Each of the films, as well as their constellation, coordinated their acceptance by the target audience through generic change, toward rooting the multidiscursivity of health films for the periphery regarding each of the three ethnic groups and the NTA.[41]

Let my people live: *Lifting the Veil of Ignorance?*

Let my people live starts with singing by the Tuskegee Institute Choir, representing one of the most important public signifiers of African American culture and its flourishing during the interwar period, the "Negro college choir."[42] At the same moment, viewers could witness the monument *Lifting the Veil of Ignorance,* by New York artist Charles Keck, dedicated to educator and African American politician Booker T. Washington, established on the campus of the University in 1927. The monument consists of the figures of two African American men, one full of power and strength, who lifts the veil from the face of other man, poised on his knees. The monument symbolizes the main idea of the film: Black elites taking responsibility for the poorer and less educated members of their community. In this way, Ulmer intends to provide an analogy between the compatible role of the Black community in the elimination of slavery and infectious diseases. Even the title of the film uses the motto of the movement by African American slaves for their abolition, only with a minor change in the last word – not "Let my people *go*" but "Let my people *live*." This motif is only stressed by the fact that there are no "white" characters in the film: everyone, including the physicians and nurses, is African American. The film thus depicts the African American periphery as a hermetically sealed space that does not need medical intervention by "superior" whites. *Let My People Live* aligns with the efforts of the Black community to cure itself and combat tuberculosis since the 1910s through spiritualizing public health.[43]

Immediately after this introduction, the physician, in the manner of a preacher, appeals to students after they finish the spiritual singing. His speech aims to mobilize young people to pay more attention to the possible symptoms of tuberculosis because "We as Negroes seem to be particularly susceptible to this disease." According to the physician, poverty is not only an obstacle to being treated in the late stages of the disease but also the reason for being at risk of infection in the first place. Immediately after, the camera focuses on George, the young protagonist and one among many other students who participate in the collective meeting. But he must abandon his peers because his mother, "who never saw a doctor," is dying of tuberculosis and his sister, Mary, has asked him to come home. His journey home is accompanied by three other spiritual psalms, among them one of the most popular, "Go down, Moses."

The focus on the brother–sister relationship references an appeal typical of African American Church communities, to one's "brother" or "sister," which transforms the interconnection between family bonds and belonging to community into the idea of a small family unit as a part of larger unit. In contrast to the other two films, the audience does not see any children or any allusion to a romantic relationship and family life in the specific role of the family unit in the fight against tuberculosis. At the same time, the consistent asexuality of film reflects the enormous efforts made by African Americans to decrease fertility rates and institutionalize various strategies of birth control.[44] The exclusion of any reference to the sexual component of relations is also consistent with the moralism of the ideology of the Black community of that period. By replacing focus on the marital couple and parents with children with siblings, Ulmer gains additional traction for differentiating the gender role of the ant person and reintroducing the patriarchal order of the periphery.

The role of the church is reinforced by the attention devoted to the male figure of the priest and the direct support for public health from the side of the church. Religiosity plays a significant role in the regime of authenticity constructed by Ulmer for African Americans who live on the periphery. Mary has made the final decision to go to the physician for a tuberculosis test after having a conversation with the local priest, who says: "I am not a doctor but I have read a lot about tuberculosis." He answers the worries of Mary that she might have symptoms: "You will be smart and go to see a doctor ... if he says no, that it's fine, if he says yes, do exactly what he tells you." We watch George as the protagonist in the narration about assessment procedures, but not Mary, who is actually sick. We observe her laying in the hospital bed, while George, despite being at risk, is full of energy. Moreover, George has had tuberculosis earlier but his organism had coped with this very primary stage of the disease. George thus forges a pathway toward vocational training (according to his uniform, as an engineer) and obviously intends to continue his career, while Mary remains a passive part of the periphery.

Undesirable patterns of behavior are attributed to the young uneducated woman, Minnie, Mary's friend who tries to persuade her not to visit the physician. But at the end of the film, they are sitting together and listening to a broadcast about tuberculosis, a direct translation concluded by one of the Hallelujah Choruses, an optimistic gospel piece performed by the Tuskegee Institute Choir.[45] Like *Stín ve světle*, *Let My People Live* underscores the role of such cultural practices in health propaganda. Ulmer has minimized the role of landscapes in *Let My People Live*, but the sunset and sunrise at the beginning and at the end of the film leave no doubt regarding the optimistic future for this community – even without showing future generations. Bringing intergenerational connections and their continuity because of the sustainable prevention of tuberculosis into focus is the main message of the films for other two minorities, *Cloud in the Sky* and *Another to Conquer.*

Cloud in the Sky: A nearly enlightened community of happy and healthy people

Cloud in the Sky not only narrates the story of young Mexican beauty Consuela, whose mother has died of tuberculosis, but also presents the Mexican community that has become enlightened through becoming educated about how to prevent tuberculosis. Among the three films produced for minorities, *Cloud in the Sky* could be seen as the most similar to *Stín ve světle* and *Ikina sudbina* in terms of the approaches to constructing the ant personality and human bondage in the peripheral community. This similarity is supplemented by various tactics aimed at presenting Latin Americans as nearly "white" but still in need of protection by professionals, and the whole society, or those who were situated on one of the highest positions of the inter-racial hierarchy.

The very first scene depicts the hard work of Latin Americans at the quarry. These very first moments are part of the introduction to the film, crafted in the style of the NO-DO newsreels, which present more than the 1.5 million US citizens whose mother tongue is Spanish as a valuable part of US American society, working in factories and defending their country by serving in the Army. In this way, presenting Latin Americans as the subjects of important news, it is possible to recognize the echo of the Ulmer's experience working as a camera operator for the *Pathé Newsreel* after his departure to New York in 1937. In the best tradition of NO-DO newsreels, this introductory scene ends with the slogan "to help these people to crush the burden of tuberculosis," which the viewers hear as they observe dozens of Latin Americans in Army uniforms, with the US flag in the background. These very first moments of the film construct the image of the ant personality, who operates in the multiple interests of the "American" nation, and who deserves to be rescued.

Ulmer frames the narration about threat and survival with the rhythmic opposition of the symbols of the sun, sunlight and a clear sky, on the one hand, and clouds, shadows, and darkness, on the other hand. At the beginning of the film, the family of Consuela wears black clothing to mourn the mother, but at the end, when whole community celebrates not only the wedding of Consuela and her fiancée, Basil, but also the absence of tuberculosis, all wear vibrant and bright colors. All the scenes shot in the sanatorium in which Consuela has been placed are full of the color white. The physician compares the tuberculosis in Consuela with a small cloud in the hellish sky. Young Basil, who is in love with Consuela, sings under the windows of the sanatorium *Cielito lindo* (literally "Cute little sky"), one of the most popular Mexican songs with a refrain that compares a girl with the sun. The very last shot of the film shows the clouds in the sky one last time, and then, they are replaced by the symbol of the international movement against tuberculosis, the Cross of Lorraine.[46] Mexicans are described by the "wise Padre," the priest who has played a decisive role in leading Consuela to the decision to be treated by the physician himself, as happy people who "work hard but enjoy life too."

As in *Ikina sudbina*, the main characters perform the *Jarabe Tapatío* (the Mexican Hat Dance) in national costumes, and Consuela, who is dancing with Basil, remains unrecognizable among other beautiful Mexican girls. Ulmer has had the opportunity to make sound films and the voices of the periphery, the music, the rhythms, the styles of communication, make the idea of a collectivity among Mexicans clear and understandable. The dance scene is accompanied by a short dialogue between the priest and the physician about the happiness of Latin Americans, who wear the old costumes, speak the old language, and who recognize how all of these things mean so much to them. The fact that unlike *Stín ve světle* or *Ikina sudbina*, it is a young woman rather than a man placed at the center of the narration does not destroy the semantics of health films for the periphery, which heavily rely on the patriarchal order as a "proper" mode of community life.

The positive role of the father visible in *Ikina sudbina* has been reinforced by attributing to the father of Consuela the role of a key local agent who educates his own community. The father not only convinces Consuela to be examined and treated, but he also remains a protagonist that transforms a "nearly enlightened" community of happy people into a "really enlightened" community of happy and healthy people – as the priest and the physician announce at both the beginning and end of the film, respectively. The most decisive scene in the film concerns a dispute between the father and his old friend, who blames the father for selling his soul to devil because he has sent his innocent daughter to an unknown, alien place, the sanatorium. In response, the father of Consuela blames his friend for his ignorance. When an angry friend spits upon the floor, the father repeats a pointed lecture on the spread of germs through spitting - previously given to him by a physician.

While the father is the most decisive in civilizing his community, Consuela remains totally passive. Not she but rather her father obtains Consuela's medical test results, and it is he who has made the decision to place her in a sanatorium. Like Mary in *Let My People Live,* only once Consuela has made her own decision to share her fears with the priest, she asserts that she is going to be a "good girl," but clearly because the priest motivates her to do so. All the other characters in the film, the nurses, the members of her family, refer to Consuela this way. The profile of the "good girl" includes a call for sexual abstinence – Consuela is in love with Basil since the very beginning of the film, but they are only married after two years of Consuela's treatment. As in *Ikina sudbina*, the prevention of infectious disease is presented hand-in-hand with the motives of sexual education aimed at persuading young people to say "no" in high-risk health situations.

Along with the human bondage built around the love story and inter-generational attachment, *Cloud in the Sky* has introduced the motif of orphanhood: the death of the mother is a departure point of narration in the film. The disease threatens individuals, families and the community through striking key figures within the community's older generation and orphaned children.[47] Moreover, through the dissemination of psychoanalysis, occurring at the time that film was produced, becoming an orphan had started to be seen as a trigger for engaging in unhealthy dependencies or human bondage in order to attract quasi-parents; such a scenario reinforces the message of Ulmer's films for the NTA.[48] This directorial move not only strengthens the role of the doctor as a proper quasi-father of the community, but also emphasizes the fragility of minorities and the need to protect them – from the risk of becoming involved in psychologically "bad" relations. In each of the five fictional films produced by Ulmer for the NTA, the loss of parents is a thread that carries through, one of the most important syntaxes which connect the ant personality, human bondage and the role of public health in overcoming it. It is notable that the nurse who regularly visits the family of Consuela during her treatment in the sanatorium is presented as a quasi-mother of the family, who supervises younger siblings and cares for the father.

Another novelty in constructing the positive role of community for emancipation from human bondage lies in the opposition of the older gen-erations, represented by Consuela, who continues trusting more in priests than in physicians, and the younger siblings, who are more interested in medical treatment. The film depicts the curiosity of Juan and Maria, the younger siblings of Consuela, and the ease with which they overcome the fear of being treated. Maria's remark, "It didn't hurt," regarding a TB skin test can be seen as another signifier of the resemblance between Latin Americans and the white middle class of US Americans, whose children are full of curiosity, just as Ulmer has shown in his film *Goodbye, Mr. Germ.*[49] This opposition between the youngest generation, most inclined toward medical progress, and the older generations, also underscores the role of racial difference: "[W]hite children absorb what adults of color need to be more actively convinced of: the scientific realities of the disease and its treatment."[50] In *The Light Ahead*, Ulmer has turned this racialized semantics in favor of reestablishing the dignity of Jews.

The Light Ahead: Moving beyond the boundaries of health films produced for the periphery

In 1939, after finishing *Cloud in the Sky* and before starting *Another to Conquer*, Ulmer filmed the story of love, desperation and escape by two young Jewish orphans, the "lame" Fischke and visually impaired Hodel, from a shtetl named either Glubsk or Glupsk. The hopeless situation for the heroes is resolved paradoxically due to the cholera epidemic. The shtetl's residents have decided to cope with the epidemic through the custom of marrying disabled people, considered "ugly," in a cemetery, which would, ostensibly multiply the frightening ugliness and drive the cholera out of the town. Fischke has become the cholera groom, and Hodel – the cholera bride. The very next day after the wedding and collecting the wedding money, they have escaped the shtetl with the assistance of a book-peddler, the wise Mendele Moykher Sforim, a main narrator of the story, who says at the very end: "Probably, there is a better future for all the Fishkes and Hodels among our people."

Formally, the film was presented for the New York public as an adaptation of the short novel *Fishke der Krumer* (*Fishke the Lame,* 1869) by Sholem Yankev Abramovitsh. But despite the audience's success, a majority of Jewish critics rejected the idea of consistency in this adaptation. Indeed, Ulmer and his wife, who actively helped write the plot, significantly revised the novel's text by introducing more romantic cliches. Those familiar with the vicissitudes of Ulmer's love story could recognize the echo of their own expulsion from Hollywood in the dramatic but universal history of exclusion of the poor by the elites, even in such strange places as Beverly Hills or the shtetl Glupsk. Along with this obvious commercialization of one of the most famous Jewish novels, Ulmer has introduced a major part of the semantics of health films for minorities produced by him for the NTA. What has motivated Ulmer to not only reinforce the role of the epidemic in contrast to the novel but to also reframe the story of Fishke with the assistance of the semantics of health films?

The novel, recounted to Ulmer because he did not read Yiddish, and the health films represented two extremes in constructing the autonomy and significance of culture. If health films were located within the social realm, and would gain power only by becoming a part of social events, the novel was an example of total analytical or abstract autonomy, which would be achieved through the ongoing separation from the pressure of events as a source of experience in favor of eternal humanistic ideals.[51] These different but powerful performances of culture challenged Ulmer, who could not resist the option to work through not only the "analytical" autonomy of Yiddish literature but also the "concrete" power of health films. The meaning-making process in *The Light Ahead* stems from the consistent deconstruction of the core of health films, tough prescriptions regarding personal profile, a desirable dependence on progress, and the patriarchal order, which allowed Ulmer to preserve the original humanistic message of the novel but to, at the same time, question the skeptical view of Abramovitsch on Western evolutionism as a suitable survival strategy for the Jews.

The story of one of the unremarkable Jewish poor, whom Abramovitsh compares to "mushrooms that appear after every rain"[52] (another metaphor compatible with the ant personality), aims to underscore the uniqueness of human beings, not because they possess outstanding qualities but because they have worked through the personal drama of loneliness.[53] The writer has reinforced the well-known artistic device to narrate the story of the unremarkable through a wise, intelligent, and trust-deserved character like Mendele Moykher Sforim, with a heavy dose of self-irony that not only questions the ability of readers to refrain from attributing labels to the characters but also inclines them to distance themselves from the expectations of "civilized" people introduced by the Enlightenment.

Mendele shares the story of Fishke with his old friend and compatriot, Alter, after Alter has finished complaining about his own troubles with his wife and children. They move together to Glupsk to sell their books and other stuff, and the exchange of such stories helps them to cope with the unbearable heat. Fishke who, according to Mendele, is situated at the bottom of social hierarchy of the shtetl, accidentally marries the visually impaired and poor Basya, which advances his position in the hierarchy of Jewish "beggars." The story of the incidental fortune of Fishke has emerged at the moment Mendele and Alter need to search for their stolen horses, and when they find them, Mendele and Alter fight with the gang of beggars to retrieve their stolen horses. In the decisive moment of this battle, Mendele takes a strong hit and loses consciousness. When he has woken up, he again encounters Fishke, who has helped Mendele and Alter to overcome the gang. They begin to travel all together, and Fishke continues his story. Under the pressure of marriage, Fishke has abandoned Glupsk and as a result of his wandering, his wife starts distancing from him. Fishke has now lost his prestigious position among the beggars. In his turn, he falls in love with a hunchbacked girl who is another scapegoat among the beggars because she refuses to accept the harassment of the head of the beggars' gang, Red, who has stolen the horses of Mendele and Alter. Fishke describes all his unsuccessful attempts to abandon the gang and rescue his hunchbacked lover, and at the very end, they realize that this girl is the daughter of Alter, who has promised to find and protect his daughter. Fishke remains with Mendele, and Alter has gone to perform his father's duty.

The novel significantly transforms the idea of human bondage and the ways to become emancipated from it, one of the pillars of modern European literature that had directly shaped the genre of the health films produced for the periphery. Fishke provides a crystal-clear description of human bondage when he explains why it was impossible for him to divorce Basya and abandon the gang for so long:

> No matter how much I suffered, no matter how much I endured, I still felt that I was addicted to her ... Glamor and nothing more! I liked her. ... I won't say that she is beautiful, but pretty. ... "Today," I thought, "today, we must put an end to this! Today, I will tell her: Divorce!" But as soon as I got closer to her, as soon as she spoke to me or put her hand on my shoulder and say: "Lead me, Fishke!" - how the language was taken away from me, and I became different.[54]

His new love for the hunchbacked girl replaced his dependence on his former wife, but Fishke has not invested in achieving self-transformation and curing himself of human bondage, like Philip in the Maugham's *Of Human Bondage*. He remains the same unremarkable Jew with a total absence of desire to be on the side of progress. At one moment in his narration, Fishke says: "For becoming a wealthy Jew one needs only a fortune. Impudence, shamelessness and other qualities then come by themselves."[55] This skeptical view on the modernist idea of possessive individualism is one of the central motifs of the entire text. The culmination of this skepticism comes in the meeting of Fishke and an unknown writer, whom Fishke assumes is a beggar. Fischke invited the writer to beg together, and for quite a long time neither the writer nor Fishke understood that they did not belong to the same profession.

In the film, it is not the gang of beggars but rather the shtetl that represents the web that ensnares Fishke and Hodel. One of the clearest messages of both the novel and the film is the categorical negation of the shtetl, not by the hubris of the gentiles but by those who try to cope with the intolerable burdens of shtetl life – poor Jews themselves. The name of the shtetl, Glupsk (literally meaning "stupidity"[56]), was one of the collective images introduced by Abramovitsch (e.g., along with town *Tunejadsk*, literally, "town of parasites") for describing shtetls. Along with it, Glu*b*sk can be heard with "b" instead of a "p" as "glu*b*inka" (literally "remote place"). The double-meaning of the name of the shtetl, Glupsk/Glubsk, where Fischke and Hodel have been born and live, is comprehensible not only for Russian-speaking Jews but also for the majority of those for whom one or another Slavic language was familiar. As in the novel, poverty is shown in the film hand-in-hand with the unsanitary conditions of Glupsk. But the absence of public care has obtained the position of one of the main signifiers of "backwardness." The never-ending debates of the inhabitants regarding the building of a hospital and introducing regular medical care, "before cholera will come next time," have not transformed into action, even after the epidemic, which only increases the feeling of desperation.

The film provides a consistent view on community life as generating psychological and social addiction. The shtetl keeps its inhabitants on an invisible tether of mendicancy as the only possible pattern of communication, regardless of the class belonging of the characters. The cascade of the dialogues between the different inhabitants of Glupsk illustrates this interdependence. Mendele, as a quasi-father, is tethered to his "children" because of their illiteracy, and he feels obliged to help them despite the meaninglessness of the attempts to educate them.[57] He is always asked to read to or inform them. The chance to help Fischke and Hodel escape makes him happy, and it is the very last moment of the film. Drabke, a bitter and rude widow who gives shelter to Hodel, cannot marry again and have children because of her memories about her deceased husband. She asks Hodel to go begging but without results. The thief Getzel and the beggar Dobe, the filmic echo of the beggars' gang in the novel, perform human bondage and try to involve Fishke and Hodel in this vicious circle of interdependence. As in the novel, in the film, Fishke and Hodel overcome human bondage together – by overcoming the fear to become the cholera groom and bride. This moment is a last stand against the patriarchal order, consistently deconstructed in the film by demonstrating the helplessness of the power wielded by men.

Step-by-step, *The Light Ahead* deconstructs each of the pedagogical messages of the health films produced for the periphery and builds a regime of authenticity, not as a process of attributing a desirable identity but by experiencing a crisis of identity. Obviously, it is possible to actualize this process through narration by Jews for Jews, but not only that way. *The Light Ahead* can be defined as an example of cultural autonomy that "fully and authentically expresses the past, present, and future aspirations of its participants,"[58] but it is not autonomous from the social contexts of the time in which it was produced, namely, the acceptance by the US American middle class of the ideals of health, including the fight against tuberculosis and other diseases, so important for the Jews in the interwar United States. In this turn, it is possible to say that *The Light Ahead* is a part of "an interconnected network of user groups and their supporting institutions, each using the genre [of health film for the periphery] to satisfy its own needs and desires."[59] Such belonging to this network only increases the concrete power of health films as a part of the social surveillance over minorities and as one of the agents of delegitimizing local culture as incompatible with "civilization." *Another to Conquer*, the most racially infiltrated film among those that Ulmer produced for the NTA, further demonstrates this point.

Another to Conquer: Become civilized at any price?

Like *Cloud in the Sky*, which addresses all Latin Americans but presents the most numerous subgroup among them, Mexicans, *Another to Conquer* seeks to address all Native Americans but in order to be "authentic," presents only one group, the Navajo. The film starts with a ritual dance around the fire. Then, the Navajo are driving a herd of wild mustangs and galloping on the prairie. This image of this "wild" life is accompanied by an introductory comment about the occupation of the land now known as the United States by Native Americans, their long history of fighting numerous enemies, including the wars between tribes and the crimes of white US Americans, and the necessity to take a step toward achieving new glory in defeating new enemies, namely, disease, and especially one of the cruelest, tuberculosis. In the next moment, the image of a half-naked young Navajo on a horse is exchanged for an image of the same man now dressed in the modern clothing of the "cowboy," and instead of mustangs, he drives sheep. The voice back at the screen says that the Navajo have not lost the courage of their fathers, and this courage will help them to conquer another enemy, disease. This introductory part ends with a collective image of seated Navajo.

The film then turns to the dramatic story of Nema and Don, whose parents died of tuberculosis, and who are brought up by their grandfather, Slow-Talker (!). In line with tradition, the family burns down the house where death has settled and moves away to find a new settlement. When they arrive, the children meet their peer Robert, who has become "an ardent admirer of Don" but falls in love with Nema. When the children become older, Robert has made the decision to go to the boarding school so he can begin "learning something to live better." Slow-Talker asserts that the departure of Robert represents the fact that he "has forsaken the ways of his people." Meanwhile, Don continues the Navajo traditions, including the rejection of any medical treatment. He repeats what Slow-Talker has said: "We die because we do not keep our customs." In this turn, the human bondage of Don and Slow-Talker look very similar to the negative dependence on a "backward" community in *The Light Ahead*.

The film presents the prevention of disease as an inseparable part of assimilation as a process of emancipation from old-fashioned and threatening prescriptions. Robert goes to boarding school and not only advances his academic competencies but also accepts "order and cleanliness as a part of his daily life." The sports exercises build his strong body and teach him to be part of a team. Robert's thirst for knowledge is one of the dominant motifs for presenting the desirable way for the Navajo to become healthy. Even in the situation when the doctor recognizes that Robert has early-stage tuberculosis, he uses this situation as a chance to know more about disease and how to prevent it. In contrast to the story of George from *Let My People Live*, who was strong enough to defeat the disease without medical treatment, the case of Robert demonstrates that looking strong and being healthy are not the same.

The film reflects the role of "white," military medicine – the medical examination of Robert is performed by a "white" surgeon. Indeed, since the second third of the nineteenth century, medical care for Native Americans was implemented by "white" military surgeons, often interpreted as an attempt to protect US military personnel from the spread of infection by the local population.[60] In contrast to *Cloud in the Sky* and *Let My People Live*, men, and not women are placed in the sanatorium, and viewers can witness Robert lying in bed and taking his medicines. This difference operates in favor of subordinating not only women but also men, the most active members of the minority at that time, to the rules of preventive medicine. But in contrast to Consuela and Mary, Robert becomes the mediator between (white) "civilization" and Native American culture because, according to the doctors, he knows his people better. Obviously, this directorial move requires more effort to provide arguments in favor of such a strategy, to "fight the enemy in bed," and the physician compares placement in the sanatorium aimed at giving damaged lungs the opportunity to rest to the bondage that fixes a damaged leg "because there is no bondage for lungs."

The long conversations with the doctor have equipped Robert with comprehensible analogies for disseminating information about tuberculosis among the Navajo. The physician does his best to convey a clear visualization of the spread of tuberculosis and the role of the sanatorium, which he compares to plots that prevent fire, and the spread of tuberculosis germs are "invisible worms" that foster the growth of weeds. The communication between Robert and the physician is unlike the quasi-parenting that occurs in the role of priests and physicians in the films produced for Latin Americans and African Americans. The major part of the communication between Robert and the physician resembles that of a teacher and his favorite gifted student, who, even lying weak in bed, cannot help but repeat the words and suggestions of his teacher.

But Slow-Talker remains skeptical and comments on Robert's stay in the sanatorium by saying: "He is just lazy and lies [in bed] all day." Don remains on the side of older generations and firstly rejects being examined even though he exhibits all the symptoms of the disease. But when he starts bleeding during the annual sheep-dipping[61] and is taken to the hospital and diagnosed, Slow-Talker makes the decision to take Nema to the hospital and have her be examined too. Blaming the "false" masculinity of Native Americans reaches an extreme when viewers realize that the main carrier of tuberculosis in his family is Slow-Talker, who has had the disease for a long time, and who "has given the disease to his family." This conclusion, which Slow-Talker has reached by himself, is met with only the slow and silent head-shaking of the physician.

In this moment, the film puts the beliefs of Native Americans and the security of lives in direct opposition: "The erroneous 'hoodooism' of the older generation is foregrounded in this pivotal exchange, its belief in the heredity and inevitable fatality of the disease systematically taken apart. A previous generation's presumed subscription to folk traditions is cautiously dismantled."[62] And the dramatic destiny of Don, who dies in the film, only reinforces the opposition between Robert as a representative of the youngest generation, and Slow-Talker, who has been labeled as responsible for the spread of disease. In the end, Robert's efforts are similar to the story of Consuela – he marries Nema, and the health of their child is the last argument for Slow-Talker to obey the rules of "new world" and sacrifice his desire to be among his people and be a part of the nature that he so loves – to stay in the sanatorium and "not to bring the enemy to the fireside." In short, the division of Native Americans into those who will prevent or treat disease and those who won't meet an intra-racial hierarchy based upon the ability to be assimilated. Don is unable to accept the choice in favor of assimilation, and he dies, but Robert gains the right to reproduction and likely, the opportunity to find a better job than the hard work of a cattle herder.

Connecting preventability with the options to move up in the social hierarchies represents the central motif for another film made by Ulmer for the NTA in the same year, *They do come back.* This film addresses urban working-class youth and tells the story of the young orphans, Julie and Roy, who work at factories and love each other. The need to fight tuberculosis leads them to the sanatorium, where Roy is not only treated but also retrained for office work as an engineer. The film links the option to move up to the middle class for those who undergo timely medical examinations and accept the assistance of the authorities. The reverberation of class and racial hierarchies in the films by Ulmer for the NTA introduce new ways to apply the semantics of health films produced for the periphery: the ant personality emancipates from unhealthy human bondage by being treated in a timely manner and eventually becoming a valuable member of their community. These new syntaxes of health films aim to differentiate communities or, in a more general meaning, peripheries, into "preventable" and "unpreventable" from the threat of "backwardness." Even more, these films provide an argument in favor of attributing these labels to the entire community or periphery.

According to Orgeron, one of the first historians who first attracted attention to the films produced by Ulmer for the NTA, one of the legacies is the missionary message that "the word can arrest the spread of the disease,"[63] which was shaped by films and later reproduced in other media. Interpreting these films as a part of the wider history of health films produced for the periphery adds one more historical concern – the issue of cultural power and cultural autonomy as a part of cultural violence and resistance to it: "Cultural violence makes direct and structural violence look, even feel, right – or at least not wrong."[64] In terms of Galtung's taxonomy of violence,[65] the health films for the periphery produced in Czechoslovakia and Yugoslavia legitimize the oppression of identity needs by calling for the resocialization of ant personalities. The films against tuberculosis produced for the NTA justify the segmentation within each of the minority communities and those who belong to lower-class social groups as a reasonable strategy – when the health of the nation is at stake. In the *Another to Conquer*, this mission substantiates the fragmentation of Native Americans and even their segregation and detention.

234 Health films for the interwar periphery

Notes

1 Rockefeller Foundation *Annual Report* 1936: p. 8 [available at https://www. rockefellerfoundation.org/wp-content/uploads/Annual-Report-1936-1.pdf retrieved 23.05.2021).
2 Ibid., p. 98.
3 Ibid., p. 99.
4 Ibid.
5 Carol R. Byerly (2013) *Good tuberculosis men: The Army Medical Department's struggle with tuberculosis* Fort Sam Houston, Texas: Office of The Surgeon General, Borden Institute, U.S. Army Medical Department Center and School, p.158.
6 Edgar Sydenstricker (1934) Health in the New Deal, *The Annals of the American Academy of Political and Social Science,* 176, 131–137, p. 132.
7 Ibid.
8 Devin Orgeron (2011) Spreading the word: race, religion and the rhetoric of contagion in Edgar G. Ulmer's TB Films in Devin Orgeron, Marsha Orgeron, Don Streible (eds.) *Learning with the Lights Off: Educational Film in the United States* Oxford: Oxford University Press, pp. 295–319.
9 Ibid., p. 301.
10 Cynthia A. Connolly and Mary E. Gibson (2011) The "white plague" and color: Children, race, and tuberculosis in Virginia 1900-1935, *The Journal of Pediatric Nursing: Nursing Care of Children and Families,* 26 3, 230–238.
11 Ibid.
12 Marion Torchia (1975) The Tuberculosis movement and the race question 1890-1950, *Bulletin of the History of Medicine,* 49, 2, 152–168, p. 160.
13 Ibid., pp. 161–162.
14 Christian Bonah and Vincent Lowy (2013) "Lorsque le regard l'emporte sur le message. Les courts-métrages de lutte contre la tuberculose d'Edgar G. Ulmer" [When visual wins over the message. Edgar G. Ulmer's short films in the fight against tuberculosis], *Alliage* 71, 46–56.
15 Connolly and Gibson, ibid.
16 Marion Torchia, ibid., p. 160.
17 Oregon, ibid., p. 300.
18 Georgina Feldberg (1995) *Disease and Class: Tuberculosis and the Shaping of Modern North American Society,* New Brunswick: Rutgers University Press, p. 6.
19 Rick Altman (1999) *Film/genre* London: British Film Institute, p. 208.
20 Feldberg, ibid., p. 7.
21 Orgeron, ibid., 296.
22 Ibid.
23 Noah Isenberg (2004) Perennial Detour: The Cinema of Edgar G. Ulmer and the Experience of Exile, *Cinema Journal,* 43, 2, pp. 3–25.
24 Jonathan Munby (1999) Heimat Hollywood: Billy Wilder, Otto Preminger, Edgar Ulmer and the criminal cinema of the Austrian-Jewish Diaspora, *David F. Good and Ruth Wodak From world war to Waldheim Culture and politics in Austria and the United States,* New York: Berghahn Books, pp. 138–164.
25 Christian Bonah and Anja Laukötter (2020) *Body, Capital, and Screens: Visual Media and the Healthy Self in the 20th Century,* Amsterdam University Press.
26 Orgeron, ibid., p. 296.
27 Kimball Young (1922) Intelligence tests of certain immigrant groups, *The Scientific Monthly,* 15, 5, 417–434, p. 418.
28 Ulmer produced a film about venereal diseases, *Damaged Lives* (1933), as a Canadian/American pre-Code exploitation film. The screenplay is based on the

French play *Les Avariés* (The damaged, 1901) by Eugène Brieux, more in Chapter 8.

29 Noah Isenberg, ibid.

30 Bonah and Lowy, ibid.

31 Hannu Salmi (2011) Cultural history, the possible and principle of plenitude, *History and Theory*, 50, pp. 171–187.

32 The Czech film *Osudná chvíle* (Fortuitous Moment, 1935), aimed at preventing syphilis, heavily relied on the style and visuality of *Damaged Lives* (1933) by Ulmer, produced for the Canadian Social Health Council; more in Chapter 8.

33 Kenneth V. Lottick (1950) Some distinctions between culture and civilization as displayed in sociological literature, *Social Forces*, 28, 3, pp. 240–250.

34 Ibid., p.244.

35 A 1939 Harvard anthropologists' textbook entitled "The races of Europa," as well as other texts of the interwar period, introduced the hierarchical order of whiteness.

36 Victoria Shmidt (2019) *Politics of disability in interwar and socialist Czechoslovakia: Segregation in the name of the nation,* Amsterdam: Amsterdam University Press, pp. 155–157.

37 Bonah and Lowy, ibid.

38 Orgeron, ibid., p. 300.

39 Altman, ibid., p. 212.

40 Jennifer L. Hochschild, Vesla M. Weaver and Traci R. Burch (2012) *Creating a new racial order*, Princeton: Princeton University Press.

41 Altman, ibid., p. 208.

42 Evelyn Davidson (1996) *White Choral music by African American Composers: A selected, annotated Bibliography,* Lanham, Md., & London: The Scarecrow Press, p. 3.

43 Torchia, ibid., pp. 152–168.

44 Jessie M. Rodrique (1992) The Black community and the birth control movement in Dorothy O. Helly and Susan M. Reverby (eds.) *Gendered Domains: Rethinking Public and Private in Women's History,* Cornell: Cornell University Press, 244–262.

45 In the 1930s, the choir regularly accompanied various U.S. American broadcasting.

46 The Cross of Lorraine was offered by the French physician Gilbert Sersiron as a symbol for combating tuberculosis during the international meeting of the phisiatricians in Berlin in 1902.

47 Orgeron, ibid., p. 302.

48 Before introducing orphanhood as an additional way to present minorities as vulnerable, Ulmer had already portrayed it when he filmed the play *Grine Felder* (Green Fields, 1916) by Peretz Hirschbein in 1937. This comedy tells the story of a Jewish student, an orphan, who after being disappointed by his studies, moved to countryside and met his true love.

49 The children, a young brother and sister, ask their father, a physician and scientist, to provide more information about germs and tuberculosis, and their father mixes entertainment and health education through interviewing Mr. Germ, one of the oldest germs of tuberculosis. This part is supplemented by the demonstration of various medical tests, more in Chapter 7.

50 Orgeron, ibid., p. 308.

51 Anne Kane (1991) Cultural Analysis in Historical Sociology: The Analytic and Concrete Forms of the Autonomy of Culture *Sociological Theory*, 9, 1, 53–69.

52 Sholem Yankev Abramovitsh (1996) *Tales of Mendele the Book Peddler: Fishke the Lame and Benjamin the Third,* Schocken Books.

53 Susanne Klingenstein (2014) Mendele der Buchhändler: Leben und Werk des Sholem Yankev Abramovitsh; eine Geschichte der jiddischen Literatur zwischen Berdichev und Odessa, 1835–1917 Wiesbaden: Harrassowitz.

54 Abramovitsh, ibid.
55 Ibid.
56 It is notable that in the same year as *Fischke der Krumer*, Mikhail Yevgrafovich Saltykov-Shchedrin published the satiric fictional chronicle, *Istorija odnogo goroda* (The history of a town, 1879), about the life in Glupovsk, an imaginary town that symbolizes the meaninglessness of provincial life in Russia.
57 Naomi Seidman (1997) *A marriage made in heaven: The sexual politics of Hebrew and Yiddish,* California: University of California Press.
58 Edward T. Silva (1980) Cultural autonomy and ideas in transit: Notes from the Canadian case, *Comparative Education Review,* 24, 1, 63–72, p. 63.
59 Altman, ibid., p. 195.
60 Abraham B. Bergman, David C. Grossman, Angela M. Erdrich, John G. Todd and Ralph Forquera (1999) A political history of the Indian Health Service, *The Milbank Quarterly,* 77, 4, pp. 571–604.
61 In the film, Ulmer used some fragments of the NO-DO newsreels made for presenting the new regulations regarding livestock, which only added pedagogical pathos to the film.
62 Ordeon, ibid., p. 304.
63 Ibid., p. 310.
64 Johan Galtung (1990) Cultural violence *Journal of Peace Research*, 27, 3, 291–305, p. 291.
65 Ibid., p. 292.

Conclusion

Health film as fantasy and event

Historicizing the health films produced in interwar Eastern Europe and beyond brings into analytical lenses the dichotomy of fantasy vs. reality. Health films intensively recruited the demonization of diseases and the sacralization of medicine, primary vehicles for constructing fantasies concerning health, yet multiple forms of skepticism regarding the historical significance of health films have arisen concerning their role in establishing global, national and local orders of health security. Our research shows that fantasy and its agents, such as health films, should not be seen as "antagonistic to social reality but its precondition or psychic glue."[1]

Deconstructing the dichotomy of fantasy vs. "real" event is decisive for an intelligible narrative about producing and disseminating health films. It is possible to say that health films represent "the imaginary relation of individuals to the real conditions of their existence."[2] Each of the health films explored in this book, along with their assemblages, is connected with various actions and events "when grouped in sequences, generate the narrative"[3] of men, women, children, populations of the periphery and entire nations. We interpret each of the films in terms of historical peculiarities, including a clear and precise definition of the places, events, visual analogies, etc., used in the films. This strategy for exploring films aligns with the core of left-leaning semiotics that scrutinizes "social and artistic productions in order to discern the cultural and ideological codes operative in them."[4]

Such subversive work of denaturalization not only prevents historical presentism but also introduces the devices of a visual analysis sensitive to the ceaseless movement of the original messages of health films into unpredictably novel contexts of meaning, resisting closure by a process of constant interpretation.[5] This approach aims at presenting a comprehensive historical reconstruction of the health film as a social and cultural practice, not only embedded in health propaganda but also operating as an agent that shapes regimes of authenticity. Incorporating these contexts and missions into health films reinforced their power to create fantasies able to serve multiple functions concerning surveillance over different populations.

Fantasies enact the fulfillment of desire and the consequences of this fulfillment,[6] and health films primarily construct their narration around the

DOI: 10.4324/9781003272267-19

boundary between "proper" and "improper" desires through depicting their consequences. Aligned with the mission of modernism, namely, to be "a whole Utopian compensation for increasing dehumanization on the level of daily life,"[7] health films blur the line between the benefits and harms of routine pleasurable practices such as making love, eating and drinking heartily, gaining recognition, achieving success in a career, and loving one's own children, in favor of public health surveillance as an instrument that ensured a clear and achievable predisposition for gaining amelioration and preventing degradation.

Health films should be seen among other producers of fantasies that aimed at masking the multiple conflicts, antagonisms, or contradictions[8] that accompanied interwar Eastern Europe.[9] Being closely connected with progressive agrarianism and the eugenic movement, health films brought back the "jouissance" stolen by political tensions, class divisions and gender disparities, through uniting people under the umbrella of public health and with its main representatives, doctors and nurses. The consistent nurturing of physicians' sex appeal and the attractive progress of medical intervention are among the artistic devices targeted at employing the libidinal energy of audiences.[10] Subjecting individuals of different ethnicities, ages, genders and classes to the power of public health reinforced the "we-versus-they construction" aimed at nuancing and deepening multiple hierarchies.

Operating as tightly compressed narratives, health films spawned fantasies of healing, happiness and well-being on the one hand, and disability, death and poverty on the other. These routine preconditions for human life have found their exclusive meaning as embedded in the intensively developed machinery of public health and social welfare – but not only that. Impressive stories that connected fantasies with recent events, such as pandemics during the Great War, campaigns against infectious diseases, or the substitute placement of children without parents, were often narrated by ambitious and gifted filmmakers who connected health films with the evolution of the film language in Eastern Europe and beyond. In this way, health films became a part of shaping a "certain doubtless vision of the world, influenced by man's relation with a technical civilization and cinema as a fruit of this civilization."[11]

Assuming the function of a herald of progress, health films participated in the historicization of Eastern Europe and rebuilt continuities and changes between its past and present. Moreover, by documenting events, health films claimed their right to be considered an authentic document of their time. Instead of dwelling on whether health films actually represent historical evidence, because of their propagandist nature, we can now ask ourselves how historicizing Eastern Europe through the lens of health films would revise the multiple narratives about the region that have been already told through the lenses of other dichotomies.

The interwar period is often presented as a historical bridge between exposing the oppression of imperial and authoritative regimes, the "two siblings of subalternity."[12] The periods before 1918 and after 1939 not only embody a predominant position in narrating the history of Eastern Europe, but also reduce the role of the interwar period to the prelude to experiencing fascism and communism as direct successors of one or another of the four empires that ruled Eastern Europe before 1918. The systematic exploration of the interwar period as an era of regimes with different degrees of democracy preserves the imaginary institutions of collective memory based upon Western values, leaving the interwar period untouchable for critical heritage studies. Measuring the deviation from the "Western" standard of political and economic development among interwar Eastern European countries mediates the role of dominant social institutions such as the state in establishing a self-secure, delineated identity of nations. These "molar" historical models, with a focus on the dichotomy of state vs. nation, are premised on the fetishization of an already present identity that exists in a nurturing social environment of nationalism and global capitalism,[13] constrains the imagination and leaves us incapable of constructing reflexive empirical models of social processes.[14] Within this narrative, health films remain untouchable heritage that symbolizes the multiplicity of national identities and the reasons underlying either national pride or national shame.

Two interrelated trends tend to attack the interpretations produced by linear narrations about Eastern Europe as filled with nations that have struggled against arbitrary states. The trend to question the leading role of nationalism and its reverse side, global capitalism, through interpreting interwar Eastern Europe as practicing national indifference and deglobalization,[15] generates binary oppositions between the global and the local, or the national and the international, which are often resolved through coupling both dichotomies within the tripartite construction of *national/regional/ international*.[16] Regional history has garnered the leading position in this construction and inclines scholars to interpret interwar Europe in terms of orders and crises that twisted and melted together various spheres of public life and economic development, including public health.[17] Not only the institutionalization of health care but also the cross-country dynamics of this process continue to be perceived as homogenous, which leads to superficial comparisons, for instance, the idea that "Yugoslavia, like Poland and Czechoslovakia, experienced a transition from relief to welfare that was closely interwoven with international collaboration."[18]

The variety of health films produced in Eastern Europe questions such "post-colonial" visions on public health and inclines scholars to differentiate not only country cases, but also the intra-country dynamic, even as it was determined by the vicissitudes of intervention from the side of international bodies. Films for the periphery provided a different range of regimes of authenticity as the main trajectories for uniting people than the films produced for the "center," which reflected different trajectories of institutionalizing public health in the different parts of the same country. In its intention to demonstrate the historical significance of interwar Eastern Europe as consisting of "small states [that] can be nodes of global order,"[19] focusing on (de)constructing the dichotomy of national vs. international is obsessed with indicating the most important events and the explanations behind them, which relegates not only fantasies but also events not relevant to this historical selection – such as health films or practicing race science to the margins of narration. Furthermore, historicizing Eastern Europe through the lenses of *national/regional/international* itself produces such fantasies – through imposing "sequential order on otherwise chaotic and contingent occurrences,"[20] with questions about the potential for negating the linearity of historical models as a source of frequent logical "fallacies."

The medicalization that has brought forth changes in medical practices imposed from above, and in the case of Eastern Europe, from the global order of health security, is an essential lens through which to examine health propaganda. However, it has its limits when it comes to answering the question posed by the problem of use, rather than the problem of meaning: How does it operate?[21] To elaborate fully the mechanisms through which health films work, which often remain hidden or unconscious, this book has utilized the lens of medical culture, an influential approach that explores "those complex ways that doctors sought to explain their socio-political universe through bio-medical language."[22] The instrumental task of applying such a lens lies in examining the complex of factors that provide the "foundation for members of a society to perceive and to interpret health and illness."[23] Listening to the historical echoes of interwar health films, which, as the book demonstrates, remains powerful to this day, is part of the challenge in understanding medical culture and the factors that drive its transformation.

A critical history of health film in Eastern Europe seems like an endless story that must be revisited under the call of new events and actions. The historicization of health films in this way could trigger a critical re-examination of narrative practices and move toward a more nuanced temporalization of public health, gender-based politics and the struggle for social justice necessary for deconstructing deeply rooted master narratives concerning the emancipation of former subalterns and ascribing greater historical responsibility to Eastern Europe.

Notes

1 Joan W. Scott (2001) Fantasy echo: History and the construction of identity, *Critical Inquiry*, 27, 2, 284–304, p. 289.
2 Louis Althusser (2001) Lenin and philosophy and other essays, New York: Monthly Review.
3 Claude Bremond and Elaine D. Cancalon (1980) The logic of narrative possibilities, *New Literary History*, 11, 3, pp. 387–411, p. 388.
4 Robert Stam, Robert Bugoyne and Sandy Flitterman-Lewis (1992) *New vocabularies in film semiotics. Structuralism post-structuralism and beyond*, London and New York: Routledge, p. 22.
5 Ibid., p. 23.

6 Scott, ibid., 288.
7 Fredric Jameson (1981) *The political unconscious,* London and New York: Routledge, p. 42.
8 Scott, ibid., 290.
9 Some recent examples of rigorous analysis in atomizing Central Eastern Europe after 1918 include: Jochen Böhler, Ota Konrád, Rudolf Kučera (2021) *In the Shadow of the Great War: Physical Violence in East-Central Europe, 1917–1923, New York:* Berghahn Books; Mark Cornwall and John Paul Newman (2016) *Sacrifice and Rebirth: the Legacy of the Habsburg Empire's Last War*, New York: Berghahn Press.
10 The male physician as a symbol of masculinity in Czech mass culture has its own longue-durée, started in the late nineteenth century, when doctors began to be affiliated with the *Sokol* movement. This symbolism endures until nowadays.
11 Colin MacCabe (2003) On impurity: The dialectics of cinema and literature in Julian Murphet and Lydia Rainford, *Literature and visual technologies Writing after cinema*, Palgrave Macmillan, 2003, pp. 15–28, p. 19.
12 Bogdan Ştefănescu (2012) *Postcommunism/postcolonialism: Siblings of subalternity,* Bucharest Editura universitätii din bucuresti.
13 Nickolas Thoburn (2006) Vacuoles of noncommunication: Minor politics? Communist style and the multitude *in* Ian Buchanan and Andrian Parr (eds.), *Deleuze and the contemporary world*, Edinburg: Edinburg University Press, pp. 42–56, p. 44.
14 Randolph Roth (1992) Is history a process? Nonlinearity, revitalization theory, and the central metaphor of social science history, *Social Science History,* 16, 2, 197–243, p. 218.
15 Tara Zahra (2008). *Kidnapped souls: National indifference and the battle for children in the Bohemian Lands, 1900–1948,* Cornell University Press; Maarten van Ginderachter and Jon Fox (2018). *National indifference and the History of Nationalism in Modern Europe: National indifference and the History of Nationalism in Modern Europe*, London: Routledge; Alexei Miller (2019). "National Indifference" as a Political Strategy? *Kritika: Explorations in Russian and Eurasian History,* 20(1), 63–72.
16 Peter Becker and Natasha Wheatley (2020) Introduction. In: Peter Becker and Natasha Wheatley (eds.), *Remaking Central Europe,* Oxford: Oxford University Press, pp. 2–15, p. 5.
17 Becker and Wheatley, ibid., p. 6.
18 Sara Silverstein (2020) Reinventing international health in East Central Europe. In: Peter Becker and Natasha Wheatley (eds.), *Remaking Central Europe*, Oxford: Oxford University Press, pp. 71–98, p. 92.
19 Becker and Wheatley, ibid., p. 15.
20 Scott, ibid., 291.
21 Gilles Deleuze and Félix Guattari (1972) *Anti-Oedipus: Capitalism and Schizophrenia,* Minnesota: University of Minnesota Press, 109.
22 Sean Quinlan (2004) Physical and moral regeneration after the terror: Medical culture, sensibility and family politics in France, 1794–1804, *Social History,* 29, 2, 139–164, 142.
23 Francisca Loetz (2010) Why change habits? Early modern medical innovation between medicalisation and medical culture, *History and Philosophy of the Life Sciences,* 32, 4, pp. 453–473, 455.

Bibliography

A National Encyclopedia of Educational Films and 16 mm Apparatus, Available in Great Britain (1935), pp. 160, 236.

A two-year-old goes to hospital: a film shown by John N. Bowlby and James Robertson (1952), *in Proceedings of the Royal Society of Medicine, Section of Paediatrics*, 46, 425–426.

Abramovitsh, Sholem Yankev (1996) *Tales of Mendele the Book Peddler: Fishke the Lame and Benjamin the Third*. New York: Schocken Books.

Alibašić, Ahmet (2020) History of inter-religious dialogue in Bosnia and Herzegovina from force-feeding to sustainability? *Interdisciplinary Journal for Religion and Transformation in Contemporary Society*, 6, 343–364.

Althusser, Louis (2001) *Lenin and Philosophy and Other Essays*, New York: Monthly Review.

Altman, Rick (1984) Semantic/syntactic Approach to Film Genre, *Cinema Journal*, 23, 3, 6–18.

Altman, Rick (1999) *Film/Genre*, London: BFI.

Armstrong, David (1995) The Rise of Surveillance Medicine, *Sociology of Health and Illness* 7, 3, 393–404.

Aschenbrenner, Susanne (1996) Dr. med. Marta Fraenkel, Generalsekretärin der Gesolei: Organisatorin und Schriftstellerin in der Gesundheitaufklärung [Doctor of medicine Marta Fraenkel: General Secretary and the author of health education] In Christoph Meinel and Monika Renneberg (eds.), *Geschlechterverhältnisse in Medizin, Naturwissenschaft und Technik [Gender patterns in Medicine, natural sciences and technique]*, Bassum Stuttgart Verlag für Geschichte der Naturwissenschaften und der Technik, 83–88, 85.

Balle, Thorstein Johannes (2014) Myten om Grundtvigs indflydelse på den danske folkeskole [The myth of Grundtvig's influence on the Danish public school], *Grundtvig Studier*, 65, 1, 65–98.

Barona, Josep L. (2019) *Health Policies in Interwar Europe: A Transnational Perspective*, London: Routledge.

Barrusse, Virginie De Luca and Catriona Dutreuilh (2009) Pro-natalism and hygienism in France, 1900–1940. The example of the fight against venereal disease, *Population*, 64, 3, 477–506.

Bartoš, August (1925) *Cestou k životu: Feuilletony vychovatelovy* [On the way to life: Feuilletons from the educator], Brno, 53.

Bartoš, Jan, Jaroslav Hloušek and Karel Kobrle (1918) *Franz. hrabě Pocci, klasik loutkových her* [Franz von Pocci: The classic of puppet plays], Chocneň: Čeněk J. Mojžíš, 17.

Becker, Peter and Natasha Wheatley (2020) Introduction. In Peter Becker and Natasha Wheatley (eds.), *Remaking Central Europe*, Oxford: Oxford University Press, 2–15, p. 5.

Bělehrádek, Jan Vladislav Růžička and Vladimír Bergauer (1934) *Obecná biologie* [General Biology], Prague: Melantrich, 19–20.

Belfast News-Letter. Educational films, p. 11. Monday 29.02.1932.

Belloc, Hilaire (1897) *More beasts (For Worse Children)*, London: Duckworth and Co.

Bergman, Abraham B., David C. Grossman, Angela M. Erdrich, John G. Todd and Ralph Forquera (1999) A political history of the Indian Health Service, *The Milbank Quarterly*, 77, 4, 571–604.

Birtija Subtitles to the film. Kinoteka of the State Archives of Croatia, Fond of Škola za narodnog zdravja, box 1.

Birth to be shown whole week again, *The Washington Herald* (Washington, District of Columbia), 5.05.1918, p. 14.

Biskup Nikolaj i Arhiđakon Ljubomir Ranković (2012) *Srpske slave i verski običaji [Serbian religious celebrations and traditions]*, available online: https://svetosavlje. org/srpske-slave-i-verski-obicaji/?pismo=lat

Bisom, Wilhelm (1928) Expozice vědy, duchové a technické kultury a škosltví vysokého na Výstavě soudobé kultury v Brně in Expozice odboru vědy, duchové a technické kultury a školství vysokého Publikace č.1 [Exposition of Science, Spiritual and Technical Culture and Higher Education at the Exhibition of Contemporary Culture in Brno in Exposition of the Department of Science, Spiritual and Technical Culture and Higher Education Publication No.1] Brno, p. 19–24.

Bjažić Klarin, Tamara (2015) *Ernest Weissmann: društveno angažirana arhitektura, 1926–1939* [Socially Engaged Architecture, 1926–1939]. Zagreb: Hrvatska Akademija Znanosti i Umjetnosti, Hrvatski muzej arhitekture.

Blekastad, Milada (1976) Probleme der Originalität in *Ze života hmyzu* der Brüder Čapek, [The issue of originality of *Ze života hmyzu* by Čapeks], *Scando-Slavica*, 22, 1, 79–91.

Bogner-Šaban, Antonina, Dalibor Foretić, Livija Kroflin, and Abdulah Seferović (1997) *Hrvatsko lutkarstvo* [Croatian puppet theatre], Hrvatski centrum Unima, p. 9. Remarkable that the heyday of puppet theatres including health puppet plays fell on the first decades of the existence of the German Democratic Republic. In 1967 the documentary that presented the history of socialist puppet theatre in health propaganda got the special prize of the International Festival of Red Cross and health films.

Böhler, Jochen, Ota Konrád, and Rudolf Kučera (2021) *In the Shadow of the Great War: Physical Violence in East-Central Europe, 1917–1923*, New York: Berghahn Books.

Bokor, Zsuzsa (2013) *Testtörténetek - A nemzet és a nemi betegségek medikalizálása a két világháború közötti Kolozsváron* [The History of bodies - The Medicalization of the Nation and Sexually Transmitted Diseases in Cluj-Napoca between the Two World Wars], Editura ISPMN, 112–114.

Bokor, Zsuzsa (2017) Kihez szól a? Egy egészségügyi kampányfilm a 20. század elejéről [Who is it for? A health campaign film from the early twentieth century]. Available online. https://filmtett.ro/cikk/a-vilagrem-egy-egeszsegugyi-kampanyfilm-a-20-szazad-elejerol

Bölsche, Wilhelm (1903) *Vom Bazillus zum Affenmenschen. Naturwissenschaftliche Plaudereien* [From the bacillus to the ape-man. Scientific conversations], Leipzig: Diederichs.

Bonah, Christian (2015) "A word from man to man". Interwar venereal disease education films for military audiences in France, *Gesnerus*, 72/1, 15–39.

Bonah, Christian and Anja Laukötter (2015) Screening diseases. Films on sex hygiene in Germany and France in the first half of the 20th century (Themenheft), *Gesnerus*, 72, 1.

Bonah, Christian and Anja Laukötter (2020) *Body, Capital, and Screens: Visual Media and the Healthy Self in the 20th Century,* Amsterdam University Press.

Bonah, Christian and Vincent Lowy (2013) "Lorsque le regard l'emporte sur le message. Les courts-métrages de lutte contre la tuberculose d'Edgar G. Ulmer" [When visual wins over the message. Edgar G. Ulmer's short films in the fight against tuberculosis], *Alliage*, 71, 46–56.

Bouřlivý úspěch filmu [The stormy success of the film] *Čech: Politický týdenník katolický*, 21.11.1921, No. 320.

Bradbrook, Bohuslava. R. (1983) A Russian Model for the Čapeks' "The Insect Play"? *The Slavonic and East European Review*, 61, 3, 411–415.

Braddock, David and Susan Parish (2001) An institutional history of disability. In Gary L. Albrecht, Katherine D. Seelman, and Michael Bury (eds.), *Handbook of Disability Studies*, Sage: London, 11–68.

Braidotti, Rosi (2006) The becoming-Minoritarian of Europe. In Ian Buchanan and Andrian Parr (eds.), *Deleuze and the Contemporary World*, Edinburg University Press: Edinburg, 79–94, pp. 79–81.

Bremond, Claude (1966) La logique des possibles narratifs, *Communications*, 8, 60–76.

Bremond, Claude (1973) *La Logique du récit*, Collection Poétique, Éditions du Seuil.

Bremond, Claude and Elaine D. Cancalon (1980) The logic of narrative possibilities, *New Literary History*, 11, 3, 387–411, p. 388.

Brett, Daniel (2018) Indifferent but mobilized: Rural politics during the interwar period in Eastern and Western Europe, *Central Europe*, 16, 2, 65–80, p.77.

Brockington, Fraser (1958) *World Health*, London: Penguin Book, 182.

Brown, Noel (2012) *The Hollywood Family Film: A History from Shirley Temple to Harry Poter*, London, New York: I.B.Tauris.

Bruckner, Záboj (1927) Příčiny a prevence slepoty v dětském věku [The causes and prevention of blindness in child ages]. In Cyril Stejskal (ed.), *Třetí sjezd pro výzkum dítěte. V Praze 30., 31. října 1. a 2. listopadu 1926* [The third congress for the studies of child. In Prague 30.10.1926-02.11.1926], Pedologický ústav: Praha, 351–390.

Brychlová, Vlasta Potřebujeme loutkové hry [We call for puppet plays], *Lidové noviny* 20.08.1950, p. 7.

Brzaković, Đura (1934) Prosvećivanje žene u selu [Enlightenment of women in the village], *Sokolska prosveta*, 4, 3–4, 122–125.

Buchenau, Artur (1924) *Kultur und Zivilisation. Eine Studie zur Geschichte der Sozialpädagogik* [Culture and civilisation. One study of the History of social pedagogy], *Natorp-Festschrift*, p. 13.

Bunton, Robin and Alan Petersen (2002) Genetics, ethics and governance, *Critical Public Health*, 12, 2, 95–102.

Burgdörfer, Friedrich (1932) *Volk ohne Jugend. Geburtenschwund und Überalterung des deutschen Volkskörpers. Ein Problem der Volkswirtschaft - der Sozialpolitik der nationalen Zukunft* [People without youth. Declining birth rates and aging of the

Germans. A problem of the national economy - the social policy of the future of nation] Berlin: Vowinckel.

Byerly, Carol R. (2013) *Good tuberculosis men: The Army Medical Department's struggle with tuberculosis*, Fort Sam Houston, Texas: Office of The Surgeon General, Borden Institute, U.S. Army Medical Department Center and School, 158.

Borowy, I. (2009) *Coming to Terms with the World's Health: The League of Nations Health Organization 1921–1946*, Frankfurt a. M. 2009, 13–15)

Cain, Victoria (2011) "An indirect influence upon industry": Rockefeller. Philanthropies and the development of educational film in the United States, 1935–1953. In Devin Orgeron, Marsha Orgeron, and Dan Streible (eds.), *Learning with the Lights Off: Educational Film in the United States*, Oxford University Press: Oxford.

Capo, Beth Widmaier (2004) Can this woman be saved? Birth control and marriage in Modern American literature, *Modern Language Studies*, 34, 1/2, 28–41.

Ćepulić, Vladimir (1940) Smjernice za suzbijanje tuberkuloze u Banovino Hrvatskoj [Guidelines for tuberculosis control in Croatia] in *Organizacija zdravstvene službe na selu Zagreb: Zbirka separatu „Liječničkog vjesnika"* [Organization of the Health Service in the Rural area Zagreb: The collection of articles of the Medical Herald], p. 1.

Černý, František (1985) "Jindřich Veselý" *Československý loutkář* [Czechoslovak Puppeteer], Vol. 12.

Česálková, Lucie (2012) Cinema outside cinema: Czech educational cinema of the 1930s under the control of pedagogues, scientists and humanitarian groups, *Studies in Eastern European Cinema*, 3,2, 175–191.

Česálková, Lucie (2014) *Atomy věčnosti. Český krátký film 30. až 50. let* [Atoms of Eternity Czech short film of the 1930s and 1950s], Prague: NFA.

Česálková, Lucie et al. (2015) Film – náš pomocník: studie o (ne)užitečnosti českého krátkého filmu 50. Let [Film – our assistant: a study of the (un) usefulness of Czech short film in the 1950s], Praha: NFA.

Childs, Donald J. (2001) *Modernism and Eugenics: Woolf, Eliot, Yeats, and the Culture of Degeneration*, Cambridge University Press.

Chloupek, Drago (1936) Subtitles to the film "Dobro za zlo". Kinoteka of the State Archives of Croatia, Fond of Skola za narodnog zdravja, box 1.

Chloupek, Drago (1952) Nacrt zdravstveno-prosvjetnog filma o trachomu [Draft script of the health-enlightening film about trachoma]. Kinoteka of the State Archives of Croatia, Fond of Skola za narodnog zdravja, box 2.

Chura, Alojz (1936) "Slovensko bez dorastu?: *sociálne-paediatrické štúdium*" [Slovakia without youth: socially-pediatric study] Bratislava.

Cífka, Stanislav (1986) *Jindřich Veselý, tvůrce moderního českého loutkářství* [Jindřich Veselý, Creator of Modern Czech Puppetry], České Budějovice: Jihočeské. nakladatelství.

Co nového v cizině [News from abroad] (1924) *Zdraví lidu Zdravotnický měsíčník Čsl. Červeného kříže*, 2, 3, 23.

Co nového ve filmu [What is new in film production] (1940) *Český deník* 29, 142, 8.

Comedy and eugenics feature films: Their mutual child. *The Omaha Daily News* (Omaha, Nebraska) 21.04.1921, p. 4; *The Morning Post* (Camden, New Jersey) · 10.03.1921, p. 3.

Connolly Cynthia A. and Mary E. Gibson (2011) The "white plague" and color: children, race, and tuberculosis in Virginia 1900–1935, *The Journal of Pediatric Nursing: Nursing Care of Children and Families*, 26, 3, 230–238.

Cornwall, Mark and John Paul Newman (2016) *Sacrifice and Rebirth: The Legacy of the Habsburg Empire's Last War*, New York: Berghahn Press.

Čudovita, Lilika [Beautiful Lilika] Tedenska tribuna Ljubljana 17.12.1970.

Dahlquist, Marina and Frykholm, Joel (2019) *The Institutionalization of Educational Cinema: North America and Europe in the 1910s and 1920s*, Bloomington, Indiana: Indiana University Press.

Damaged lives coming to the Lido *WestMiddlesex Gazette,* 25.11.1933.

Danet, Joël (2015) Representation of Dangerous Sexuality in Interwar Non-Fiction Sex Hygiene Films: A Franco-German Comparison, *Gesnerus*, 72/1, 39–55.

Das Staatsministerium des Innern 1933 Der Brief an die Filmoberprüfstelle [The letter to Film supervision office] Berlin. Betreff: Widerruf des Bildstreifens "Geschlecht und Leben; die Gesund der Frau" [Subject: Revocation of the cutting the images in the film "Sex and Life: the health of the woman"] BayHStA.

Davidson, Evelyn (1996) *White Choral Music by African American Composers: A Selected, Annotated Bibliography*, Lanham, Md., & London: The Scarecrow Press.

Debay, Auguste (1908) *Muž a žena v manželství* [Men and women in marriage], Praha: I.L. Kober.

Deleuze, Gilles (1998) *Essays Critical and Clinical*, Verso, 42.

Děti a zdravotně výchovná jednotka Čs.Červeného kříže [Children and the mobile unit of Czechoslovak Red Cross], *Měsíčník dorostu Červeného kříže* [Monthly magazine of the Red Cross for youth], 1923, 3, 7, 4.

Dnistrjanskyj, Stanislav Severynovič (1927) Kultur, Zivilisation und Recht, [Culture, civilization, and right], *Archiv für Rechts- und Wirtschaftsphilosophie*, 21, 1, 1–17.

Doležalová, Antonie and Hana Moravcová (2020) Czechoslovak film industry on the way from private business to public good (1918–1945), *Business History*, DOI: 10.1 080/00076791.2020.1751822

Dom Narodnog Zdravja u Mostaru [House of people's health in Mostar] (1929) Ministarstvu socialne politike i narodnog zdravja. Sanitske odelenje u Beogradu Kredit od 50000 dinar iz Kralevog Fonda za izgradnu vodenich objekata u Hercegovini [The Letter to the Ministry of social policy and public health. The Department of Hygiene in Belgrade. Credit of 50000 dinars for building water supply system in Hercegovina] Andrija Štampar, HR-HDA-831 Andrija Štampar, box 1.

Dom Narodnog Zdravja u Plevlu [House of people's health in Plevel] (1929) Ministarstvu socialne politike i narodnog zdravja. Higienicke odelenje [The letter to the Ministry of Social Policy and Public Health. The Department of Hygiene] Andrija Štampar, HR-HDA-831 Andrija Štampar, box 1.

Dopis Ministerstvu sociální péče v Praze [Letter to the Ministry of Social affairs in Prague] Opatření proti trachomu v státních a statem subvenovaných sociálních ústavech pro mládež na Slovensku [Measures against trachoma in the state and by state supported social institutions for the youth in Slovakia] 24.01.1924 Protitrachomová akcia školské děti, skolníci [Anti-trachom action, school children] 1010-27. Box 107 Expositura Ministerstva veřejného zdravotnictví SNA.

Dopis Referátu ministerstva školství a národnej osvety v Bratislave Obezník č.135 [The Letter to the Board of the Ministry of Education and People's enlightenment in Bratislav] Bratislava 22.IX.1927, box 107 Expositura Mnisterstva veřejného zdravotnictví SNA.

Đorđević, Vojin (1933) *Filmski almanah* [Film Year Book], Belgrade: Arfa.

Douglas, Mary (ed.) (1987) *Constructive Drinking: Perspectives on Drink from Anthropology*, London and New York: Routledge.

Drakić, Gordana (2011) Prekid trudnoche prema krivichnom zakonu kraljevine Jugoslavije i proektima koji su ga prethodni [Abortion Under the Criminal Code of the Kingdom of Yugoslavia and the Projects that Preceded it], *Zbornik radova Pravnog fakulteta Novi Sad* [The collection of works of the Faculty of Law of the University Novi Sad], 45, 3, 533–542.

Driml, Karel (1923) Puppet plays teach health to Czechoslovak children, *The Nation's Health*, 7/6, 464–465.

Driml, Karel (1921) Náš společný nepřítel [Our common enemy], *Měsíčník dorostu Červeného kříže*, 1, 4, 8.

Driml, Karel (1922) Zdravotnické táčky, *Měsíčník dorostu Červeného kříže*, 5, 13.

Driml, Karel (1924) *Král Asinus*, Choceň: Loutkář.

Driml, Karel (1927) *Čarodějka Špindimůra*, Choceň: Loutkář.

Driml, Karel (1927) Přednaška pro učitele škol přihlášených k dorostu Československého Červeného Kříže [Lecture for teachers of schools engaged with the Czechoslovak Red Cross], *Příručky dorostu Československého Červeného Kříže No. 8* [Czechoslovak Red Cross youth manuals], Prague: Zdravotnická výchova na školách [Health Education at schools], 17.

Driml, Karel (1927) Zdravotní výchova loutkovým divadlem. (Proč jsem je angažoval?) [Puppet theatre for health education, *Why have I engaged?*] *Česká osvěta [Czech enlightenment]*, 2, 3.

Driml, Karel (1928) Propagace a boj proti tuberkulose na podkladě statistik a evidence [Propagation and the struggle against tuberculosis on the grounds of statistic data and evidences], *Věstník Masarykovy ligy proti tuberkulózy*, IX, 8.

Driml, Karel Otroci I loutky [Slaves and puppets] Fond Veselý Jindřich undated document, *LA PNP*.

Druick, Zoë (2007) The International Educational Cinematograph Institute, reactionary modernism, and the formation of film studies, *Canadian Journal of Film Studies*, 16, 1, 80–97.

Drzhavna filmska centrála [The State film Board] (1934) *Izveschtaj drzhavne filmske centrale o prometu i snimanju filmova i broju bioskopa u Kraljevni Yugoslavii u 1933 god.* [The report of the state film Central Committee about the dissemination and production of films and the number of cinemas in the Kingdom of Yugoslavia] Kinoteka of the State Archives of Croatia, Fond of Škola za narodnog zdravja, box 3.

Duara, Prasenjit (1998) The regime of authenticity: timelessness, *Gender, and National History in Modern China History and Theory*, 37, 3, 287–308.

Dugac, Željko (2005) *Protiv bolesti i neznanja: Rockefellerova fondacija i međuratnoj Jugoslaviji* [Against Disease and Ignorance: The Rockefeller Foundation and Interwar Yugoslavia], Zagreb: Srednja Europe.

Dugac, Željko (2010) "Like Yeast in Fermentation": Public Health in Interwar Yugoslavia. In Christian Promitzer, Sevasti Trubeta and Marius Turda. Budapest (eds.), *Hygiene, Health and Eugenics in Southeastern Europe to 1945*, CEU Press: New York, 193–232, 201–204.

Dugac, Željko (2010) *Kako biti čist i zdrav. Zdravstveno prosvjećivanje u međuratnoj Hrvatskoj* [How to be clean and healthy. Health education in interwar Croatia], Zagreb: Srednja Europa, 109–114.

Durić, Dejan (2012) Patrijarhat, rod i pripovijetke Dinka Šimunovića [Patriarchat, gender, short stories by Dinko Šimunović], *Croatica et Slavica Iadertina*, 8, 1, 259–276.

Ehrlich, Vera (1964) *Obitelj u transformaciji: studija u tri stotine jugoslavenskih sela* [Family in transformation: study in three hundred Yugoslav villages], Zagreb: Naprijed, 140–144.

Enyedi, Delia (2021) Janovics' Menace: inquiries Into a duplicated silent film script, *Studies in Eastern European Cinema*, 12, 1, 1–12.

Epstein, Sonia Shechet (2019) The way they move, available online https://lareviewofbooks.org/article/the-way-they-move/

Evening Public Ledger (Philadelphia, Pennsylvania) · 27.10.1921, p. 11.

Feldberg, Georgina (1995) *Disease and Class: Tuberculosis and the Shaping of Modern North American Society*, New Brunswick: Rutgers University Press, 6.

Fernandez, Juan (2020) Story makes history, theory makes story: developing Rüsen's *Historik* in logical and semiotic directions *History and Theory*, 57, 1, 75–103, 91–92.

Fifth Festival of Czechoslovak short films (1964) *Československý film*, No. 4, 14–18, p. 17.

Filmová industrie - Josef Kokeisl (1927) Zpravodaj Zemského Svazu kinematografů v Čechách, [Newsletter of the Union of filmmakers in Bohemia], 7, 10.

Filmová kartotéka: týdeník pro kulturní využití filmu [Film archive: a weekly magazine for the cultural use of film], 1940 3, p. 2.

Filmový kurýr [Film courier] 01.09.1928, p. 12.

Films restored by the National Archives of Canada Montreal, 1993, 62; Canadian Film Research AMPAS Personal collection of Edgar Ulmer folder 62.

Fraenkel, Marta (07.12.1932) The Letter to An. Štampar HR-HDA-831 Andrija Štampar, box 9.

Frederic, J. (13.05.1916) Haskin Better Care for Babies, *Altoona Tribune* (Altoona, Pennsylvania), 8.

French, Martin and Cavin Smith (2013) 'Health' Surveillance: new modes of monitoring bodies, populations, and polities, *Critical Public Health*, 23, 4, 383–392.

Fuchs, Brigitta (2016) Škerljevo, Frenjak, Syphilis: Constructing the Ottoman origin of not sexually transmitted venereal disease in Austria and Hungary, 1815–1918. In Jörg Vögele, Stephanie Knöll and Thorsten Noack (eds.), *Epidemien und Pandemien in historischer Perspektive/Epidemics and Pandemics in Historical Perspective*, Springer: Geneve.

Fügner, Hynek and Karel Hübschmann (1934) *Osudná chvíle. Námět.* [Fortuitous Moment. Draft] Filmová industrie Josef Kokeisl [Film production by Josef Kokeisl] NFA.

Galtung, Johan (1990) Cultural violence, *Journal of Peace Research*, 27, 3, 291–305, p. 291.

Gard, Walter S. (1921) Playing a great game, *Junior Red Cross News*, March, 101–103.

Garner, Kenneth (2012) Seeing is knowing: The educational cinema movement in France, 1910–1945, Doctoral Thesis, University of Michigan.

Gastelum, Bernardo J. (1930) The cinema and hygiene propaganda, *International Review of Educational Cinematography*, 3, 155, 2.

Gertiser, Anita (2013) *Falsche Scham: Strategien der Überzeugung in Aufklärungsfilmen zur Bekämpfung der Geschlechtskrankheiten 1915–1935* [False shame: The strategies of persuading and educating within the struggle against sexually transmitted diseases between 1915 and 1935], University of Zurich, Faculty of Arts p. 26.

Ginderachter, Maarten van and Jon Fox (2018). *National indifference and the history of nationalism in Modern Europe: national indifference and the history of nationalism in Modern Europe*, London: Routledge.

Giroux, Henry (2002) Neoliberalism, corporate culture, and the promise of higher education: The university as a democratic public sphere, *Harvard Education*, 72, 2.

Godioli, Alberto (2015) *Laughter from realism to modernism: misfits and humorists in Pirandello, Svevo, Palazzeschi, and Gadda*, London and New York: Routledge.

Goldscheid, David (1909) *Darwin als Lebenselement unserer modernen Kultur* [Darwin as a decisive part of our contemporary culture], Wien und Leipzig, Hugo Heller, 99.

Goodman, Charlotte (1983) The Lost Brother, the Twin: Women Novelists and the Male-Female Double Bildungsroman, *Novel: A Forum on Fiction,* 17, 1, 28–43, p. 30.

Grace, Whitney (2017) *Lotte Reiniger Pioneer of Film Animation*, Jefferson, Horth Carolina: McFarland & Company, 185.

Gradmann, Christoph (2014) Exoticism, Bacteriology and staging of the dangerous. In Thomas Rütten and Martina King (eds.), *Contagionism and Contagious Diseases: Medicine and Literature 1880–1933*, De Gruyter: Berlin, Boston.

Greimas, Algirdas Julien (1988) *Maupassant: The Semiotics of Text. Practical Exercises*, Amsterdam: John Benjamins Publishing Company.

Grieveson, Lee (2017) *Cinema and the Wealth of Nations: Media, Capital, and the Liberal World System*, California: University of California Press, 3.

Guattari, Félix (2009) *Soft subversions: Texts and interviews 1977–1985*, Los Angeles: Semiotexte, 37–38.

Hájek, Viktor (1967) Jak jsem reklamu dělal [How I made advertisement], Part 1, *Propogace*, 5, 105–107.

Hájek, Viktor (1967) Jak jsem reklamu dělal [How I made advertisement] Part 2, 6, *Propogace*, 132–133.

Hannan, Barbara (1997) Love and Human Bondage in *Maugham*. In Roger E. Lamb (ed.), Spinoza and Freud *Love analyzed*, Routledge: New York.

Hansen, Miriam (1991) *Babel and Babylon: Spectatorship and American Silent Film*, Cambridge, MA: Harvard University Press, 77.

Hanuš, Otakar (1940) Manželství pod drobnohledem, *Filmový kurýr*, 14, 3, 5.

Hanuš, Otakar (1914) *Portréty milenek* [Portraits of mistresses], Královské Vinohrady: Přerod, 92–102.

Harrison, Rodney (2013). *Heritage: Critical Approaches*. New York: Routledge, 98.

Hazemann, Robert Henri The letter to A.Štampar 22.12.1937, HR-HDA-831 Andrija Štampar, box 10.

Hes, Milan (2017) *Dandy nezná lásky k ženě: Tragické příběhy českých dekadentů* [Dandy knows no love for women: tragic stories of Czech decadents], Prague: Epocha, 58–59.

Higijenska izložba [Hygienic exhibition] ŠNZ 1929 Subtitles to the film. Kinoteka of the State Archives of Croatia, Fond of Škola za narodnog zdravja, box 1.

Hochschild, Jennifer L., Vesla M. Weaver and Traci R. Burch (2012) *Creating a New Racial Order*, Princeton: Princeton University Press.

Hofer, Veronika (2002) Rudolf Goldscheid, Paul Kammerer und die Biologen des Prater-Vivariums in der liberalen Volksbildung der Wiener Moderne [Rudolf Goldscheid, Paul Kammerer and the biologists of Prater-Vivariums in liberal education for all in modern Vienna]. In Mitchell G. Ash and Christian H. Stifter (eds.), *Wissenschaft, Politik und Öffentlichkeit* [Science, Politics and Openless], WUV: Vienna, 149–184.

Hoffmann, David (2000) Mothers in the motherland: Stalinist Pronatalism in its Pan-European context, *Journal of Social History*, 34, 1, 35–54.

Honzáková, Anna (1936) Úsilí žen o vysokoškolském vzdělání [Women's efforts in higher education] PNR Fond Honzáková Anna, 1875–1940 Č.Inv. 93 22/76. *LA PNP*.

Hübl, Adolf (1931) *Dritte internationale Lehrfilm-Konferenz in Wien* [The Third conference of educational film in Vienna] Wien: Österreichische Bildspielbund.

Hurley, Neil (1960) The Social Philosophy of Charlie Chaplin, *Studies: An Irish Quarterly Review*, 49, 165, 313–320, p. 316.

Hutcheon, Linda (2006) *A Theory of Adaptation*, London: Routledge.

Hvězda československých paní a dívek, 22.6.1935, No. 25, p. 2

Inspekcioni izveshtaj: Odelenje za smeshtaj duševno zaostale dece Velika Gorica [The report for the Department of the protection of the mentally retarded child in Velika Gorica] Fond 39 Ministarstvo socijalne Politike a narodnog zdravlja 1919–1945, FAS 7 AJ.

International Union Save the children, Vergleichende Übersicht über einiger Ausdrucke der Kinderfürsorge. Attachment to the letter to Yugoslav Union for Child Protection of 22.08.1935 Fond 39 Ministarstvo Socijalne Politike a narodnog zdravlja 1919–1945, box 7, folder 2 AJ.

Isenberg, Noah (2004) Perennial Detour: The Cinema of Edgar G. Ulmer and the Experience of Exile, *Cinema Journal*, 43, 2, 3–25.

Isenberg, Noah (2014) *Edgar G. Ulmer: A filmmaker at the margins*, California: University of California Press, 47.

Ivanov, Ivan (1935) Brak i triper [Marriage and gonorrhea], *Narod i potomstvo* [People and offsprings], 01.02.1935.

Jak Vašíček přišel k nohám *Čas,* 23.11.1921, No 274, p. 3.

Jak Vašíček přišel k nohám Školní kinematografie časopis pro uvedení filmu jakožto výchovné učební pomůcky [School cinematography magazine for the introduction of film as an educational teaching aid] 26.11.1921, p. 11.

Jakobson, Roman (1963) Russkiy istochnik cheshskoy komedii [Russian source of the Czech comedy], *Ricerche slavistiche*, I, 331–335.

Jameson, Fredric (1981) *The Political Unconscious*, London and New York: Routledge.

Jazbinsek, Dietmar (2000) *Gesundheitskommunikation:* Medien in der Medizin - Medizin in den Medien! [Communication within public health: Mass media in medicine and medicine in mass-media], VS Verlag für Sozialwissenschaften.

Jirásková, Marie and Pavel Jirásek (2011) *Loutka a moderna: vizualita českého loutkového rodinného divadla, spolkového divadla a uměleckých scén v první polovině 20. století jako osobitý odraz avantgardních a modernistických snah českých výtvarných umělců* [Puppet and modernity: the visuality of Czech puppet family theater, amateur's theater and art scenes in the first half of the 20th century as a distinctive reflection of the avant-garde and modernist efforts of Czech visual artists], Řevnice: Arbor Vitae, 301.

Jones, Kathleen W. (1980) Mother's Day: The Creation, Promotion and Meaning of a New Holiday in the Progressive Era, *Texas Studies in Literature and Language*, 175–196.

Joravsky, David (2019) *Great nations of the West: Conflicting mind-sets*, Unpublished manuscript, 128.

Jović, Bojan (2018) *Avangardni mit Čaplin* [Avantgarde-Mythos Chaplin], Beograd: Službeni glasnik, 236–237.

Jugoslovenski prosvetni film [Yugoslav enlightening film] Ministerstvu prosvete opshte odelenie [Letter to the Ministry of Education. The Department of General Issues] 29.09.1931 1930 Arhiv Jugoslavije fond 66 fascikle 92.

Junior Red Cross (1945), Design, 47, 3, 19.

Jusová, Iveta and Jiřina Šiklová (eds.) (2016) *Czech Feminisms: Perspectives on Gender in East Central Europe*, Indiana: Indiana University Press.

Kahn, Rachel (2019) *Best Common Enemies: Disease Campaigns in America*, Oxford: Oxford University Press, 24.

Kane, Anne (1991) Cultural analysis in historical sociology: the analytic and concrete forms of the autonomy of culture, *Sociological Theory*, 9, 1, 53–69.

Kaser, Karl (2018) *Hollywood auf dem Balkan Die visuelle Moderne an der europaischen Peripherie (1900–1970)*, Wien: Böhlau Verlag.

Kaufmann, Eric and Oliver Zimmer (1998) In Search of the Authentic Nation: Landscape and National Identity in Canada and Switzerland, *Nations and Nationalism*, 4, 4, 483–510, p. 496.

Kim, Grace "Where Are My Children? (1916)". In *Embryo Project Encyclopedia* (26.05.2017), available online: https://embryo.asu.edu/pages/where-are-my-children-1916

King, Martina (2013) Anarchist and Aphrodite: On the literary history of germs. In Thomas Rütten and Martina King (eds.), *Contagionism and Contagious Diseases: Medicine and Literature 1880–1933*, Berlin: De Gruyeter, 101–130, p. 106.

Kisić, Dubravka (2014) *Škola narodnog zdravlja "Andrija Štampar" 1926–1939. Arhitektura i sanitarna tehnika u službi napredka* [The School of Public Health "Andrija Štampar" 1926–1939. Sanitary Engineering in the Mission of progress], Zagreb: Hrvatska Akademija Znatnosti i Umjetnosti Hrvatski Muzej Arhitekture.

Klingenstein, Susanne (2014) *Mendele der Buchhändler: Leben und Werk des Sholem Yankev Abramovitsh; eine Geschichte der jiddischen Literatur zwischen Berdichev und Odessa, 1835–1917*, Wiesbaden: Harrassowitz.

Kocourek, Franta (1929) Institut für Kulturforschung [Institute for cultural research], *Nová svoboda*, 6 24, 375–377, p. 375.

Komarac (1929) The sketches for the film. Kinoteka of the State Archives of Croatia, Fond of Skola za narodnog zdravja, box 1.

Kurka, Vladislav (1911) *Pohlavní zdravověda a sebeochrana* [Sexual health knowledge and selfprotection], Kladno: K. Stejskal.

Kurs o boji proti tyfu pro úťední lékaťe na Slovensku porádaný v Košicích v únoru 1933 [Retraining for the district physicians about the struggle against endemic typhus organized in Kosice in February 1933] HR-HDA-831 Andrija Štampar, folder Vaček, box 14.

Kyjundžić, M. (16.10.1970) Gledamo u bioskopima. Tuga iygublenog detinstva [We look at lost childhood in cinemas], *Dnevnik Novi Sad*.

Lahire, Bernard (2019) Sociological biography and socialisation process: a dispositionalist- contextualist conception, *Contemporary Social Science*, 14, 3–4, 379–393.

Lakoff, George (1987) *Women, Fire, and Dangerous Things What Categories Reveal About the Mind Chicago*, University of Chicago Press; Dedre Gentner, Keith J. Holyoak and Boicho N. Kokinov. Kokinov (2001) *The Analogical Mind: Perspectives from Cognitive Science*, Cambridge, MA: MIT Press.

Langmeir, Josef and Zděnek Matějček (1963) *Psychická deprivace* [Mental deprivation]. Prague: SZN.

Laukötter, Anja (2021) *Sex – richtig! Körperpolitik und Gefühlerziehung im Kino des 20. Jahrhunderts* [Sex – right! Bodypolitics and education of feelings in the films of the twentieth century], Göttingen: Wallstein Verlag, 67.

Lawrence Daily Journal-World (Lawrence, Kansas), 25.12.1920, p. 5.

Lebas, Elizabeth (1995) 'When Every Street Became a Cinema'. The Film Work of Bermondsey Borough Council's Public Health Department, 1923–1953, *History Workshop Journal*, 39, 1, 42–66.

Lebas, Elizabeth (2011) *Forgotten Futures: British Municipal Cinema 1920–1980*, London: Black Dog Press.

Lefebvre, Thierry (1995) Représentations cinématographiques de la syphilis entre les deux guerres: séropositivité, traitement et charlatanisme [Representations of syphilis in the film between the two wars: seropositivity, treatment and charlatanism], *Revue d'histoire de la Pharmacie*, 83, 306, 267–278.

Lewis, Jane and Barbara Brookes (1983) A Reassessment of the Work of the Peckham Health Centre 1926–1951, *Health and Society*, 61, 2, 307–350, p. 329.

Lilika Branka Pleshe dobar posao [*Lilika* by Branka Pleše does her job well] Јутарње новости Београд 18.VII. 1970.

Loetz, Francisca (2010) Why Change Habits? Early Modern Medical Innovation Between Medicalisation and Medical Culture, *History and Philosophy of the Life Sciences*, 32, 4, 453–473.

Logan, Cheryl (2013) *Hormones, Heredity, and Race*, New Brunswick, NJ: Rutgers University Press, 113–116.

Logan, William and Gamini Wijesuriya (2015) The new heritage studies and education, training, and capacity-building. In William Logan, Máiréad Nic Craith, and Ullrich Kockele (eds.), *A Companion to Heritage Studies*, John Wiley and Sons: Malden, MA, 557–573. p. 569.

Lord, Alexandra M. (2010) *Condom Nation: The U.S. Government's Sex Education Campaign from World War I Baltimore*, The Johns Hopkins University Press.

Lorusso, Lorenzo, Thierry Lefebvre and Béatrice de Pastre (2016) Jean Comandon Neuroscientist, *Journal of the History of the Neurosciences*, 25, 1, 72–83.

Lottick, Kenneth V. (1950) Some distinctions between culture and civilization as displayed in sociological literature, *Social Forces*, 28, 3, 240–250.

Luczak Ewa, Barbara (2021) *Mocking Eugenics: American Culture against Scientific Hatred*, Routledge, 23.

MacCabe, Colin (2003) On impurity: The dialectics of cinema and literature in Julian Murphet and Lydia Rainford, *Literature and Visual technologies Writing after cinema*, Palgrave Macmillan, 15–28 p. 19.

Machule, Dittmar Olaf Mischer, and Arnold Sywottek (1996) *Macht Stadt krank?: vom Umgang mit Gesundheit und Krankheit* [Does the city make sick? Treating Health and disease], Hamburg: Dölling und Galitz Verlag, 146.

Majcen, Vjekoslav (1995) *Filmska djelatnost škole narodnog zdravlja "Andrija Štampar": (1926–1960)* [Film activities of the School of Public Health Andrija Štampar" 1926–1969], Zagreb: Hrvatski državni arhiv, 46, 107.

Majcen, Vjekoslav (1995) *Filmska djelatnost škole narodnog zdravlja "Andrija Štampar": (1926.–1960.)* [Films' activities of the School of Public Health Andrija Štampar" 1926–1969], Zagreb: Hrvatski državni arhiv.

Malík, Jan (1950) Bacilínek IV. Výdaní Umění lidu Moderní loutková scéna, 6, 1.

Malý, Karel (1916) *Žena, její krása a život pohlavní (ženy sebeochrana a pohlavní zdravově*da) [Women, her beauty and sexual life: Self-protection and sexual health knowledge for women], Prague: Rudilf Storh.

Many fail to clean alleys. Inspection shows germ breeding places yet untouched warning issued. The Republican News Journal (Newkirk, Oklahoma), 28.04.1922, p. 1.

Manželství pod drobnohledem (1937) *Film Orgán Svazu kinematogr. industrie ČSR v Praze* [Film Organization of the Union of cinematography in Czechoslovak Republic, Prague], 17, 20, 3.

Marcus, Laura (2003) How newness enters the world: the birth of cinema and the origins of man, in Julian Murphet and Lydia Rainford, *Literature and Visual Technologies Writing after Cinema*, Palgrave Macmillan, 29–48, 32.

Marinchevska, Nadezhda (2001) *Bylgarsko animacionno kino 1915–1995* [Bulgarian animation between 1915 and 1995], Sofia: Kolibri.

Marjanović, Milan (1927) Filmska Industrie [Film industry], *Vijenac*, 3–4, 85–88, p. 88.

Marjanović, Milan (1927) Filmska tehnika [Film techniques], *Vijenac*, 6, 155–157.

Marsh, Bill (2010) Visual Education in the United States and the 'Fly Pest' Campaign of 1910, *Historical Journal of Film, Radio and Television*, 30, 1, 21–36.

Marvan, Miroslav and Josef Chaloupecký (1993) *Dějiny pojišťovnictví v Československu* [The history of insurance companies in Czechoslovakia] Volume 2: Dějiny pojišťovnictví v Československu (1918–1945), Bratislava: Alfa Konti, 206–207, p. 345.

McBride Stetson, Dorothy (2001) *Abortion Politics, Women's Movements, and the Democratic State: A Comparative Study of State Feminism*, Oxford: Oxford University Press.

McCallum, Robyn (2018) *Screen Adaptation and the Politics of Childhood*, Palgrave, 22.

McCarthy, Anna (2011) Screen culture and Group discussion in postwar race relations. In Devin Orgeron, Marsha Orgeron, and Dan Streible (eds.), *Learning with the Lights Off: Educational Film in the United States*, Oxford University Press: Oxford, 397–423, p. 398.

Megu idniti domakinki [Among future housewives] Subtitles to the film. Kinoteka of the State Archives of Croatia, Fond of Škola za narodnog zdravja, box 2.

Měsíčník dorostu Červeného kříže [Monthly magazine of the Red Cross for youth], Vzpominky na pana Broučka [Memories about pan Brouček], Dorost Čs. Červeného křiže obecné školy v Knyku [Youth of the Red Cross of the secondary school in Knyk] (1924) 4, 5, p. 67.

Meška, Aleš (1922) Poznámka k boji proti pohlavním chorobám mezi našimi krajany v cizině [The remark to the struggle against venereal diseases among our compatriots abroad], *Dermatologie*, 7, 9, 2–4.

Michl, Susanne (2014) Mapping the war: gender, health, and the medical profession in France and Germany, 1914–1918, *Medicine, Conflict and Survival*, 30, 4, 276–294.

Miller, Alexei (2019). "National indifference" as a political strategy?, *Kritika: Explorations in Russian and Eurasian History*, 20, 1, 63–72.

Milovanović, Aleksandra and Mila Turajlić (2017) Balkanski film na raskršću: Evropeizacija vs. regionalizacija [Balkan film on the crossroad: Europeanization vs. regionalization], *Casopis Instituta za pozorishte, film, radio i televiziju*, 32, 119–137.

Ministarstvo inostranih dela Kralevine Srba, Chrvata i Slovenaca [Ministry of foreign affairs of the Kingdom of Serbs, Croats, and Slovenes] Miniserstvu Prosvete [The letter to the Ministry of education] 29.01.1930 Arhiv Jugoslavije fond 66 fascikle 92.

Ministarstvo inostranih dela Kralevine Srba, Chrvata i Slovenaca [Ministry of foreign affairs of the Kingdom of Serbs, Croats, and Slovenes] Miniserstvu Prosvete [The letter to the Ministry of education] 30.01.1930 Arhiv Jugoslavije fond 66 fascikle 92.

Ministarstvo inostranih dela Kralevine Srba, Chrvata i Slovenaca [Ministry of foreign affairs of the Kingdom of Serbs, Croats, and Slovenes] Miniserstvu Prosvete [The letter to the Ministry of education] 30.04.1930 Arhiv Jugoslavije fond 66 fascikle 92.

Ministarstvo inostranih dela Kralevine Srba, Chrvata i Slovenaca [Ministry of foreign affairs of the Kingdom of Serbs, Croats, and Slovenes] Miniserstvu Prosvete [The letter to the Ministry of education] 30.05.1930 Arhiv Jugoslavije fond 66 fascikle 92.

Ministarstvo inostranih poslova Ministerstvu prosvete Mezhdunarodni institut za vospitni bioskop: izdanje mezhdunarodnog kataloga pouchnih filmova [Letter to the Ministry of Education: International Educational Cinematographic Institute: Publication of the international catalogue of educational films] 08.09.1931 1930 Arhiv Jugoslavije fond 66 fascikle 92.

Ministarstvo prosvete Kraljevine Yugoslavie [Ministry of Education of the Kingdom of Yugoslavia] Ministarstvu inostranih poslova [The letter to the Ministry of foreign affairs] 24.08.1930 Arhiv Jugoslavije fond 66 fascikle 92.

Ministarstvo prosvete Kraljevine Yugoslavie [Ministry of Education of the Kingdom of Yugoslavia] Ministarstvu inostranih poslova [The letter to the Ministry of foreign affairs] 12.12.1930 1930 Arhiv Jugoslavije fond 66 fascikle 92.

Ministerstvo veřejného zdravotnictvi a tělesné výchovy (1923) [Ministry of health and physical culture] Poučení o pohlavních chorobách [The instruction about venereal diseases] Fond EMVZ 97 SNA.

Motýl, Ivan (2018) Tulák Charlie a jeho české stopy [The Tramp Charlie and his Czech traces], *Týden*, 25, 2, 38–41.

Mr. Cash looks forward to workless doctors Derby *Daily Telegraph* – Wednesday 18.06.1930, p. 3.

Muir, W. A., George H. Green, and G. F. Buchan (1938) *Health and Cleanliness: A Textbook for Teachers*, London: Health and Cleanliness Council.

Munby, Jonathan (1999) Heimat Hollywood: Billy Wilder, Otto Preminger, Edgar Ulmer and the criminal cinema of the Austrian-Jewish Diaspora, *David F. Good and Ruth Wodak From World War to Waldheim Culture and Politics in Austria and the United States*, New York: Berghahn Books, 138–164.

Narodna čitanka o zdravljiu [National book about health] (1930). Zagreb: Škola narodnog zdravlja u Zagrebu.

Nový český film z oboru hygeny [New Czech film in the field of hygiene] (1925) *Zdraví lidu: Zdravotnický měsíčník Čsl, Červeného kříže*, 9, 3, 71.

Nowak, Kai (2012) Mütterlichkeit und Mutterschaft. Der Filmskandal um "Frauennot-Frauenglück" (1929/30) [Motherliness and Motherhood. The scandal around The Misery and Fortune of Women (1929/30)], *Ariadne. Forum für Frauen- und Geschlechtergeschichte*, 27, 62, 32–40.

O filmové naději bez drobnohledu [About film hope without microscope] (1940) *Expres* 102, 3.

O'Connor, John (1990) *Image as Artifact. The Historical Analysis of Film and Television*, Florida: Malabar Robert E. Krieger Publishing Company.

Object of the month: Bacilínek https://muzeum.nlk.cz/2021/01/predmet-mesice-leden-2021

Okresný úřad v Turčianskom Sv. Martine [Local authority office, Turčiansky svatý Martin] 25.07.1925 Vlád. Nariadenie k zákonu o potieraní pohlavných nemoci. Prievodný výnos k nemu. Zriadenie venerického oddelenia a Wassermannovej stanice při žup. Nemocnici v Turč. Sv. Martine. [Governmental guidance on implementing the Law about the combat of venereal diseases. Supplementing information. The establishment of venreal subdepartment in Wassermann station at the district hospital in Turčiansky svatý Martin] Fond EMVZ 97 SNA.

Okresný úřad v Turčianskom Sv. Martine [Local authority office, Turčiansky svatý Martin] 10.01. 1927 Výročná zpráva o prevádzaní zákona o potieraní pohlavných nemoci [Annual report about implementing the Law on Combating Sexual Diseases] Fond EMVZ 97 SNA.

Orachovats, D. (1942) Pismo do gospodin Lange Glaven sekretar' na Bylgaro-germanskoto druzhestvo [Letter to the Lange, chief-secretary of the Bulgaraina-German society], Sofiya 21.03.1942, CDA Fond Bylgarsko druzhestvo Cherven krst 156 207.

Orgeron, Devin, Marsha Orgeron, and Dan Streible (2011) Introduction. In Devin Orgeron, Marsha Orgeron, and Dan Streible (eds.), *Learning with the Lights Off: Educational Film in the United States*, Oxford University Press: Oxford, 3–15.

Orgeron, Devin (2011) Spreading the word: race, religion and the rhetoric of contagion in Edgar G. Ulmer's TB Films. In Devin Orgeron, Marsha Orgeron, and Don Streible (eds.), *Learning with the Lights Off: Educational Film in the United States* Oxford University Press: Oxford, 295–319.

Osudná, chvíle (1935) *Film a diapositiv v osvětové práci a ve škole*, 13, 1, 4.

Otis, Laura (1995) The Language of Infection: Disease and Identity in Schnitzler's, *Reigen, The Germanic Review: Literature, Culture, Theory*, 70, 2, 65–75.

Quinlan, Sean (2004) Physical and Moral Regeneration after the Terror: Medical Culture, Sensibility and Family Politics in France, 1794–1804, *Social History*, 29, 2, 139–164.

Patton, Paul (2006) The event of colonialisation. In Ian Buchanan and Andrian Parr (eds.), *Deleuze and the Contemporary World*, Edinburg University Press: Edinburg, 108–124.

Perica, Vjekoslav (2002) *Balkan Idols: Religion and Nationalism in Yugoslav states*, Oxford: Oxford University Press, 19–20.

Pernick, Martin (1999) *The Black Stork: Eugenics and the Death of "Defective" Babies in American Medicine and Motion Pictures since 1915*, Oxford: Oxford University Press, 14.

Petešić, Ćiril (1991) Kamilo Brössler – naš Pestalozzi: pedagoško-socijalni rad i bibliografija objavljenih i neobjavljenih članaka, knjiga i filmova K. Brösslera [Kamilo Brössler is our Pestalozzi: pedagogical-social work and bibliography of known and unknown articles, books and films by K. Brössler] *Zbornik za povijest školstva i prosvjete*, 24, 145–165.

Petrović, Alexandar (1934) *Male Pčelice: tuberkuloza i narodna medicina* [Tuberculosis and folk medicine in Male Pčelice], Belgrade: Štamparija Centralnog Higijenskog Zavoda, 36.

Petrungaro, Stefano (2019) The medical debate about prostitution and venereal diseases in Yugoslavia (1918–1941), *Social History of Medicine*, 32, 1, February, 121–142, p. 128.

Philips-Krug, Jutta and Cecilia Hausheer (1997) *Frankensteins Kinder. Film und Medizin*, Zurich: Hatje Cantz Verlag.

Pictures in the service of the Red Cross (1982) *International Review of the Red Cross*, 4, 120–126.

Pocci, Franz von (2008) *Lustiges Komödienbüchlein* [The book of funny comedies], Vol. 3, Edition Monacensia, Allitera Verlag.

Pocci, Franz von (2010) *Lustiges Komödienbüchlein* [The book of funny comedies], Vol. 5, Edition Monacensia, Allitera Verlag.

Polanská, Jitka (2017) *Děti bez lásky*: film, který změnil pohled na jesle [Children without love: a film that changed the way we look at the nursery] available online: https://www.eduzin.cz/skola-a-ucitele/predskolni-vzdelavani/laska-na-pridel/

Policejní ředitelství v Bratislave [Police Headquarters in Bratislava] 24.03.1922 Dopis Zdravotnímu oddělení města Bratislavy [The Letter to the Department of Public Health, Bratislava] Fond EMVZ 97 SNA.

Popova, Kristina (2011) Combating infant mortality in Bulgaria Welfare activities, national propaganda, and the establishment of pediatrics 1900–1940. In Christian Promitzer, Sevasti Trubeta and Marius Turda (eds.), *Health, Hygiene and Eugenics in Southeastern Europe to 1945*, CEU Press: Budapest, 143–164.

Posner, Miriam (2011) Communicating disease: tuberculosis, narrative, and social order in Thomas Edison's red cross seal films, in Devin Orgeron, Marsha Orgeron and Dan Streible, *Learning with the Lights Off: Educational Film in the United States*, Oxford University Press, 90–106.

Posner, Miriam (2018) Prostitutes, charity girls, and the end of the road: hostile worlds of sex and commerce in an early sexual hygiene film. In Bonah Christian, Cantor David, and Laukötter Anja (eds.), *Health education films in the twentieth century*. Rochester, NY University of Rochester Press, 173–187.

President Woodrow Wilson's Mother's Day Proclamation, source: U.S. National Archive and Records Administration https://www.archives.gov/global-pages/larger-image.html?i=/historical-docs/doc-content/images/mothers-day-proc-l.jpg&c=/historical-docs/doc-content/images/mothers-day-proc.caption.html

Presidium Československého vojenského ředitelství v Bratislavě [Central Committee of Czechoslovak Military Headquarters in Bratislava] Dopis Ministerstvu národní obrany [Letter to the Ministry of Defence] 18.11.1920 Fond EMVZ 97 SNA.

Pressa Filmová tisková služba [Pressa: Film Press Service], 1939, 11, 218, p. 1.

Proctor, Robert (1999) *The Nazi War on Cancer*, Princeton: Princeton University Press.

Programmer for Child welfare week. *Buffalo Morning Express* and *Illustrated Buffalo Express* (Buffalo, New York), 21.09.1919.

Ragonese, Cody, Tim Shand, and Gary Barker (2019) *Masculine Norms and Men's Health: Making the Connections*, The Movember Foundation.

Rare Edward G. Ulmer Unknown newspaper AMPAS Personal collection of Edgar Ulmer folder 62.

Reagan, Leslie J., Nancy Tomes, Paula A. Treichler (eds.) (2007) *Medicine's Moving Pictures: Medicine, Health, and Bodies in American Film and Television*, University Rochester Press.

Retzlaff, Steffen (2017) Der tschechoslowakische Märchenspielfilm (1920–1989). In Claudia Ute Dettmar, Maria Pecher and Ron Schlesinger (eds), *Märchen im Medienwechsel: Zur Geschichte und Gegenwart des Märchenfilms*, J.B. Metzler Verlag: Stuttgart, 229–250.

Reynolds, Siân (1996) *France Between the Wars: Gender and Politics*, London: Routledge.

Richard, Howells and Robert W. Matson (2009) *Using Visual Evidence*, Berkshire Open University Press.

Richards, Jeffrey (2000) 'Rethinking British Cinema', paper given at 'Cinema, Identity, History: An International Conference on British Cinema', held at the University of East Anglia in July 1998. Published. In Justine Ashby and Andrew Higson (eds), *British Cinema, Past and Present* (London 2000), 21–34.

Roberts, Mary Louise (1994) *Civilization Without Sexes: Reconstructing Gender in Postwar France, 1917–1927*, Chicago: The Chicago University Press, 120–121.

Rockefeller Foundation *Annual report* 1936: p. 8 [available at https://www. rockefellerfoundation.org/wp-content/uploads/Annual-Report-1936-1.pdf retrieved 23 .05. 2021].

Rodrique, Jessie M. (1992) The Black Community and the Birth Control Movement. In Dorothy O. Helly and Susan M. Reverby (eds.) *Gendered Domains: Rethinking Public and Private in Women's History*, Cornell: Cornell University Press, 244–262.

Roos, Julia (2010) *Weimar through the Lens of Gender: Prostitution Reform, Woman's Emancipation, and German Democracy, 1919–33*, Ann Arbor, MI: University of Michigan.

Rost, Karl Ludwig (1987) *Sterilisation und Euthanasie im Film des "Dritten Reiches"*[]. Husum; Karl Ludwig Rost (1988): Propaganda zur Vernichtung "unwerten Lebens" durch das Rassenpolitische Amt der NSDAP [Propaganda for extermination of unvaluable lives through the Race polotic Department of NSDAP]. *1999* 3, 46–55.

Roth, Karl-Heinz (1988) Filmpropaganda für die Vernichtung der Geisteskranken und Behinderten im "Dritten Reich" [Film propaganda for extermination of mentally disabled people in the Third Reich]. In Gütz Aly, Karl Friedrich Masuhr, and Maria. Lehmann (eds.) *Reform und Gewissen. Euthanasie im Dienst des Fortschritts* [Reform and conscience: Euthanasie in the service of progress], Berlin: Rotbuch Verlag, 125–193.

Roth, Randolph (1992) Is history a process? Nonlinearity, revitalization theory, and the central metaphor of social science history, *Social Science History*, 16, 2, 197–243, p. 200.

Rožánek, Otakar (1903) *Pud pohlavní a prostituce vývoj a poruchy pudu pohlavního* [Sexual instinct and prostitution: development of sexual disorders], Praha: Hejda a Tuček, 135.

Rožánek, Otakar (1906) *Choroby pohlavní u muže a ženy* [Venereal diseases of men and women], Prague: B.Koči.

Rugby Advertiser – Friday 15 November 1929, p. 4.

Rus, Richard (1924) Kašpárek ve službách pokroku: loutkářská příručka s Kašpárkovými besídkami pro sokolské a lidovýchovné malé i velké pracovníky [Kašpárek in the service of progress: a puppet guidance with Kašpárek's plays for small and big educators in Sokol and people's initiatives], Pardubici: Vzdělání lidů.

Salmi, Hannu (2011) Cultural history, the possible and principle of plenitude, *History and Theory*, 50, 171–187.

Sa zbora župskih prosvetara [News from the meeting of local educators] (1934) *Sokolska Prosveta*, IV 5, 218.

Scaglia, Ilaria (2020) *The Emotions of Internationalism: Feeling International Cooperation in the Alps in the Interwar Period (Emotions in History)*, Oxford University Press.

Schaefer, Eric (2011) Exploitation as education. In Devin Orgeron, Marsha Orgeron and Dan Streible (eds.), *Learning with the Lights Off: Educational Film in the United States*, Oxford University Press, 316–337, p. 319.

Schlegelmilch, Sabine (2017) Film als medizinhistorische Quelle / Film sources in medical history Author(s): Medizinhistorisches Journal, 2017, Bd. 52, H, 2/3 (2017), 100–115.

Schmidt, Ulf (1995) Der medizinische Film in der historischen Forschung, *Mitteilungen aus dem Bundesarchiv*, 3, 82–84.

Schmidt, Ulf (2000) *Medical Research Films, Perpetrators, and Victims in National Socialist Germany 1933–1945*, Husum.

Schwarz, Ori (2016) The Symbolic Economy of Authenticity as a Form of Symbolic Violence: The Case of Middle-class Ethnic Minorities *Distinktion*, 17, 1, 2–19.

Scott, Joan W. (2001) Fantasy echo: History and the construction of identity, *Critical Inquiry*, 27, 2, 284–304, p. 289.

Seidman, Karmenlara (2004) The call of the wise baby in Chaplin's the kid women and performance, *A Journal of Feminist Theory*, 14, 1, 117–136, pp. 131–132.

Seidman, Naomi (1997) *A Marriage Made in Heaven: The Sexual Politics of Hebrew and Yiddish*, California: University of California Press.

Senica [District Senica] 19.01.1928Výročná zpráva o prevádzaní zákona o potieraní pohlavních nemocí [Annual report about implementing the Law on Combating Sexual Diseases] Fond EMVZ 97 SNA.

Shapira, Michal (2013) *The War Inside: Psychoanalysis, Total War and the Making of the Democratic Self in Postwar Britain*, Cambridge: Cambridge University Press, 212–213.

Shepherd-Barr, Kirsten (2015). *Edwardians and Eugenicists. In Theatre and Evolution from Ibsen to Beckett*, Colombia: Columbia University Press, 168.

Shmidt, Victoria (2015) *Child Welfare Discourses and Practices in the Czech Lands: The Segregation of Roma and Disabled Children During the Nineteenth and Twentieth Centuries*, Brno: Muni Press.

Shmidt, Victoria (2019) *Politics of Disability in Interwar and Socialist Czechoslovakia: Segregation in the Name of the Nation*, Amsterdam: Amsterdam University Press.

Shmidt, Victoria (2019) When National Female Bildungsroman Meets Global Fantasies about Nazis: Historical Roots and Current Troubles in *Lída Baarová*, 4, 61–78, p. 63.

Shmidt, Victoria (2020) Female Bildungsroman in Czech Conduct Periodicals: The Inception of the Genre, *History of Education & Children's Literature*, XV, 2, 407–428.

Shmidt, Victoria (2020) Race science in Czechoslovakia: Serving Segregation in the Name of the Nation Studies, *History and Philosophy of Science Part C: Studies in History and Philosophy of Biological and Biomedical Sciences*, 83. DOI:10.1016/j.shpsc.2019.101241. https://www.sciencedirect.com/science/article/pii/S1369848618301365?via%3Dihub

Shmidt, Victoria and Bernadette Nadya Jaworsky (2020) *Historicizing Roma in Central Europe: Between Critical Whiteness and Epistemic Injustice*, London: Routledge, 36–37.

Shmidt, Victoria (2018) Public Health as an Agent of Internal Colonialism in Interwar Czechoslovakia: Shaping the Discourse about The Nation's Children, *Patterns of Prejudice*, 52, 4, 355–387.

Silva, Edward T. (1980) Cultural Autonomy and Ideas in Transit: Notes from the Canadian Case, *Comparative Education Review* 24, 1, 63–72, p. 63.

Silverstein, Sara (2013) Man of an Impossible Mission? Andrija Štampar's Separation of Politics and Healthcare in Yugoslavia and the World Health Organization available online: https://www.issuelab.org/resources/27898/27898.pdf?download=true

Silverstein, Sara (2020) Reinventing International Health in East Central Europe, In Peter Becker and Natasha Wheatley (eds.), *Remaking Central Europe*, Oxford University Press: Oxford, 71–98.

Šimunović, Dinko (1873–1933) was a Croatian teacher and writer famous for his overtly patriarchal views and their promotion in fiction and public activities.

Širola, Mladen (1927) *Marionetsko kazalište u službi zdravstvenog prosvjećivanja* [Puppet theatre in serving the mission of health enlightenment], Zagreb: Tisak Jugoslovenske štampe.

Skalarjeva, Elza (1934) Jugoslavenska žena u sokolskoj organizaciji [Yugoslav woman in the Socol organization], *Sokolska prosveta*, 4, 3-4, 125–129.

Škrabalo, Ivo (1998) 101 godina filma u Hrvatskoj, 1896–1997. [101 years of film in Croatia] Zagreb, Nakladni zavod Globus.

Smetáček, Zdeněk (1925) Bergson a Chaplin [Bergson and Chaplin], *Přítomnost*, 12, 03, 136–138, p. 138.

Sobotková, Josefina (1928) Nemanželské dětí [Children born outside of marriage] in *Výroční zpráva o činnosti okresní péče o mládež a ostatních humanních spolků v Holešově* [Annual report about the activities of local authorities concerning youth care and other charity unions in Holešov], Halašov: Tiskarna Balatka a Šrámak.

Šobová, Marie (1945) Moje vzpomínky na MUDr. A.Honzákovou [My memories of MUDr. A.Honzáková] PNR Fond Honzáková Anna, 1875–1940, Č.inv. 134-135 22/76, p. 1 *LA PNP*.

Sociálně právní ochrana [Social protection for youth] Den matek [Social protection: Mother's day] 1949, box 6, folder 423/49, State Regional Archives in Kroměříž.

Sojka, Jaroslav (1996) *Komenšti* [The successors of Jan Komenius], Brno, 3.

Sokolska prosveta, 1934, IV 3-4 p.150.

South Yorkshire Times and Mexborough & Swinton Times – Friday 19.10.1934, p. 12.

Spinoza, Benedict de (1883) *The Ethics*, Part IV Of Human Bondage, or the Strength of the Emotions available online: https://www.sacred-texts.com/phi/spinoza/ethics/eth04.htm

Spode, Hasso (1993) *Die Macht der Trunkenheit: Kultur- und Sozialgeschichte des Alkohols in Deutschland* [The power of drunkeness: Cultural and social history of alcohols in Germany], Opladen: Leske und Budrich.

Spoločnost československoho červeného kríža [The Red Cross] (1926), Soznam filmov pre deti [List of the films for children], Fond of Košická župa 1923–1928, II. ZV, box 522.

Springer, Jenny (1911) Die Ärztin im *Hause* [The Doctor at home], Dresden: Max Otto Groh.

Stam, Robert, Robert Bugoyne and Sandy Flitterman-Lewis (1992) *New vocabularies in film semiotics Structuralism post-structuralism and beyond*, London and New York: Routledge.

Štampar, Andrija (1932) Rural Hygiene: The Draft of the Report to the League of Nation. HR-HDA-831 Andrija Štampar, box 3.

Štampar, Andrija (1913) Izvešće o pošasti Kolere u Kotaru Novogradiškom [The report about Cholera epidemic in Nova Gradiška] Ditrict HR-HDA-831 Andrija Štampar, HR-HDA-831 Andrija Štampar, box 1.

Štampar, Andrija (1919) *Narodna čitanka o alkoholu* [People's manual about alcohol] Knižnica protiv alkoholu [Library collection against alcohol], Zagreb: Društvo apstinenata u Hrvatskoj i Slavoniji [Union of the abstinents of Croatia and Slovenia], 31.

Štampar, Andrija (1920) O socijalnoj terapiji [About social therapy] Glasnik Ministarstva narodnog zdravlja [Newslatter of the Ministzr of Public health], 7, 261–271.

Štampar, Andrija (1911) Socijalna medicina [Social medicine], *Zora*, 3, 126–131.

Štampar, Andrija (1919) O zdravstvenoj politici Jugoslavenska [About public health in Yugoslavia], *Njiva*, 29–31, 1–29.

Štampar, Andrija (1925) *Socijalna medicina. Uz saradnju jugoslovenskih socijalnih lekara* [Social medicine: From the experinece of Yugoslav physicians], First volume, Zagreb: Institut za socijalnu medicinu.

Štampar, Andrija (1926) *Pet godina socijalno-medicinskog rada u Kraljevini Srba, Hrvata i Slovenaca* [Five years of social-medical work in the Kingdom of Serbia, Croatia and Slovenia], Zagreb, 3.

Štampar, Andrija (1928) Naša ideologija [Our ideology], *Nova Evropa* [Our Europe], 229–231.

Štampar, Andrija (1931) Hygiene auf dem Lande: Aufteilung des Programms Štampar in einzelne Darstellungen [Hygiene in the rural areas: texts' supplement of the Štampar's program to special exhibition] HR-HDA-831 Andrija Štampar, HR-HDA-831 Andrija Štampar, box 14.

Štampar, Andrija (1937) Visit to the State Institute for Maternal and Child Protection, Moscow HR-HDA-831 Andrija Štampar, box 3.

Štampar, Andrija (undated document) Maternal and child welfare in Yugoslavia the draft of the presentation, Undated document HR-HDA-831 Andrija Štampar, box 3.

Štampar, Andrija (10.12.1932) The letter to Marta Fraenkel HR-HDA-831 Andrija Štampar, box 9.

Štampar, Andrija The letter To Alice Masaryková 01.03.1933, HR-HDA-831, Andrija Štampar, HR-HDA-831 Andrija Štampar, box 11.

Štampar, Andrija Untitled and undated text 9.1.3.2 HR-HDA-831 Andrija Štampar, HR-HDA-831 Andrija Štampar, box 7.

Štampar, Andrja Letter to Vacek 11.01.1933 HR-HDA-831 Andria Štampar, box 14.

Stark, James F. and Catherine Stones (2019) Constructing Representations of Germs in the Twentieth Century, *Cultural and Social History*, 16, 3, 287–314, p. 289.

Stationary and moving pictures for hygiene propaganda (1930) *International review of educational cinematography*, 1, 53–54, p. 54.

Statistički podaci o stanovništvu: skarlatina, variola vera, morbilli, dysentiria, difteria et croup, typhus abdominalis, typhus exanthemanticus [Population statistics: scarlet fewer, measles, dysentery, diphtheria and croup, abdominal typhus, asthmatic typhus], Fond 39 Ministarstvo Socijalne Politike a narodnog zdravlja 1919-1945, box 6, folder 15, AJ.

Štebi, Alojz (1935) Les devoire et la collaboration des *banovinas*, des districts, et des autres institutions administratives et autonomes pour la protection des enfants de la campagne [The oblugations and collaboration of banovinas, districts, and other administrative and autonomous institutions for the protection of rural children]. Resume to the presentation at the First Balkan Congress on Child Development Fond 39 Ministarstvo Socijalne Politike a narodnog zdravlja 1919-1945, box 7, folder 2, AJ.

Ştefănescu, Bogdan (2012) *Postcommunism/Postcolonialism: Siblings of Subalternity*, Bucharest: Editura universitätii din bucuresti.

Stepan, Nancy Ley (2012) *Eradication: Ridding the World of Diseases Forever?* London: Reaktion Books.

Stewart, Jez (2021) *The Story of British Animation*, London: The British Film Institute, 55–56.

Stones, Catherine James Stark, Sophie Rutter and Colin Macduff (2020) The visual representation of germs: a typology of popular germ depictions, *Visual Communication*, 10.1177/1470357219896055

Stopes, Marie Carmichael (1918) *Married Love: A New Contribution to the Solution of Sex Difficulties*, London: A.C. Fifield.

Streible, Dan Roepke, Martina and Anke Mebold (2007) Nontheatrical Film, *Film History*, 19, 339–343.

Sudović, Zlatko (1978) *Pedeset godina crtanog filma u Hrvatskoj 1922–1972* [Fifty Years of Cartoon Film in Croatia, 1922–1972], Zagreb.

Světozor: časopis pro zábavu i poučení [*Světozor:* a magazine for entertainment and instruction] 1940, 40.

Sydenstricker, Edgar (1934) Health in the New Deal, *The Annals of the American Academy of Political and Social Science*, 176, 131–137.

Szelągowska, Grażyna (2019) Lutheran Revival and National Education in Denmark: The Religious Background of N. F. S. Grundtvig's Educational Ideas, *Scandinavica*, 58, 1, 6–30.

Tadić, Zoran (2004) Zaboravljeni Chloupek [Forgotten Chloupek] Dokumentarni film – uvod: škola Narodnog Zdravlija available online: https://www.matica.hr/vijenac/279/Zaboravljeni%20Chloupek/

Takové jsou: Sestry z Okresního ústavu národního zdraví v Holešové [Such are: Nurses from the District Institute of Public Health in Holešov] (1956) *Zdravotnická pracovnice. Časopis pro střední a nižší zdravotnické pracovníky* [*Journal for Middle and Lower Level Healthcare Professionals*], 6, p. 20.

Taylor, Alan J.P. (2001) *English History 1914–1945*, Oxford: Oxford University Press, 313.

Taylor, Rex and Annelie Rieger (1984) Rudolf Virchow on the typhus epidemic in Upper Silesia: an introduction and translation, *Sociology of Health and Illness*, 6, 2, 201–217.

Tekovský župan Zlaté Moravy [District Tekov, Zlata Morava](10.06.1922) Policajný dohlaď nad prostitucí na Slovensku [Police surveillance over prostitution in Slovakia] Fond EMVZ 97 SNA.

Tells of Life's pitfalls, *The Baltimore Sun (Baltimore, Maryland)*, · 29.06.1919, p. 54.

The draft of the leaflet Škola narodnog zdravija u Zagrebu NDH 1940 3/517.

The first Bulgarian animated film "Villains", *Dyga* 30.11.1936, 170, p. 6.

The League of Red Cross Societies Geneva Switzerland (1921) *Conditions concernant le prêt des films par la Ligue des societies de la Croix-Rouge* [Prerequisites for loaning films by the League of Red Cross Societies], EMVZ, box 106, SNA.

The Rockefeller Foundation, A review for 1919 Public health and Medical education in many lands, p. 25–26.

Thoburn, Nickolas (2006) Vacuoles of Noncommunication: Minor Politics? Communist Style and the Multitude. In Ian Buchanan and Andrian Parr (eds.), *Deleuze and the Contemporary World*, Edinburg: Edinburg University Press, 42–56.

Todd, Wider (1990) The positive image of the physician In American cinema during the 1930s, *Journal of Popular Film and Television*, 17, 4, 139–152.

Torchia, Marion (1975) The tuberculosis movement and the race question 1890–1950, *Bulletin of the History of Medicine*, 49, 2, 152–168, p. 160.

Toshkov, Alex (2019) *Agrarianism as Modernity in 20th-century Europe: The golden Age of the Peasantry*, London: Bloomsbury, 10.

Trbojević, Mica (1935) La paysanne – gardienne de l'enfant étranger [Peasants as guardians for alien children] Congrès balkanique de protection de l'Enfance [The first Balkan child-welfare congress] Fond 39 Ministarstvo socijalne politike a narodnog zdravlja 1919-1945 [Ministry] box 7, folder 2, AJ.

Trbojević, Mica (1935) Le rôle de la paysanne dans le placement familial rural des infants [The role of rural women in the substitute family palcement of infants] Congrès balkanique de protection de l'Enfance, Archiv of Yugoslavia Fond 39 Ministarstvo Socijalne Politike a narodnog zdravlja 1919-1945, box 7, folder 2.

Večer lidový denník *Jak Vašíček přišel k nohám: film o nejubožejších a nejzapominanějších* [Jak Vašíček přišel k nohám: a film about the poorest and most forgotten], 20.07.1921, No. 162, p. 12.

Velde, Th. H., and Van De (1928) *Ideal Marriage: Its Physiology and Techniques*, London: William Heinemann.

Verma, Surya P. and Binod Mishra (2021) The Art of Survival: Understanding Charlie Chaplin's the Little Tramp through the Lens of Little Narrative, *Quarterly Review of Film and Video*, 38, 5, 400–413.

Vidović, Miljenko (1926) Dolaze sunčani ljudi [Sun people are coming], *Novi čovjek*, 2, 1.

Vidović, Miljenko (1927) Ognjeni ljudi [Fiery people], *Novi Čovjek*, 62, 1.

Vidović, Miljenko (1927) *Ideje i problemi: članci i rasprave* [Ideas and issues: articles and discussions], Sarajevo: Obod.

Vidović, Miljenko (1927) Tražite čovjeka [Look for a man], *Uzgajatelj*, 2, 1.

Vignaux, Valérie (2007) *Jean Benoit-Lévy ou le corps comme utopie* [Jean Benoit-Lévy or the body as utopia] Paris: AFRHC.

Vignaux, Valérie (2011) *Entertainment and Instruction as Models in the Early Years of Animated Film: New Perspectives on Filmmaking in France in Animation*, SAGE Publications, 6, 177–192.

Vintrová, Marie (2004) Rodiná krnonika z periferie (žánrová inovace v nejrozšířenějším ženském týdeníku První republiky [Family chronicle from the periphery (genre innovation in the most widespread women's weekly of the First Republic]. In Michak Jareš, Pavel Janáček, and Petr Šámal (eds.), *Povídka, roman a periodický tisk v 19. a 20.století* [Short story, novel and periodical in the 19th and 20th centuries] Sborník příspěvků ze sympozia pořádaného oddělením pro výzkum literární kultury ÚČL AV ČR v Praze 13.-14.11 2004 [Collection of the contributions to the symposium of the research of literal culture of the Institute of Czech literature, Academy of Science: Prague, 194–200.

Vlasta 1964, 18, 13, pp. 10–12.

Vleugels, An (2013) *Narratives of Drunkenness: Belgium, 1830–1914*, London and New York: Routledge, 14.

Výstava soudobé kultura v Československu: Odbor pro vědu, duchovou a technickou kulturu a školství vysoké [the Exhibition of Contemporary Culture in Czechoslovakia: The Board of science, spiritual and technical culture and higher education] Vladimír Úlehla Personal collection B 57, box 18, folder 888, AMU.

Výstava soudobé kultura v Československu: Odbor pro vědu, duchovou a technickou kulturu a školství vysoké [Exhibition of Contemporary Culture in Czechoslovakia: Department of Science, Spiritual and Technical Culture and Higher Education] Vladimír Úlehla, Personal collection B 57, box 18, folder 888, AMU.

Vzorná zdravotní demonstrace v okresu Turč. Sv. Martin [Exemplary public health demonstration in the district Turč. Sv. Martin] M.U.Dr. M. Šulc 1927 p. 9, box 107, Expositura Ministerstva veřejného zdravotnictví Slovenský narodný archiv [Slovak National Archive SNA].

Vzorná zdravotní demonstrace v okresu Turč. Sv. Martin [Exemplary public health organization in the district of Turčiansky sv. Martin] M.U.Dr. M. Šulc 1927, p. 7, box 107, Expositura Mnisterstva veřejného zdravotnictví SNA.

Vzpomínky dětí na zdravotně-výchovnou jednotku [The memories of children about the health education unit meeting], *Měsíčník dorostu Červeného kříže* (1925), 5, p. 59.

Waling, Andrea (2019) Problematising 'toxic' and 'healthy' masculinity for addressing gender inequalities, *Australian Feminist Studies*, 34, 101, 362–375.

Walzer, Michael (1987) *Interpretation and Social Criticism*. Cambridge, MA: Harvard University Press.

Warriner, Doreen (1959) Urban thinkers and peasant policy in Yugoslavia, 1918–59, *The Slavonic and East European Review*, 38, 90, 59–81.

Weindling, Paul (1995) Social medicine at the League of Nations Health Organization and the International Labour Office compared in Colin Jones, Paul Weindling, and Charles Rosenberg (eds.), *International Health Organisations and Movements, 1918–1939*, Cambridge University Press: Cambridge, 134–149, p. 135.

Weindling, Paul (2007) Ansteckungsherde. Die deutsche Baktereiologie als wissenschaftlicher Rassismus 1890–1920 [The sources of infection: German bacteriology as scientific racism in the 1890s and 1920s]. In Philipp Sarasin, Silvia Berger, Marianne Hänseler, and Myriam Spörri (eds) *Bakteriologie und Moderne. Studien zur Biopolitik des Unsichtbaren 1870–1920* [Bacteriology and moderne. The studies of biopolotics concerning invisible in the 1870s and 1920s], Frankfurt am Main: Suhrkamp, 2007, 354–374.

Westminster Gazette – Tuesday 05.07.1927, p. 7.

Whitehead, Stephen M. (2021) Toxic masculinity: curing the virus: making men smarter, healthier, safer, AG Books.

Winkler, Anita (2015) Debating sex: education films and sexual morality for the young in post-war Germany, 1945–55, *Gesnerus*, 72, 1, 77–93.

Witcomb, Andrea and Kristal Buckley (2013). Engaging with the future of 'critical heritage studies': looking back in order to look forward. *International Journal of Heritage Studies*, 19, 6, 562–578.

Wolff, Tamsen (2009) *Mendel's Theory: Heredity, Eugenics, and Early Twentieth-century American Drama*, Palgrave, 5.

Woodbridge, Benjamin Mather (1922) Maupassant's realism, *Texas Review*, 8, 1, 7–20, p. 16.

Yeomans, Rory (2008) Fighting the White plague: demography and abortion in the independent state of Croatia, 1941–1945. In Christian Promitzer, Sevasti Trubeta, and Marius Turda (eds.), *Health, Hygiene and Eugenics in Southeastern Europe to 1945*, CEU Press: Budapest, 385–426.

Young, William (1850) *Beranger: Two Hundred of his Lyrical Poems*, New York: Georg P. Putnam, 249.

Young, Kimball (1922) Intelligence Tests of Certain Immigrant Groups, *The Scientific Monthly*, 15, 5, 417–434, p. 418.

Záběr zblízka [Close up shot] *Kino*, 1970 25 19, p. 14.

Za Liliku specijalne predstave [Special performance of Lilika] *Veherne новости Београд* 5.06.1971.

Zahra, Tara (2008). *Kidnapped Souls: National Indifference and the Battle for Children in the Bohemian Lands, 1900–1948*. Cornell University Press.

Zavlékání nakazlivých němoci ze Slovenska v Brně [Dissemination of infectious diseases in Brno] 10.04.1926 Protitrachomová akcia školské děti, skolníci [Antitrachom action, school children] 1010-27, box 107, Expositura Ministerstva veřejného zdravotnictví SNA.

Zdravstevni odsjek za Hrvatsku Slavoniju i Medjimurje i Zagreb [The Department of public health at Slavonia, Međimurje and Zagreb] (1922) Gradskom školskom nadvorništvu [The letter to the Department of education] Arhiv Jugoslavije Ministarstvo socijalne politike i narodnog zdravlje Kraljevine Yugoslavie Broj fond 39, Broj fasikle 2.

Zdravstveno-prosvjetni rad [Health education] (1935) *Kniga za sokolsko selo [Book about Sokol village]*, 1, 8-9, 29.

Zipes, Jack (2012) *The Irresistible Fairy Tale: The Cultural and Social History of a Genre*, Princeton: Princeton University Press, 67.

Župný úrad v Turč. Sv. Martine [District authorities in Turčiansky Svätý Martin] Organizovanie vzorného okresu na Slovensku [The organization of an exemplary district of public health in Slovakia] Číslo 51.555/125 07.11.1925, box 107, Expositura Mnisterstva veřejného zdravotnictví SNA.

Župný uřad Zvolen [District authorities of Zvolen] 29.05.1923 Dopis Expositúre ministerstva verejného zdravotníctva a telesnej výchovy v Bratislave [The letter to the Ministry of Health and Physical Culture] Zatvorenie nevestincov [Closing brothels], Fond EMVZ 97 SNA.

Žužić, Đorđe (1934) Ministerstvu socialnoj politiky i narodnogo zdorovjy Alexandrovi Zemun Referentu za abnormalu decu [To the Ministry of Social Policy and National Health Alexander Zemun Referent for abnormal children] folie 475-484 Fond 39 Ministarstvo socijalne politike a narodnog zdravlja 1919-945, box 7, AJ.

Filmography to the book

1 *A two-year-old goes to the hospital* (by John Robertson 1952)
2 *Another to conquer* (by Edgar Ulmer, 1941)
3 *Arvák imája* (The prayer of orphans, by János Fröhlich 1922)
4 *Birth* (for Eugenic film company, 1917)
5 *Birtija* (The pub, by Drago Chloupek 1929)
6 *Blago kući gdje se žena uči* (Wellbeing of home where women are learning, by Stevan Mišković 1936)
7 *Borba protiv bolesti putem filma* (Fighting disease with the help of film, 1934)
8 *Bringing it home* (N/A 1919)
9 *Bunny backslide* (by George D. Baker, 1914)
10 *Campek nevaljalac* (Naughty Champek, by Mladen Širola, 1929)
11 *Čarobnjaci* (Wizards, by Mladen Širola, 1928)
12 *Clara cleans her teeth* (by Walt Disney, 1927)
13 *Cloud in the sky* (by Edgar Ulmer, 1939)
14 *Dačko ljetovalište Martinščica* (Resort for children Martinščica by Milan Marjanović 1927)
15 *Damaged lives* (by Edgar Ulmer 1933)
16 *Děti bez lásky* (Children without love, by Kurt Goldberger 1963)
17 *Diagnostic procedures in tuberculosis (1940, by Edgar Ulmer)*
18 *Die Biene Maja und ihre Abenteuer* (The adventures of Maya the bee, 1926)
19 *Dluh – Jedličkův ústav* [Our debt to Jedličkův ústav, by Libuše Hájková 1968]
20 *Dobro za zlo* (Good for evil, by Drago Chloupek 1936)
21 *Drei entscheidende Jahre* (Three decisive years, by Kurt Goldberger, 1971)
22 *Dva brata: film o sušuci* (Two brothers: A film about tuberculosis, by Kamilo Brössler 1931)
23 *Dvije seke: film o njezi dojenčadi* (Two sisters: A film about caring for infants, 1932)
24 *Es werde Licht* (It will be light, by Richard Oswald, 1918)

25 *Eugenics baby* (N/A, 1914)

26 *Eugenics vs. love* (by Harry A. Pollard, 1914)

27 *Falsche Scham* (False shame 1925 /1926 by Rudolf Bierbach)

28 *Frauennot-Frauenglück* (The misery or fortune of women, by Eduard Tissé and Grigory Alexandov, 1929)

29 *Giro fast and loose* (sponsor: Health and Cleanliness Council, 1935)

30 *Giro the germ*, episodes 1–2 (sponsor: Health and Cleanliness Council, 1927)

31 *Gonorröa iseravimise ohtlikkus* (The danger in self-treatment of gonorrhea, N/A about film director, 1986, Tallinfilm)

32 *Goodbye, Mr. Germ* (1940 by Edgar Ulmer)

33 *Griješnice: Macina i Ankina sudbina* (Sinners: Maca and Anka's destiny, by Joza Ivakić, 1930)

34 *Ikina sudbina* (Ika's destiny, by Kamilo Brössler, 1933)

35 *Il était une fois trois amis* (Once upon a time there were three friends, by Jean Benoit-Lévy 1927)

36 *Ivin zub, Macin nos* (Iva's tooth, Masa's nose, by Petar Papp and Milan Marjanović, 1928)

37 *Izmjena liječnika Lige naroda* (The transformation of the physician in the League of Nations, by Milan Marjanović, 1928)

38 *Jak Vašíček přišel k nohám* (How Vašíček got his legs, by Antonín Jiroušek, 1921)

39 *Jerry's eugenic marriage* (by Milton J. Fahrney, 1917)

40 *Jinks*, (N/A about film director, Bray Studios 1918)

41 *Kašparek a Bodulínek* (The clown and Bodulínek, by Josef Kokeisl, 1927)

42 *Kašpárek kouzelníkem* (Magic medicine, by Josef Kokeisl, 1927)

43 *Kolja* (Kolya, by Jan Svěrak, 1996)

44 *Komarac a njegov razvoj* (The mosquito and his development, by Petar Papp and Milan Marjanović, 1929)

45 *Kukačka v temném lesu* (Cuckoo in a dark forest, by Antonín Moskalyk, 1985)

46 *Let my people live* (by Edgar Ulmer 1938)

47 *Lidé* (Humans, by Kurt Goldberger 1964)

48 *Lilika* (by Branko Pleša, 1970)

49 *Lječilište Topolšica* (Sanatorium Topolšica, by Milan Marjanović, 1927)

50 *Malarija* (Malaria, by Stevan Mišković 1931)

51 *Manželství pod drobnohledem* (Marriage under the microscope, by Josef Kokeisl, 1940)

52 *Marian* (by Petr Václav, 1995)

53 *Martin u nebo Martin iz neba* (Martin goes to heaven and back, by Petar Papp and Milan Marjanović, 1929)

54 *Megu idniti domakinki* (Among the future housewives, by Stevan Mišković 1931)

55 *Na sonce i vzduch* (In the sun and the air, by Stevan Mišković 1931)

56 *Nell's eugenic wedding* (by Edward Dillon, 1914)

57 *Neúplné zatmení* (Incomplete eclipse, by Jaromil Jires, 1983)

58 *O Popelce* (About Cinderella, by Josef Kokeisl, 1929)

59 *On doit le dïre* (It must be said, by Marius O'Galop 1918)

60 *Osudná chvíle* (Fortuitous moment, by Josef Kokeisl, 1935)

61 *Our children* (N/A, 1921)

62 *Pakostnitsi* (Villains, by Vasil Bakyrdzhiev and Stoyan Venev, 1936)

63 *Parentage* (by *Hobart Henley,*1919)

64 *Peter and the Moon Man* (sponsor: Health and Cleanliness Council, 1929)

65 *Počátek nového období veřejného zdravotnictví* (The inception of a new era in public health, by Josef Kokeisl, 1925)

66 *Pomoć u pravi čas* (Help at the right time, by Mladen Širola 1930)

67 *Pošast: film o tifusu* (Pestilence: A film about typhus, 1931)

68 *Pramen lásky* or *Láska kvete v každém věku* (The seed of love/Love blossoms at any age, by Josef Kokeisl, 1929)

69 *Procitnuí ženy* (Recognizing the Woman, by Josef Kokeisl, 1925)

70 *Requiem pro panenku* (Requiem for a maiden, by Filip Renč 1991)

71 *Seljačko sveučilište Škole narodnog zdravija: ženski tečaj (*Peasant's university of the School of Public Health: Women's course, by Milan Marjanović 1929)

72 *Spas male Zorice* (The rescue young Zorka, by Mladen Širola 1929)

73 *Státní epidemická kolona* (The state epidemiological mobile service, by Josef Kokeisl, 1925)

74 *Stín ve světle/Tvrdošíjný Juro/Slepý Juro/Tvrdohlavý Jura* (The Shadow in the Light/Stubborn Juro/Blind Juro/Hardheaded Juro, by Josef Kokeisl, 1928)

75 *Terenska sestra* (Visiting nurse, by Milan Marjanović 1929)

76 *The end of the road* (by Edward H. Griffith, 1919)

77 *The fly pest*, (by David Aylott, 1911)

78 *The kid* (by Charlie Chaplin, 1921)

79 *The light ahead* (by Edgar Ulmer, 1939)

80 *Where Are My Children?* (by Lois Weber and Phillips Smalley, 1916)

Index